Palgrave Macmillan Studies in Family and Intimate Life

Series Editors

Lynn Jamieson
University of Edinburgh
Edinburgh, UK

Jacqui Gabb
Faculty of Arts & Social Sciences
Open University
Milton Keynes, UK

Sara Eldén
Lund University
Lund, Sweden

Chiara Bertone
University of Eastern Piedmont
Alessandria, Italy

Vida Česnuitytė
Mykolas Romeris University
Vilnius, Lithuania

'The Palgrave Macmillan Studies in Family and Intimate Life series is impressive and contemporary in its themes and approaches'
– Professor Deborah Chambers, Newcastle University, UK, and author of *New Social Ties*.

The remit of the Palgrave Macmillan Studies in Family and Intimate Life series is to publish major texts, monographs and edited collections focusing broadly on the sociological exploration of intimate relationships and family life. The series encourages robust theoretical and methodologically diverse approaches. Publications cover a wide range of topics, spanning micro, meso and macro analyses, to investigate the ways that people live, love and care in diverse contexts. The series includes works by early career scholars and leading internationally acknowledged figures in the field while featuring influential and prize-winning research.

This series was originally edited by David H.J. Morgan and Graham Allan.

Magdalena Żadkowska
Marta Skowrońska
Christophe Giraud • Filip Schmidt
Editors

Reconfiguring Relations in the Empty Nest

Those Who Leave and Those Who Stay

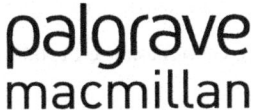

Editors
Magdalena Żadkowska
Social Sciences Department (Institute
of Sociology)
University of Gdańsk
Gdańsk, Poland

Centre de recherche sur les liens
sociaux (CERLIS, UMR 8070)
Université Paris Cité
Paris, France

Marta Skowrońska
Faculty of Sociology
Adam Mickiewicz University
Poznań, Poland

Filip Schmidt
Faculty of Sociology
Adam Mickiewicz University
Poznań, Poland

Christophe Giraud
Centre de recherche sur les liens
sociaux (CERLIS, UMR 8070)
Université Paris Cité
Paris, France

ISSN 2731-6440   ISSN 2731-6459   (electronic)
Palgrave Macmillan Studies in Family and Intimate Life
ISBN 978-3-031-50402-0   ISBN 978-3-031-50403-7   (eBook)
https://doi.org/10.1007/978-3-031-50403-7

This Palgrave Macmillan imprint is published by the registered company Springer Nature
Switzerland AG.
The registered company address is: Gewerbestrasse 11, 6330 Cham, Switzerland

Paper in this product is recyclable.

ACKNOWLEDGMENTS

Above all, we want to express our gratitude to our research participants for sharing their personal stories, experiences, and perspectives.

Special thanks go to the students from the University of Gdańsk (BA Sociology 2020–2023, "Sociology of Family Life") and Université Paris Cité (3rd year of Licence of Social Sciences, "Sociology of Family") whose interviews made a significant contribution to our research.

We want to acknowledge the support of our colleagues who agreed to review the chapters of this book. We appreciate all valuable comments and suggestions that helped improve the quality of the manuscript: Rita Gouveia PhD, Instituto de Ciências Sociais da Universidade de Lisboa (ICS-UL); Paweł Jurek PhD, University of Gdańsk; Saba Safdar, University of Guelph; Prof. Sandra Gaviria, Université Le Havre; Emmanuelle Maunaye PhD, Université de Rennes; Prof. Natasza Kosakowska-Berezecka, Prof. Dorota Rancew-Sikora, Prof. Radosław Kossakowski, and Magdalena Anita Gajewska PhD, University of Gdańsk.

We would like to thank all the members of the team who contributed to the different stages of this research in Poland and France. The work on this volume was greatly enhanced by team meetings and debates in Poland, in France, and online.

We would also like to express our gratitude to Professor Emeritus François de Singly, who has been involved in this study since the beginning and has accompanied us through all its stages. His vast experience, his critical eye, and his theoretical ideas have greatly inspired our work on this volume. He always said: "Empty Nest?"—let's study it together!

We also take this opportunity to acknowledge and remember Beate Collet, a great scholar and colleague at the Sorbonne Université and a specialist in interethnic couples, who generously agreed to review chapters of the book but passed away suddenly in April 2023. She is deeply missed.

We are grateful to receive funding provided by the National Science Centre (NCN) in Poland, which made our research for this book possible. This study has been supported by NCN under the research project "Till death do us part ... Everyday life practices of 50–64 y.o. couples with at least 20 years of common life experience" (UMO-2018/30/E/ HS6/00159). We also thank the help of the laboratory CERLIS (Université Paris Cité), which helped to finance our meetings in Paris and welcomed our discussions.

We also thank Jeremy Pearman for assisting with proofreading and Marianna Kostecka for the final edition.

CONTENTS

1 Introduction: The Empty Nest in Poland and in France   1
Magdalena Żadkowska, Christophe Giraud, Marta
Skowrońska, and Filip Schmidt

2 The Value of "Empty Nest Syndrome" in Sociology   27
François de Singly

Part I   The Family in 'The Empty Nest'   37

3 Reconfiguration of the Mother's Role After the Departure
of the Children   39
Magdalena Herzberg-Kurasz, Christophe Giraud, Magdalena
Anita Gajewska, Sophie David–Goretta, and François de Singly

4 The Empty Nest as a Phase of Fatherhood   65
Christophe Giraud, Radosław Kossakowski,
Magdalena Żadkowska, and Bogna Dowgiałło

5 Adult Children's Bedrooms and the Emptying Nest:
Mechanisms of Transition   91
Marta Skowrońska, Filip Schmidt, Emmanuelle Maunaye,
Marianna Kostecka, and Cyrano Andre–Vieille

6   Adult Children's Visits to Their Parents: Recomposition
     and Renegotiation of Family Roles and Responsibilities   115
     Marta Skowrońska, Emmanuelle Maunaye, Dorota Rancew-
     Sikora, and Cyrano Andre–Vieille

7   Return to the 'Full Nest'—Re-Cohabitation in Times of
     the Pandemic in France and Poland   141
     Sandra Gaviria, Magdalena Herzberg-Kurasz, and
     Magdalena Żadkowska

8   Animals in the Empty Nest: Recomposition of Family
     Roles   159
     Magdalena Anita Gajewska, François de Singly,
     Magdalena Żadkowska, Christophe Giraud,
     Marianna Kostecka, and Sophie David–Goretta

Part II   The Couple in 'The Empty Nest'   179

9   Redefining a Couple's Relationship in the Empty Nest:
     The New Honeymoon   181
     Filip Schmidt, Marta Skowrońska, Magdalena Żadkowska,
     and Christophe Giraud

10   Redefining a Couple's Relationship in the Empty Nest:
     Together Apart   209
     Marta Skowrońska, Filip Schmidt, Christophe Giraud, and
     Magdalena Żadkowska

11   Recoupling Transitions in the Empty Nest: Women's
     Perspective   239
     Magdalena Żadkowska and Christophe Giraud

Part III   The Self in 'The Empty Nest'   263

12   Without Children at Home: Transition to Herplaces and
      Hisplaces   265
      Marianna Kostecka, Magdalena Żadkowska,
      Bogna Dowgiałło, and Sophie David–Goretta

13   Navigating Emotional Terrain: Women's Experiences of
      Loss and Gain   291
      Bogna Dowgiałło, Christophe Giraud, and
      Magdalena Herzberg-Kurasz

14   Struggling with Limitations, Creating New Possibilities:
      Perspective of Men Experiencing the Empty Nest   309
      Radosław Kossakowski, Natasza Kosakowska-Berezecka, and
      Sophie David–Goretta

Appendix: Characteristics of Participants   327

NOTES ON CONTRIBUTORS

Cyrano André–Vieille has a BA in Social Sciences from the University of Paris Cité (UPC) and is pursuing MA in Investigative Sociology at the UPC. He is working on family leisure and shared family moments under the supervision of Elsa Ramos (CERLIS). His thesis examines the exploration of the forbidden catacombs of Paris as a family.

Sophie David–Goretta has two bachelor's degrees in psychology (Université Côte d'Azur) and social sciences (Université Paris-Cité – UPC) and is now an MA student in sociology at the Université Paris-Cité (UPC). Her work focuses on privacy, couple life processes, and the representation of homosexuality.

François de Singly is Professor Emeritus of sociology (two doctorates in sociology) at the University of Paris Cité and a researcher at CERLIS. He works on family, couple, education, and sociology of an individual. He has published thirty books and a hundred academic articles and chapters. He is currently working on a sociological analysis of pets in families.

Bogna Dowgiałło is an assistant professor at the Institute of Sociology at the University of Gdańsk. Her research focuses on everyday life, sociology of emotions, and qualitative methodology. She is also a psychotherapist.

Magdalena Anita Gajewska, PhD, is an assistant professor and tutor at the University of Gdańsk, Institute of Sociology. She works in the fields of the sociology of gender, the sociology of body, and the sociology of interspecies relations. She studies educational and hypnotherapeutic activities with horses.

Sandra Gaviria is a professor of sociology at the University of Le Havre Normandy and a researcher at the UMR IDEES. Her work and publications focus on the emancipation of young people in France and Spain and the relationship between young people and their work. Her book *Revenir vivre en famille. Éditions au bord de l'eau* was published in France in 2020. She regularly publishes in France, Spain, and Canada. She is currently working on how young people face social or professional vulnerabilities in France, Spain, and Belgium.

Christophe Giraud is a professor of sociology at the University of Paris Cité and a researcher at CERLIS. He works on family and couple and intimate relationships at different ages. His latest book entitled *L'amour réaliste* was published in 2017. He is now working on new intimate relationships after the age of 50.

Magdalena Herzberg-Kurasz has an MA in sociology and is a PhD student at the Doctoral School of Humanities and Social Sciences at the University of Gdańsk. She is a scholarship holder and researcher in a National Science Center research project devoted to the empty nest phase that is led by Magdalena Żadkowska. She has worked as a researcher in several international research projects and has authored various scientific articles. Her doctoral dissertation focuses on the experiences of women whose adult children have left their family home, relating directly to the role of the mother.

Natasza Kosakowska-Berezecka works as an associate professor and head in the Division of Cross-Cultural Psychology and Psychology of Gender at the University of Gdańsk (Poland). Her main area of research and practice is cross-cultural psychology of gender and her special interests are social change and cultural cues fostering gender equality within societies across the world. Currently she is a principal investigator in two exciting projects: Towards Gender Harmony project, in which over 100 collaborators in 62 countries have collected data on the contemporary understanding of masculinity and femininity, and EQUAMAN, analyzing how adolescent boys and men understand gender equality in different cultural contexts. More information about her projects is available at www.towardsgenderharmony.ug.edu.pl.

Radosław Kossakowski is an associate professor of sociology at the University of Gdańsk. His research focuses on the sociology of sport, football studies, qualitative research, and masculinity studies. His articles have been published in many well-recognized journals: *Sport in Society, Sociology of Sport Journal, International Review for the Sociology of Sport, East European Politics and Societies, Revista de Psicología del Deporte, Soccer & Society, Problems of Post-Communism.*

Marianna Kostecka has a BA from the Faculty of Polish and Classical Philology (AMU) and is an MA student at the Faculty of Sociology (AMU). She is a researcher in a National Science Center research project on the Empty Nest Phase, led by Magdalena Żadkowska, and in a National Science Center research project on Travel Behaviour in Polish Cities: Causality, Behavioural Changes, and Climate Impacts, led by Michał Czepkiewicz.

Emmanuelle Maunaye is a sociology lecturer at the University of Rennes and a researcher at Arènes. She works on young people's transitions to adulthood and intergenerational relations. Her research focuses on young people's access to independent housing.

Dorota Rancew-Sikora is an associate professor at the Institute of Sociology at the University of Gdańsk. In her research, she uses conversation analysis, multimodal analysis, and discourse analysis. She is interested in family communication, human–nature relationships, interaction rituals, hospitality, and other traditional practices. She has published in the *Journal of Pragmatics, Discourse Studies, Sociological Research Online,* and Polish academic journals.

Filip Schmidt, PhD, is an assistant professor at the Adam Mickiewicz University Poznań, Faculty of Sociology, focusing on the everyday lives of couples at different stages of relationship development and in relation to materiality. His doctoral thesis dealt with the transformations of ways of experiencing the moment of moving in together as a couple and was awarded by the Polish Sociological Association and the Polish Prime Minister. He is also involved in studies on mobility and travel behaviour.

Marta Skowrońska, PhD, is an assistant professor at the Department of Social Practice Research and Theory at the Faculty of Sociology, Adam Mickiewicz University Poznań. Her research focusses on everyday life, particularly in the context of home and dwelling. She is the author of two books, one of them about the secondhand goods market as a social phenomenon and the other about the relations between dwelling and comfort.

Magdalena Żadkowska, PhD, is an assistant professor at the Institute of Sociology at the University of Gdańsk, Poland. Her research interests include the sociology of everyday life, intimate couple relations and gender differences in the family, the workplace, migration processes, and academia. She was awarded a French government grant (Bourse de Stage BGF) for a study stay at CERLIS Centre de Recherche sur les Liens Sociaux, Université Paris Cité (UMR 8070) in 2017 and developed Polish-French cooperation during a visiting researcher stay at CERLIS in 2021 and 2022. She is the principal investigator of "Till death do us part … Everyday life practices of 50–64 year old couples with at least 20 years of shared life experience," funded by Sonata Bis 8 NCN grant, UMO-2018/30/E/HS6/00159.

LIST OF FIGURES

Fig. 1.1   Average age at which young people leave the parental
             household, women have their first child and women marry for
             the first time in 2020 in Poland, France and the EU. Source:
             Eurostat   8
Fig. 1.2   Average age at which young men and women leave the
             parental home and average age at which men and women
             marry for the first time in Poland and France. Source: Eurostat   8
Fig. 1.3   Period of residential independence without children and
             without being married in France and Poland. Source: Eurostat   9
Fig. 9.1   Characteristics of the "new honeymoon" scenario   188
Fig. 10.1   Characteristics of the "together apart" scenario   212

LIST OF TABLES

Table 1.1   Characteristics of the interviews   12
Table 9.1   Empty nest as the transformation of interdependencies:
             Four model scenarios   186

CHAPTER 1

Introduction: The Empty Nest in Poland and in France

Magdalena Żadkowska, Christophe Giraud,
Marta Skowrońska, and Filip Schmidt

Families grow and decrease in size, and adjust to new situations during the life course. One of the most significant changes that leads to a reconfiguration of familial roles and interactions is the process of emptying the nest,

M. Żadkowska (✉)
Social Sciences Department (Institute of Sociology), University of Gdańsk, Gdańsk, Poland

Centre de recherche sur les liens sociaux (CERLIS, UMR 8070), Université Paris Cité, Paris, France
e-mail: magdalena.zadkowska@ug.edu.pl

C. Giraud
Centre de recherche sur les liens sociaux (CERLIS, UMR 8070), Université Paris Cité, Paris, France
e-mail: christophe.giraud@parisdescartes.fr

M. Skowrońska • F. Schmidt
Faculty of Sociology, Adam Mickiewicz University, Poznań, Poland
e-mail: marta.skowronska@amu.edu.pl; fschmidt@amu.edu.pl

1

M. Żadkowska et al. (eds.), *Reconfiguring Relations in the Empty Nest*, Palgrave Macmillan Studies in Family and Intimate Life, https://doi.org/10.1007/978-3-031-50403-7_1

that is, the time when adult children leave the family home. The term is sometimes confused or associated with "empty nest syndrome". The latter term was coined in 1940s and 1950s in psychology to denote the feelings of loss, grief and depression which were supposed to accompany the parents when the child was no longer present, and popularised in the 1970s (Mitchell, 2010). However, confusing or equating empty nest with such experiences seems unfounded (Raup & Mayers, 1989; Bouchard, 2014; Mitchell, 2010). Research on empty nest syndrome has been criticised for biased methodology (Mitchell, 2010) and the fact that in vast majority of the studies, only mothers were examined (Bouchard, 2014). Moreover, the syndrome was mainly ascribed to women who were believed to suffer a major role loss in contrast to their husbands, preoccupied with work rather than family matters. Nowadays, however, women tend to engage in multiple roles, which provide them with sources of self-definition other than being a parent, while the children tend to pursue nonmarital pathways (Mitchell & Lovegreen, 2009).

Although the socio-political context and the role of women have changed considerably since the time when empty nest was mainly analysed in terms of women's loss, the importance of the parental relationship with the child has increased, counteracting the autonomisation of the relationship between the partners. First, the child becomes an object of intense emotional and financial investment and a key "life project" (Kaufmann, 2001; Szlendak, 2010). Second, the parental support of grown children has significantly increased (Fingerman et al., 2012). This is to a large extent a consequence of children completing their education, finding a job, leaving home at a later age on average in many countries (Cherlin et al., 1997; Seiffge-Krenke, 2013; Beaupré et al., 2018; cf. EUROSTAT, 2022), while the situation in the job and housing market and economic crises are helping to sustain this trend (Ostrovsky-Berman & Litwin, 2019). Of course, the extent of children independency and parental support depend strongly on the socio-political contexts and cultural roles in which young people and parents evolve. For example, according to the Survey of Health, Ageing and Retirement in Europe, 50% of parental transfers in Poland and Spain are related to covering basic needs and securing housing, while it is only 20% in Switzerland and Czech Republic (Isengard et al., 2018). But even in a country like the United States (US), where most young people leave home around the age of 18–19, they tend to remain closely connected to their parents for at least the next decade, according to a representative survey of parents with at least one child aged

18–29 (Arnett & Schwab, 2013). Majority of parents report contacting with their emerging adult every day or almost every day, support the children financially (directly or by family cell phone plan, health insurance, car repair, etc.), while 43% are "concerned that their child might never find a stable job".

While many psychological studies have investigated empty nest as a period of the family life cycle (Duvall, 1971; Feeney et al., 1994; Liberska, 2014), sociological studies of this phenomenon are less common. In psychology, a large body of literature has analysed whether the empty nest phase results in increased or decreased psychological well-being, particularly in the context of role-strain and role-loss theory (Bouchard, 2014). Marital adjustment and satisfaction have often been discussed, primarily based on quantitative psychological surveys (Harper et al., 2000; Heiman et al., 2011). Most studies, however, focused on dichotomic questions, such as whether the empty nest brings the risk of marital dissolution or whether it is a chance to renew the relationship between the spouses (Dennerstein et al., 2002; Schmidt et al., 2004; Mitchell & Lovegreen, 2009).

Our project provides an analysis that replaces the dichotomic approach to the empty nest phase of family life with a more nuanced and processual perspective. We do not aim to establish whether or not there is 'empty nest syndrome', or how severe it is, but to present the entire spectrum of experience that this life stage involves. Instead of asking whether the transition to post-parenthood increases or decreases marital satisfaction, we demonstrate how couples adapt to the changes brought about by their children's departure and how these changes impact their roles and relations. Our research shows that the commonly contradicted perspectives of role-strain and role-loss (Borland, 1982; Bouchard, 2014; Bouchard & McNair, 2016; Thibodeau & Bouchard, 2020) should not be treated as mutually exclusive, as the transition to the empty nest phase is accompanied by many ambivalences. Parental involvement and support coexist with the growing individualisation of parents who want to pursue their own interests. A sense of loss is usually accompanied by a sense of relief. In addition, while most research focuses either on the parent–children relationship or the marital quality in the empty nest phase, our book combines both perspectives: being a parent and being a spouse, and it demonstrates their interrelation.

In this book, we compare how the children's transition to independence and adulthood is experienced by Polish and French parents. Poland

and France are two European countries where family values are very important, but they understand this term differently due to their different cultural-political-historical-social contexts. We show that there is great variation in how the empty nest challenges are experienced, contributing to the studies on couplehood, and intergenerational relationships. While the vast majority of studies devoted to the empty nest phase are based on quantitative data, we use qualitative interviews, which better capture the complexity of the process of transition to the empty nest: mixed emotions, nuanced attitudes, contradictions and dissonance. We also include new themes, such as the COVID-19 pandemic, which demonstrated to be an important factor that even complicated the process of emptying the nest and brought unexpected returns. Finally, our book "gives voice" to the "supporting actors" of the transition process: animals and material objects.

Based on qualitative research conducted in Poland and France between 2019 and 2021, we aim to answer the following research questions:

1. How do parent–child relations reconfigure in the empty nest phase of the family life course?
2. What challenges and opportunities does transition to the empty nest phase in the family life course bring to the couple's relationship?
3. How do men and women use time and space to reorganise their personal lives in the empty nest phase?

LEAVING THE NEST IN FRANCE AND POLAND

Comparing five traditional markers of adulthood (Modell et al., 1976; Arnett, 2000): completing education (1), getting a first job (2), moving out of the family home and running an independent household (3), getting married (4) and/or having a child (5), nowadays such events take place at an increasingly older age (and sometimes do not occur), consequently stretching and changing the process of becoming an adult (Arnett, 2014). In the traditional model, the changes were sequential; they happened one by one and were irreversible (Galland, 1997, 2003; Arnett, 2000). Life events related to an economic and residential independence arrived at the same time. Today, however, the order and significance of these markers is no longer clear. Studies show that moving out, one of the traditional five markers of adulthood can be reversed. Young adults are "boomeranging" (Mitchell, 2006; Gaviria, 2020; Olofsson et al., 2020). The other markers are fragmented, diverse and can be regressed. According to Arnett (2000, 2007), the developmental stage of emerging adulthood is marked by psychological experiences such as experiencing possibilities, instability, exploration, self-focus and feeling in-between. Today we rather speak of negotiated adulthood (Mary, 2014), partial or emerging adulthood (Arnett, 2007) and established adulthood (Eisenberg et al., 2015).

In many aspects, changes in dynamics of the transition to adulthood in Poland and in France are similar to situations observed elsewhere in Europe and the US (Arnett, 2000; Galland, 2003; Benson & Furstenberg, 2006; Gillespie, 2020; Van de Velde, 2008). What differs among countries is the average age of the adult children's departure and the type of welfare state (Esping-Andersen, 1990) they represent. Comparing the children's departure in two European countries (Poland and France) implies putting family phenomena in the context of the welfare state differences.

France has a conservative-corporatist social system that encourages young people to become independent at an early age and has put in place several support schemes. University residences make it possible to accommodate, on the basis of social criteria, a large number of students whose families live far from university centres. This early departure constitutes an early experience of residential independence that can easily be repeated later. The second housing assistance scheme is the APL (*aide personnalisée au logement*). Based on the income of the young person and their family, this aid is paid out of the family allowance funds and helps to finance a significant part of the rent for students or young workers. Finally, the State has introduced a tax deduction for families whose children are economically dependent on their family. Children may live in the parental home or outside.

In contrast to Northern European countries, however, the means granted by the French state are limited (Van de Velde, 2008). Young people remain dependent on their families for a long time and are often obliged to find a part-time job alongside their studies. For young adults who are not studying, the difficulty to enter the job market and find a stable job and the scarcity of public help, implies a longer dependence from the family: they leave home now later than students (Robert & Sulzer, 2021).

The pattern of transition into adulthood of young adults in France who choose to go to University is in two phases. The first is 'relative residential independence'. Young people leave the family home relatively early compared to Poland (i.e. 24 years old vs. 28 years old), but they do so with financial support from their parents (and the state). In this first stage, young adults decohabitate mainly because of their studies, but they remain "integrated" into the family of orientation from which they receive various forms of support. They return regularly to their parents' home, sometimes every week, to do their laundry, find their belongings, their friends, and incidentally their parents. As Gaviria (2020), Despalins and de Saint Pol (2012) note, many return to their parents' home at the end of every academic year, and particularly when they do not yet have a job. The return is a normal experience in this first phase as young people are still closely connected to the family. They are "absent but integrated". Parents are still "parents" even if they no longer necessarily have a daily role.

The second and later phase of departure consists of complete independence from parents. The young people have a stable job and can have their own accommodation which they finance themselves. Returns have the sense of an "accident" in the course of their lives, always possible in a context where access to a stable position with a permanent contract requires a significant number of years and varied professional experience. The parents' work is less important in this phase when the young person is "absent and no more integrated" into the family.

Poland and other countries in Central and Eastern Europe have not always been included in typologies of welfare regimes (Esping-Andersen, 1990; Korpi, 2000). The typologies of "youth transition regimes" (cf. Walther et al., 2003; Walther, 2006; Van de Velde, 2008) also focus on Western Europe. In a typology used for describing the division of labour among European Couples by Bühlmann et al. (2009), all Central-East European countries, including Poland are classified as "post-communist" (Bühlmann et al., 2009: 7) with characteristics that relate only to parental leave policies. Also according to Polish scholars, Poland is representative of a post-communist European welfare state (Furmańska-Maruszak & Suwada, 2021), where we can observe a shift from implicit familialism, in which the family is responsible for caring for children and is not supported in this task to explicit familialism, in which the family still provides care personally but is supported by instruments such as paid leave and childcare benefits (Szelewa, 2017; Furmańska-Maruszak & Suwada, 2021). That is why, in Poland the transition to an empty nest is often characterised as a 'family matter', which means that young adults in Poland are dependent on the support of their parents and on insufficient youth policies (Szafraniec, 2017). With existing Western European models Poland is considered to be a mixture of 'old' (sequential—Arnett, 2000; Galland, 2003) and 'new' (prolonged/emerging/reversable) patterns to becoming an independent adult (Szafraniec, 2017; Pustułka et al., 2022). Poland is also seen as a 'northeastern' regime characterised by unfavourable market opportunity structures, an underdeveloped private rental sector, a lack of coherent youth or housing policies, and retrenched expenditure for social protection (Szafraniec, 2017).

According to the FYS2021 study, 50% of young people (between 18 and 29 years old) in Poland live with at least one parent, and 32.5% live with a partner, 9.1% of respondents live alone, and 3.7% with friends (Kajta & Mrozowicki, 2023). Almost one-third of young people (30.7%) between 25 and 29 years old still live with their parents. Compared to French young people, difficulties in achieving full financial autonomy during their studies result in a longer duration of living with their parents (Pustułka et al., 2022). The Polish welfare state is based on the "long-term dependency", which is also observed in southern European countries. The so-called delay syndrome (Slany, 2006) characterises past few decades of Polish family life.

THE EVENTS OF RESIDENTIAL AUTONOMY AND OF THE FAMILY SETTLEMENT

Back in the 1970s, 1980s and even 1990s, people left home, got married, and had children at an earlier age. For example, almost 80% of those born in France in 1950, more than 60% of those born in 1960 and 35% of those born in 1970 were married by the age of 26 (INSEE, 2021). In Poland, moving in together was synonymous with getting married and the average age of marriage fell to 22 in the 1960s, the lowest ever recorded (Schmidt, 2015). As a result, many parents whose children are now leaving home, and who were the main participants in the studies described in this book, experienced their own departure very differently.

The process of adult children moving out of the family home differs between Poland and France (see Figs. 1.1 and 1.2). In Poland, in 2020, the average age at which women leave home was 27 (29 for males), while in France it was 23 (25 for males), and it has barely changed in the last decade. As a result, according to EU-SILC in 2020, 72% of the French aged 20–24 and as many as 92% of Poles of the same age lived with their parents. The difference is even more pronounced among people aged 25–29, with just one-fourth of the French and 60% of their Polish counterparts living with their parents. Moreover, in Poland, the mean

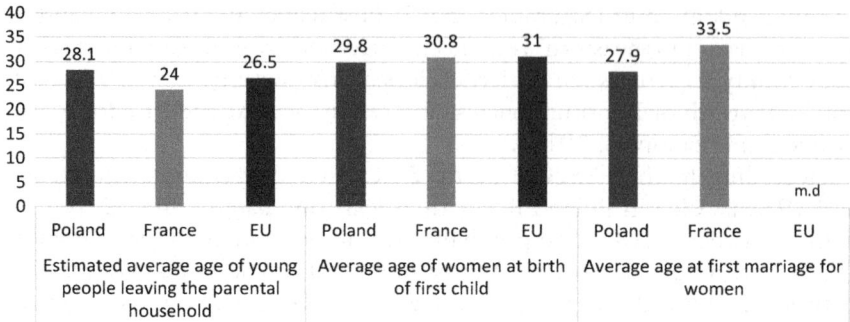

Fig. 1.1 Average age at which young people leave the parental household, women have their first child and women marry for the first time in 2020 in Poland, France and the EU. Source: Eurostat

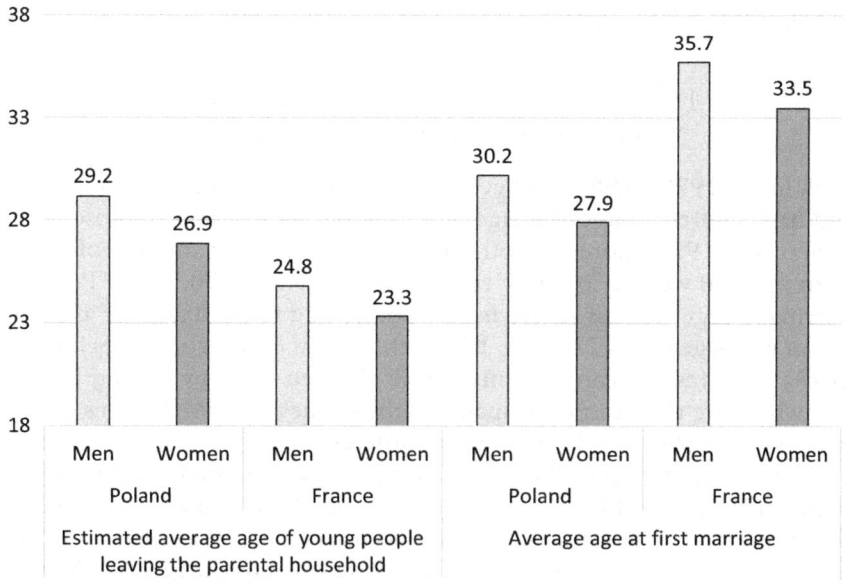

Fig. 1.2 Average age at which young men and women leave the parental home and average age at which men and women marry for the first time in Poland and France. Source: Eurostat

difference between the age of women leaving home and giving birth to the first child is just two years, while in France it is about eight years. French women leave home earlier than Polish women, but have their first child later, at around 31.

There are even greater differences between the two countries in the average duration of time between leaving home and getting married. While in Poland the average age of marriage is similar to the age of having the first child, this is not the case in France. In France the two events are separated by around 10 years on average (see Fig. 1.3).

All these elements show that departure from the family home in Poland is still closely connected to a marital and family project, whereas in France departure is more often synonymous with having space for other individual projects before settling down. In Poland, marriage is either a condition for becoming independent or at least one of the important steps in the process of becoming "fully adult" (Schmidt, 2015). As a result, the time spent living as a couple without children is relatively short (one year on average). In France, on the other hand, people leave their parental home much earlier and it is closely associated with tertiary education or starting to work and being independent of parents rather than settling down as a couple or starting a family (Van de Velde, 2008). Referring to "markers" of adulthood, we can say the order of some markers and the sense of leaving home is different according to the country. In Poland, being financially independent from the parents precedes leaving home. In France,

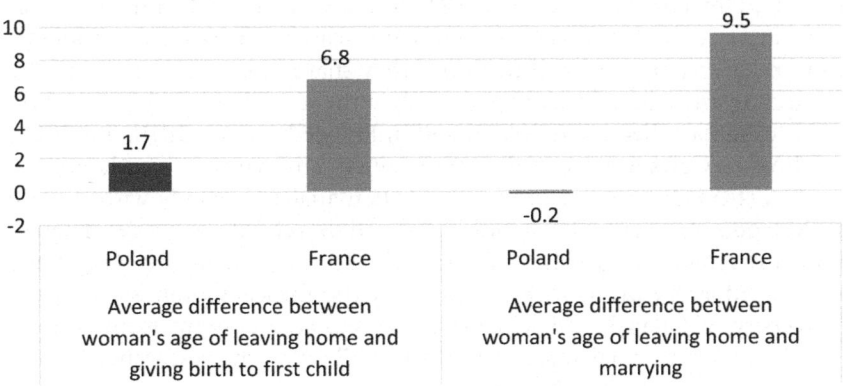

Fig. 1.3 Period of residential independence without children and without being married in France and Poland. Source: Eurostat

leaving the parental home is often a situation that precedes gaining financial independence. French young adults gain early independence (compared with Poles) but they are still financially dependent on their parents.

These differences are not related to the proportion of the population having completed tertiary education: according to Eurostat in 2020, the proportion of 30–34year olds having completed tertiary education is similar in France (49%) and Poland (47%).

In summary, the statistics described above show that children leave parental home earlier in France than in Poland and that the typical nature of adult children leaving home is different. Whereas in France the child's departure marks the beginning of a long period of education and/or work that precedes possible marriage and the arrival of children, in Poland leaving parental home, marriage and the birth of a child are more likely to occur, on average, at similar times (although there are of course different patterns and lifestyles in the two countries that are masked by the use of averages).

PROJECT DESCRIPTION

The project "Till death do us part... Everyday life practices of 50–64 year old couples with at least 20 years of common life experience" (Sonata Bis 8, UMO-2018/30/E/HS6/00159), founded by the National Science Centre in Poland was realised by the University of Gdańsk, Adam Mickiewicz University Poznań and Centre de Recherche sur les Liens Sociaux, Université Paris Cité (CERLIS) consisted of 261 in-depth qualitative interviews. The Polish and French research efforts were not identical in their assumptions and tools but they shared many of them, and the research teams worked together to analyse the data. Our book is based on empirical data collected in Poland and in France between 2019 and 2022.

The interviews were recorded, transcribed, anonymised, translated into English (from Polish and French) and then analysed mainly with the use of Maxqda software. The audio and video recordings were deleted. Standard ethical rules (Mizielińska et al., 2018) used in sociology were introduced as the project was accepted by the Ethical Commission of the University of Gdańsk. Participants either signed a consent form or gave verbal consent to participate in the study, allowing the researchers to use anonymised quotes in publications.

Data analysis was carried out using thematic analysis (Braun et al., 2017; Braun & Clarke, 2021). The project as such was not a comparative study. However, many chapters discuss how French and Polish contexts and findings are similar or different. This book is to be read as a series of independent analyses carried out by members of the Polish and French research teams. They were not based on one theoretical framework. The authors of each chapter were responsible for outlining the theoretical assumptions used in their analysis.

The data is organised in five corpuses described in Table 1.1. Throughout the book, when quoting an interview, we use a reference that indicates the corpus to which an interview belongs (letters A-E), the country (PL for Poland and FR for France), its number and the region, where available (P for Poznań and Wielkopolskie Voivodeship, G for Gdańsk, Gdynia, Sopot and Pomorskie Voivodeship). For example, B_PL_9P indicates the ninth interview in corpus B, collected in Poland in Wielkopolskie Voivodeship.

Corpus A consists of DDIs with parents of adult children in a long-term relationship, whose children have left home in recent months or years, or who are about to leave. A year later we visited many of them again to interview each parent separately (most part of the corpus B). We also conducted additional 20 IDIs with parents (mostly mothers) of adult children, whose children have left home in recent months or years, or who are about to leave, but whose spouses did not want to participate in the study (the remaining part of the corpus B). Then the study was expanded to include interviews with mothers whose relationship had ended before the children left home (corpus C). Finally, additional interviews about the impact of the pandemic on the return home (corpus D) and the role of pets in the empty nest phase (corpus E) were conducted by the students of Poznań and France. For the participants in the main study (corpuses A and B), we collected socio-demographic data, which are described below and in the appendix.

CHARACTERISTICS OF PARTICIPANTS

Poland

Participants of the main part of the study (corpus A and half of the corpus B) are married heterosexual couples who have been in a relationship together for more than 20 years and whose children have left home in recent months or years, or who are about to leave. As the population of Poland became nearly entirely ethnically homogeneous after the Second World War, the sample lacked ethnic diversity. The interviewees were a

Table 1.1 Characteristics of the interviews

Corpus	Type of interview	Quantity	Participants	Where?	When?	Focus of the interview
A	DDI	26	Parents of adult children in a long-term relationship, whose children have left home in recent months or years, or who are about to leave	Poland, urban setting, in person	2019–2020	Experiencing the Empty Nest Transition
		33		France, urban setting, in person	2020	
		16		Poland, rural setting, in person	2021	Experiencing the Empty Nest Transition Personal experiences of children's departure
B	IDI	24	Mothers of adult children, in a long-term relationship, who participated in the DDIs listed in corpus A (2nd interview, after 1 year)	Poland, urban setting, online	2020–2021	Personal experience of children's departure
		23	Fathers of adult children, in a long-term relationship, who participated in the DDIs listed in corpus A (2nd interview, after 1 year)	Poland, urban setting, online		
		18	Mothers of adult children in a long-term relationship	Poland, urban & rural setting, online	2020–2021	Experiencing the Empty Nest Transition
		2	Fathers of adult children in a long-term relationship	Poland, urban setting, online		Personal experiences of children's departure
C	IDI	20	Mothers of adult children, widowed, separated, divorced, often in recoupling	France, urban setting, in person	2019	Experiencing the Empty Nest Transition
		17	Mothers of adult children in a long-term relationship	Poland, urban & rural setting, online	2020–2021	Personal experiences of children's departure
D	IDI or DDI	14	Parents of adult children with experience of the return caused by the COVID19 pandemic	Poland, urban setting, online & in person	2021	Boomeranging during the COVID-19 pandemic
		53		France, urban setting, online & in person		
E	IDI or DDI	15	Parents of adult children who have a dog/cat	France, urban setting, in person	2022	Empty Nest Transition and animals

little more educated than the average for Poland, but still varied in terms of education; 12% had finished primary or vocational school, 34% secondary school, and 54% had tertiary education. The youngest interviewee was 44, the oldest 69 and the average age was 54 (52 for women, 55 for men). Their children were on average 26 (25.7 for daughters and 27 for sons). Almost one-third of the couples had one child, 43% had two children, 18% had three children and 8% had four or more. In a few cases, a child was still living at home with the intention of moving out or had moved out once but returned and had the intention of moving out again. Thus we tried to catch the floating nature of the empty nest with possible boomeranging children. The average time since the children's departure was three years.

For other participants (part of the corpus B, and corpuses C and D) we did not collect socio-demographic data.

France

In Corpus A, in France (married heterosexual couples who have been in a relationship together for more than 20 years), the mothers had an average age of 53 and the fathers 54.5. 14 of the couple had an upper class position, 17 had a middle class position. Only 2 couples had a working class position. Two couples included people with migration experience. The children were mainly in the first phase of departure: they had left home for school and returned regularly (which is a normal feature of this phase). Their children were 23.6 years old on average (22.8 for daughters and 24.3 for sons), three of the couples had one child, 16 had two children, 11 had three children and three had four or more. In some cases (11), a child was still living at home with the intention of moving out or had moved out once but returned and had the intention of moving out again. The average time since the children's departure was three years.

For other participants (corpuses C, D, and E) we did not collect socio-demographic data.

Overview of the Volume

In Part I, "Family in the Empty Nest", we focus on the reconfiguration of relationships between parents/spouses and their offspring in the empty nest phase. The departure of adult children from the family home presents challenges and often leads to a radical reconfiguration of parental roles. In seven chapters, we show the complexity of this process, which involves different actors, perspectives and relationships: mothers, fathers, children, animals and the material environment of the home.

Chapter 2 provides a theoretical overview of research on the empty nest phenomenon. François de Singly looks at the "nest" metaphor, tracing it through history, literature, film, and finally, the humanities and social sciences. Analysing a variety of themes and meanings associated with the "empty nest", de Singly lists the key questions that researchers should seek to answer: Is the transition to the empty nest difficult, and how so? To what extent does it create the conditions for a recomposition of identity, leaving more room for other roles, especially the marital role? To what extent does this transformation constitute a new phase of life? Which dimensions of the parental repertoire are retained and which are abandoned?

In Chap. 3, Magdalena Herzberg-Kurasz, Christophe Giraud, Magdalena Anita Gajewska, Sophie David–Goretta and François de Singly explore the reconfiguration of the maternal role in its material and relational aspects. The authors show that this role does not disappear when children leave home, but is prolonged and adapted to new family circumstances and settings, and can be expressed in new practices. They also argue that relinquishing maternal responsibilities is not an easy task. While reducing parental burdens is a considerable relief for mothers, some feel guilty about being relieved. Moreover, mothers do not stop caring—even if the practices of care evolve and change. As the study shows, mothers are heavily involved in 'distant' relational work, which is a balancing act between the need to protect the child who has left and not interfering with adequate autonomy.

Mothers are generally perceived as the primary caregivers, and the cultural image of the 'good mother' strongly shapes women's lives. In contrast, the concept of fatherhood receives relatively less social attention; it is less hegemonic or ideological. In the context of the empty nest transition, men, unlike women, are not at risk of being judged as bad parents if they experience the empty nest period as joyful (Sheriff & Weatherall, 2009). At the same time, studies show that men's involvement in the care and upbringing of children has increased and has become more meaningful in men's personal lives (Castelain-Meunier, 2005; Banchefsky & Park, 2016). Christophe Giraud, Radosław Kossakowski, Magdalena Żadkowska and Bogna Dowgiałło decided to take a closer look at fathering and how it changes when adult children move out. In Chap. 4, the authors find that, similar to mothers' roles, fathers' roles do not disappear but change.

Nevertheless, there are general differences between mothers and fathers in how they perform and experience their changing roles. Despite the less authoritarian nature of the father–child relationship, fathering still has a certain traditional character—men are often seen as responsible for "practical" or "technical" matters rather than emotional work. However, in addition to providing practical support, the interviewed fathers also take the opportunity to transform the relationship with their adult child into a more partner-like one, becoming their "buddy" and advisor.

The relationship between parents and their adult children can be interpreted as a balance between autonomy and proximity. As shown in Chaps. 3 and 4, parents are still involved in their adult children's lives, even if their roles are changing. Chapter 5 traces the details of this involvement in the materiality of children's bedrooms. Marta Skowrońska, Filip Schmidt, Emmanuelle Maunaye, Marianna Kostecka and Cyrano Andre–Vieille analyse the process of change in the use and decoration of children's bedrooms, and the changes in the parent–child relationship that accompany it. The study shows that the nature and pace of spatial transformation is related to the changing agency and identity of children and parents, on the one hand, and to contextual factors (housing conditions and uncertainty/certainty of departure), on the other hand. Transition is slowed or hindered when children can still decide about their (former) room, and accelerated when parents take control over its function or aesthetics. Change is also hindered when parents stick to their role and believe that children need to be looked after. Housing conditions can also impact the pace and intensity of change. All these factors interact and sometimes collide, with some facilitating change and others inhibiting it. This can lead to conflict between parents and children, for example, if the room change is perceived as too fast or too abrupt. They can also cause cognitive dissonance. The complexity of this process shows that the transition to the empty nest is a process that can take a long time, change direction and pace and create tension.

The authors of Chap. 6 also look at the transformation of the parent–child relationship, this time focusing on a specific practice: domestic visits. In Chap. 6, Marta Skowrońska, Emmanuelle Maunaye, Dorota Rancew-Sikora and Cyrano Andre–Vieille show the empty nest as a stage for domestic hospitality as well as a trigger of family roles and a display of family ideology (Finch, 2007; James & Curtis, 2010). The authors interpret adult children's visits as a meeting of two culturally distinct patterns of interaction. The first pattern relates to intimate family relationships characterised by close ties, reciprocity, dependence and imbalance. The other refers to the situation of a visit, characterised by politeness and ritual exchange rules. Combining these two logics helps study parents and their children as a continuation of their family relationships and as new roles. The different ways of organising and experiencing adult children's visits presented in this chapter show that the relationship between parents and their children is nuanced and constantly evolving.

The complex and processual nature of the empty nest transition is further illustrated in Chap. 7. Sandra Gaviria, Magdalena Herzberg-Kurasz and Magdalena Żadkowska examine the characteristics of returning home during COVID-19. The COVID-19 pandemic affected many families around the world. Along with the pandemic restrictions, young adults who had been living on their own returned to live in the family home. The authors observe this process by analysing changes in the home and in domestic practices. They show how the period of independent living had accelerated the children's transition to adulthood, their growing need for autonomy, privacy and independence as young adults. The chapter also explores how parents changed—developing new habits and new spaces in the home, either for themselves (see Chap. 12) or for the couple (see Chap. 9). The change in both parties made the returns a challenging task. The analysis shows that the main challenge for parents is to respect their children's growing independence and to accept the additional housework associated with their return. While parents felt burdened with additional work and the need to reorganise space and habits, they also enjoyed their children's temporary return to the full nest.

The final piece of the changing family puzzle is animals. Many recent sociological studies of couples highlight the role of animals in their lives (Carter, 2015; Owens & Grauerholz, 2019; Gouveia & Castrén, 2021). In Chap. 8, Magdalena Anita Gajewska, François de Singly, Magdalena Żadkowska, Christophe Giraud, Marianna Kostecka and Sophie David–Goretta show how animals are important actors in the family structure and how the relationship with them changes when children leave home. The authors show that pets fill the gap left by the absence of children—they are companions that bring comfort and joy, and they structure the daily routine, providing satisfaction and fulfilment. Most importantly, by assigning this role to an animal, couples whose attachment style was mediated by an object of mutual concern can protect their relationship from crisis and continue their existing intimate lifestyle by sharing responsibility for the animal.

Part II, "The Empty Nest Couple", focuses on the post-parenting couple whose children have left home and who are now living alone. This transition presents considerable challenges and opportunities for the relationship. In all three chapters, we analyse the reconfiguration of the couple's roles and practices (and the meanings attached to them) in the process of transition to the empty nest. We also look at the degree of child-centredness as an important modifying factor and examine what couples choose to display. As the chapters are closely related and based on the same principles, they are preceded by an introduction that summarizes their theoretical background and research questions regarding the transition of parental and marital bonds. The authors combine the perspectives of child–parent and parent–parent (couple) relationships, observing how the reconfiguration of couplehood differs according to the level of child-centredness of the parents. When children leave home, child-centred care practices decrease significantly and decisions no longer need to be child-centred. The transition to the empty nest phase may vary depending on the level of child-centredness of the couple. Regardless of the level of interdependence and child-centredness and the nature of the couple's attachment, a couple is involved in the process of "displaying" some aspects of couplehood/family to others (Finch, 2007).

In Chap. 9, Filip Schmidt, Marta Skowrońska, Magdalena Żadkowska and Christophe Giraud examine the couples who have redirected the resources released into strengthening the marital bond after their interdependence with their children has weakened. This scenario of the couple's trajectory in the empty nest phase is called the "new honeymoon" to emphasise the strengthening of the marital bond. Some couples begin the 'new honeymoon' immediately after their children have left home. In other cases, a couple has to learn or relearn how to be together. A couple may have a low level of interdependence after the children leave, but develop it over time by adopting new practices. On the other hand, the 'new honeymoon' may only be a period after which the partners gradually begin to fall apart. The authors analyse the factors that facilitate or hinder the emergence of this scenario and show that relearning how to be a couple after many years of focusing on children can be a challenging task.

A reverse trajectory of a post-parental couple is presented in Chap. 10, Filip Schmidt, Christophe Giraud and Magdalena Żadkowska reveal the stories of couples with low levels of interdependence who lead parallel rather than shared lives. Parenthood united the couple and gave them a sense of purpose and a common project. The empty nest phase revealed how little they had in common beyond that. The authors show, however, that these couples, like those united by a strong bond, experience the empty nest phase as a combination of sadness and relief. Even together apart couples, who rarely derive satisfaction from marital practices, may experience enjoyment in the empty nest phase due to their increased time to develop personal interests and reduced conflict and tension. The chapter presents typical trajectories of together apart couples and shows how their relationship continues despite difficulties. Four important aspects of a together apart couple maintaining their relationship are presented: reproducing daily practices, displaying couplehood/family, housing or financial issues and fear of staying alone.

Chapter 11 examines families that have experienced separation, divorce or the death of a partner prior to the empty nest transition. Magdalena Żadkowska and Christophe Giraud analyse the empty nest event as a possible trigger for women to choose a new partner or to decide on the form of a current relationship. The chapter aims to show the impact of the children's departure on the possible reconfiguration of women's intimate lives after the end of the relationship with the child's father. Using Anderson and Green's "Nine potential transitions model in postdivorce re-partnering" (Anderson & Greene, 2005), the authors present five types of transition trajectories. The empty nest is a turning point in mothers' private lives, as it changes their private commitments and provides an opportunity for them to reflect on themselves. For some, it is the moment to enter into new sentimental relationships that they had previously forbidden themselves. For others, it is a time to develop hidden LAT arrangements, love affairs or informal relationships, or to give them a new character thanks to greater independence from commitments to children.

Part III of the book is devoted to the reconfiguration of personal life that comes with an empty nest. In this part, we analyse the strategies of reconstruction of personal life in their temporal, spatial and emotional aspects. In three chapters the authors investigate how individuals reconfigure their identity, emotions and use of home space in the process of their life-course transition.

Chapter 12 examines how the children's departure influences the creation of individual space at home. Marianna Kostecka, Magdalena Żadkowska, Bogna Dowgiałło and Sophie David–Goretta observe the new use of the home space, paying particular attention to gender differences in the desire to have one's own place. While the most striking change is the decision to renovate or redecorate one's home, the authors identify other, more subtle practices that help increase the sense of privacy and intimacy. New ways of using common areas and new rituals (long baths, taking a nap) provide a sense of relaxation and comfort. Like other chapters in this volume, Chap. 12 highlights the difficulties and ambivalence that accompany parents, especially mothers, in the transition to an empty nest. The relief and relaxation experienced by women contradict the oppressive model of motherhood based on the idea of self-sacrifice.

The theme of women's emotions is continued and analysed in detail in Chap. 13 by Bogna Dowgiałło, Christophe Giraud and Magdalena Herzberg-Kurasz. Taking a sociological perspective on emotions, the authors examine how women feel, but also the emotional rules that dictate what they should and should not feel. Social expectations about the empty nest transition can have a significant impact on how women frame this experience. In their analysis, the authors distinguish five emotional patterns that emerge from women's narratives: grief, frustration, pride/guilt, relief and joy. Importantly, these emotions are often intertwined and lead to ambivalence, which can be interpreted as a consequence of conflicting societal norms and values that women have acquired.

The last chapter in our volume, Chap. 14 provides an analysis of male feelings and experiences. Radosław Kossakowski, Natasza Kosakowska-Berezecka and Sophie David–Goretta, present men as torn between the traditional model of "breadwinner" and a new model of an emotional and caring father. The authors observe that the experience of an empty nest coincides with other important aspects in men's lives: ageing, assessment of achievements and acceptance of limitations. While Chap. 4 focuses on the transition to fatherhood, Chap. 14 examines the reconstruction of masculine identity. The authors analyse the extent to which men in the empty nest phase of their lives follow traditional norms of masculinity or the new, more emotional models.

Summary

The empty nest phase proves a complex and multifaceted period in the lives of parents and families. It involves significant reconfigurations of family dynamics, relationships, roles, and emotions. The departure of adult children from the family home is a transformative event that impacts not only the parents but also the children themselves. Parents, particularly mothers, find themselves still involved in their adult children's lives, albeit in evolving roles that give rise to a complex mix of emotions, including relief, guilt, and pride. This phase also offers couples the opportunity to reconfigure their marital relationships, with some experiencing a "new honeymoon" marked by redirected attention to each other, while others may maintain more parallel lives with weaker bonds. When the bond with children continues to be strong, couples may experience relatively little change and the transition to empty nest feels smooth. Gender norms and societal expectations play a significant role in shaping individuals' experiences, with men grappling with changing identities and roles, and women navigating societal pressures related to motherhood. Emotions during this transition are multifaceted, often intertwined, and include grief, frustration, relief, pride and joy, reflecting the ambivalence stemming from societal norms and personal experiences. Moreover, empty nesters tend to reconfigure their personal identities and home spaces, involving redecoration, the creation of personal spaces, and the embrace of newfound privacy and relaxation. Throughout these changes, family relationships, even among couples with weak bonds, tend to persist, undergoing transformation as individuals adapt to shifting dynamics.

We also wish to highlight the methodology employed in our project, with a particular emphasis on its longitudinal approach, which we consider highly effective for capturing the dynamics of everyday life changes. Throughout our study, we had the privilege of reengaging with select participants after one year, enabling us to conduct individual interviews. These follow-up interviews, in combination with initial dyadic interviews, provided a fresh perspective on the new phase of family life and its evolving relationships. We strongly advocate for and recommend this research methodology (Żadkowska et al., 2018) as it allows us to comprehensively understand the experiences and perspectives of various individuals as mothers, fathers and spouses.

Furthermore, our study was a collaborative effort between Poland and France, with each chapter presenting research findings from both countries and analyses conducted by Polish–French research teams. This collaborative approach allowed us to paint a broader and more comprehensive picture of the phenomenon under investigation, transcending national boundaries and specificities. Interestingly, despite differences in cultural contexts, the emotions and experiences related to the empty nest phase in both Poland and France exhibited striking similarities.

Finally, it is crucial to acknowledge that this project coincided with the COVID-19 pandemic (2020–2022) and its far-reaching implications, which likely influenced family dynamics, particularly concerning adult children's decisions to return to their family homes after living independently. The phenomenon of 'pandemic returns' has the potential to reshape the way we perceive adult children coming back home, potentially becoming a commonplace occurrence in the family life course. Our analysis has revealed that, although parents often found themselves burdened with additional housework and the necessity to adapt their living conditions and routines, they also derived significant satisfaction from the temporary return of their adult children. These reunions provided parents with invaluable opportunities to reestablish connections with their children and cultivate new, fulfilling relationships, thereby equipping them emotionally for the eventual departure of their adult offspring.

In conclusion, the empty nest phase is a transformative period that challenges and reshapes family dynamics, identities, emotions, and relationships. It highlights the interplay between personal experiences and societal expectations and underscores the resilience and adaptability of individuals and families as they navigate this pivotal stage of life.

REFERENCES

Anderson, E. R., & Greene, S. M. (2005). Transitions in parental repartnering after divorce. *Journal of Divorce & Remarriage, 43*(3–4), 47–62. https://doi.org/10.1300/J087v43n03_03

Arnett, J. J. (2000). Emerging adulthood: A theory of development from the late teens through the twenties. *American Psychologist, 55*(5), 469–480. https://doi.org/10.1037/0003-066X.55.5.469

Arnett, J. J. (2007). Emerging adulthood: What is it, and what is it good for? *Society for Research Child Development, 1*(2), 68–73.

Arnett, J. J. (2014). *Emerging adulthood: The winding road from the late teens through the twenties* (2nd ed.). Oxford University Press.

Arnett, J. J., & Schwab, J. (2013). *Parents and their grown kids: Harmony, support, and (occasional) conflict.* The Clark University Poll of Emerging Adults.

Banchefsky, S., & Park, B. (2016). The "new father": Dynamic stereotypes of fathers. *Psychology of Men & Masculinity, 17*(1), 103–107. https://doi.org/10.1037/a0038945

Beaupré, P., Turcotte, P., & Milan, A. (2018). When is junior moving out? Transitions from the parental home to independence. *Canadian Social Trends, 11, 7.*

Benson, J. E., & Furstenberg, F. F. (2006). Entry into adulthood: Are adult role transitions meaningful markers of adult identity? *Advances in Life Course Research, 11,* 199–224.

Borland, D. C. (1982). A cohort analysis approach to the empty-nest syndrome among three ethnic groups of women: A theoretical position. *Journal of Marriage and Family, 44*(1), 117–129. https://doi.org/10.2307/351267

Bouchard, G. (2014). How do parents react when their children leave home? An integrative review. *Journal of Adult Development, 21*(2), 69–79. https://doi.org/10.1007/s10804-013-9180-8

Bouchard, G., & McNair, J. L. (2016). Dyadic examination of the influence of family relationships on life satisfaction at the empty-nest stage. *Journal of Adult Development, 23*(3), 174–182. https://doi.org/10.1007/s10804-016-9233-x

Braun, V., & Clarke, V. (2021). One size fits all? What counts as quality practice in (reflexive) thematic analysis? *Qualitative Research in Psychology, 18*(3), 328–352. https://doi.org/10.1080/14780887.2020.1769238

Braun, V., Clarke, V., & Gray, D. (2017). *Collecting qualitative data: A practical guide to textual, media and virtual techniques.* Cambridge University Press.

Bühlmann, F., Elcheroth, G., & Tettamanti, M. (2009). The division of labour among European couples: The effects of life course and welfare policy on value–practice configurations. *European Sociological Review, 26*(1), 49–66. https://doi.org/10.1093/esr/jcp004

Carter, M. (2015, June 19). What's so wrong with 'pet parenting'? *HuffPost.* Retrieved from https://www.huffingtonpost.co.uk/marie-carter/pet-parenting-whats-so-wrong-with-it_b_7079174.html

Castelain-Meunier, C. (2005). *Les métamorphoses du masculine.* PUF.

Cherlin, A. J., Scabini E., & Rossi, G. (1997). Still in the nest: Delayed home leaving in Europe and the United States. *Journal of Family Issues, 18*, 572–575. https://doi.org/10.1177%2F019251397018006001

Dennerstein, L., Dudley, E., & Guthrie, J. (2002). Empty nest or revolving door? A prospective study of women's quality of life in midlife during the phase of children leaving and re-entering the home. *Psychological Medicine, 32*(3), 545–550. https://doi.org/10.1017/S0033291701004810

Despalins, R., & de Saint Pol, T. (2012). L'entrée dans la vie adulte des bacheliers sous l'angle du logement. *Études et Résultats, 813.*

Duvall, E. M. (1971). *Family development.* Lippincott.

Eisenberg, N., Eggum-Wilkens, N. D., & Spinrad, T. L. (2015). The development of prosocial behavior. In D. A. Schroeder & W. G. Graziano (Eds.), *Oxford handbook of prosocial behavior* (pp. 114–136). Oxford University Press.

Esping-Andersen, G. (1990). *The three worlds of welfare capitalism.* Princeton University Press.

EUROSTAT. (2022). Retrieved from https://ec.europa.eu/eurostat/statistics-explained/index.php?title=Educational_attainment_statistics

Feeney, J., Peterson, C., & Noller, P. (1994). Equity and marital satisfaction over the family life cycle. *Personal Relationships, 1*(1), 83–99. https://doi.org/10.1111/j.1475-6811.1994.tb00056.x

Finch, J. (2007). Displaying families. *Sociology, 41*(1), 65–81. https://doi. org/10.1177/0038038507072284

Fingerman, K. L., Cheng, Y. P., Wesselmann, E. D., Zarit, S., Furstenberg, F., & Birditt, K. S. (2012). Helicopter parents and landing pad kids: Intense parental support of grown children. *Journal of Marriage and the Family, 74*(4), 880–896. https://doi.org/10.1111/j.1741-3737.2012.00987.x

Furmańska-Maruszak, A., & Suwada, K. (2021). Familialisation of care in European societies: Between family and the state. In A.-M. Castrén, V. Česnuitytė, I. Crespi, J.-A. Gauthier, R. Gouveia, C. Martin, A. M. Mínguez, & K. Suwada (Eds.), *The Palgrave handbook of family sociology in Europe* (pp. 205–221). Palgrave Macmillan.

Galland, O. (1997). Leaving home and family relations in France. *Journal of Family Issues, 18*(6), 645–670. https://doi.org/10.1177/019251397018006005

Galland, O. (2003). Adolescence, post-adolescence, youth: Revised interpretations. *Revue Française de Sociologie, 44*, 163–188.

Gaviria, S. (2020). *Revenir vivre en famille. Devenir adulte autrement.* Éditions du Bord de l'eau.

Gillespie, B. J. (2020). Adolescent intergenerational relationship dynamics and leaving and returning to the parental home. *Journal of Marriage and Family, 82*(3), 997–1014. https://doi.org/10.1111/jomf.12630

Gouveia, R., & Castrén, A. M. (2021). Redefining the boundaries of family and personal relationships. In A.-M. Castrén, V. Česnuitytė, I. Crespi, J.-A. Gauthier, R. Gouveia, C. Martin, A. M. Mínguez, & K. Suwada (Eds.), *The Palgrave handbook of family sociology in Europe* (pp. 259–277). Palgrave Macmillan.

Harper, J. M., Schaalje, B. G., & Sandberg, J. G. (2000). Daily hassles, intimacy, and marital quality in later life marriages. *American Journal of Family Therapy, 28*(1), 1–18. https://doi.org/10.1080/019261800261770

Heiman, J. R., Long, J. S., Smith, S. N., Fisher, W. A., Sand, M. S., & Rosen, R. C. (2011). Sexual satisfaction and relationship happiness in midlife and older couples in five countries. *Archives of Sexual Behavior, 40*(4), 741–753. https://doi.org/10.1007/s10508-010-9703-3

INSEE. (2021). Demographic balance sheet 2021 – Retrospective tables. *INSEE.* Retrieved April 30, 2023, from https://www.insee.fr/en/statistiques/6039904

Isengard, B., König, R., & Szydlik, M. (2018). Money or space? Intergenerational transfers in a comparative perspective. *Housing Studies, 33*(2), 178–200. https://doi.org/10.1080/02673037.2017.1365823

James, A., & Curtis, P. (2010). Family displays and personal lives. *Sociology, 44*(6), 1163–1180. https://doi.org/10.1177/0038038510381612

Kajta, J., & Mrozowicki, A. (2023). *Young people in Poland - Report of FES international youth studies.* Retrieved from https://library.fes.de/pdf-files/id/19162.pdf

Kaufmann, J. C. (2001). *Ego. Pour une sociologie de l'individu.* Nathan.

Korpi, W. (2000). Faces of inequality: Gender, class, and patterns of inequalities in different types of welfare states. *Social Politics: International Studies in Gender, State & Society, 7*(2), 127–191. https://doi.org/10.1093/sp/7.2.127

Liberska, H. (2014). Rozwój rodziny i rozwój w rodzinie. In I. Janicka & H. Liberska (Eds.), *Psychologia rodziny* (pp. 221–240). Wydawnictwo Naukowe PWN.

Mary, A. A. (2014). Re-evaluating the concept of adulthood and the framework of transition. *Journal of Youth Studies, 17*(3), 415–429.

Mitchell, B. A. (2006). *The boomerang age transitions to adulthood in families.* Routledge.

Mitchell, B. A. (2010). Happiness in Midlife Parental Roles: A Contextual Mixed Methods Analysis. *Family Relations, 59*(3), 326–339. http://www.jstor.org/stable/40864543

Mitchell, B. A., & Lovegreen, L. D. (2009). The empty nest syndrome in midlife families: A multimethod exploration of parental gender differences and cultural dynamics. *Journal of Family Issues, 30*(12), 1651–1670. https://doi.org/1 0.1177/0192513X09339020

Mizielińska, J., Stasińska, A., Żadkowska, M., & Halawa, M. (2018). Ethical dilemmas in research on intimate couples. Experiences from the fieldwork. *Studia Socjologiczne, 3*(230), 41–69. https://doi.org/10.24425/122472

Modell, J., Furstenberg, F. F., & Hershberg, T. (1976). Social change and transitions to adulthood in historical perspective. *Journal of Family History, 1*(1), 7–32. https://doi.org/10.1177/036319907600100103

Olofsson, J., Sandow, E., Findlay, A., & Malmberg, G. (2020). Boomerang behaviour and emerging adulthood: Moving back to the parental home and the parental neighbourhood in Sweden. *European Journal of Population, 36*(5), 919–945. https://doi.org/10.1007/s10680-020-09557-x

Ostrovsky-Berman, E., & Litwin, H. (2019). *21. Financial and non-financial transfers from parents to adult children after the economic crisis. W 21. Financial and non-financial transfers from parents to adult children after the economic crisis* (pp. 207–216). De Gruyter. https://doi.org/10.1515/9783110617245-021

Owens, N., & Grauerholz, L. (2019). Interspecies parenting: How pet parents construct their roles. *Humanity and Society, 43*(2), 96–119. https://doi.org/10.1177/0160597617748166

Pustułka, P., Sarnowska, J., & Buler, M. (2022). Resources and pace of leaving home among young adults in Poland. *Journal of Youth Studies, 25*(7), 946–962. https://doi.org/10.1080/13676261.2021.1925638

Raup, J. L., & Myers, J. E. (1989). The Empty Nest Syndrome: Myth or Reality? *Journal of Counseling & Development, 68*(2), 180–183. https://doi.org/10.1002/j.1556-6676.1989.tb01353.x

Robert, A., & Sulzer, E. (2021). Quitter le domicile parental: un processus très lié au parcours scolaire et professionnel. *INSEE*. Retrieved April 5, 2023, from https://www.insee.fr/fr/statistiques/4797666?sommaire=4928952

Schmidt, F. (2015). *Para, mieszkanie, małżeństwo. Dynamika związków intymnych na tle przemian historycznych i współczesnych dyskusji o procesach indywidualizacji*. Wydawnictwo Naukowe UMK.

Schmidt, P. J., Murphy, J. H., Haq, N., Rubinow, D. R., & Danaceau, M. A. (2004). Stressful life events, personal losses, and perimenopause-related depression. *Archives of Women's Mental Health, 7*(1), 19–26. https://doi.org/10.1007/s00737-003-0036-2

Seiffge-Krenke, I. (2013). "She's Leaving Home …" Antecedents, Consequences, and Cultural Patterns in the Leaving Home Process. *Emerging Adulthood*. https://doi.org/10.1177/2167696813479783

Sheriff, M., & Weatherall, A. (2009). A feminist discourse analysis of popular-press accounts of postmaternity. *Feminism & Psychology, 19*(1), 89–108. https://doi.org/10.1177/0959353508098621

Slany, K. (2006). Socjo-demograficzne aspekty "syndromu opóźniania" i jego konsekwencje dla polityki społecznej. *Roczniki Socjologii Rodziny, XVII*(2006), 13–25.

Szafraniec, K. (2017). Entering adulthood - from diagnoses of youth to social policies towards them: In search of specificity of transition countries. *Vietnam Social Sciences, 3*, 1–20.

Szelewa, D. (2017). From implicit to explicit familialism: Post-1989 family policy reforms in Poland. In D. Auth, J. Hergenhan, & B. Holland-Cunz (Eds.), *Gender and family in European economic policy. Developments in the new millennium* (pp. 129–156). Palgrave Macmillan.

Szlendak, T. (2010). *Socjologia rodziny*. Wydawnictwo Naukowe PWN.

Thibodeau, J., & Bouchard, G. (2020). Attachment and satisfaction at the empty-nest stage: An actor–partner interdependence model. *Journal of Adult Development, 27*(3), 212–223. https://doi.org/10.1007/s10804-019-09341-0

Van de Velde, C. (2008). *Devenir Adulte: Sociologie comparée de la jeunesse en Europe*. PUF.

Walther, A. (2006). Regimes of youth transitions: Choice, flexibility and security in young people's experiences across different European contexts. *Young, 14*, 119–139. https://doi.org/10.1177/1103308806062737

Walther, A., Blasco, A. L., & McNeish, W. (2003). *Young people and contradictions of inclusion: Towards integrated transition policies in Europe*. Policy Press.

Żadkowska, M., Olcoń-Kubicka, M., Gądecki, J., Mizielińska, J., Stasińska, A., Schmidt, F., & Halawa, M. (2018). Metodologiczne aspekty jakościowych badań par - synteza doświadczeń terenowych. *Studia Socjologiczne, 3*(230), 41–69.

CHAPTER 2

The Value of "Empty Nest Syndrome" in Sociology

François de Singly

The notion of an "empty nest" is an example of analogous reasoning. If instead of using the expression "childless house" to refer to the phase of family life when children leave their parents, we use the notion of a "nest", we can go beyond the descriptive register. What does this analogy mean?

THE NEST AS A FAMILY'S COSY SPACE

The nest (empty or not) evokes the cosiness of a family place where the whole family keeps itself warm.[1] This refers, explicitly or not, to the history of the family home, at the end of the nineteenth century, when the family

---

[1] In La chaleur du foyer. Analyse du repli domestique (1988), Jean-Claude Kaufmann stresses that the family is associated in the social imagination with a warm atmosphere created by the family home, like a nest.

F. de Singly (✉)
Centre de recherche sur les liens sociaux (CERLIS, UMR 8070), Université Paris Cité, Paris, France
e-mail: francois@singly.org

© The Author(s), under exclusive license to Springer Nature Switzerland AG 2024
M. Żadkowska et al. (eds.), *Reconfiguring Relations in the Empty Nest*, Palgrave Macmillan Studies in Family and Intimate Life, https://doi.org/10.1007/978-3-031-50403-7_2

folds into itself, when the husband is asked to return home as soon as possible in the evening, and when the wife, for this particular reason, is expected to prepare a comfortable and attractive interior (Murard & Zylberman, 1976; Perrot, 1987). The analogy with the nest becomes possible when family life seeks to become "private", intimate (this is the time when servants will have to live separately, e.g. in the maid's rooms [*chambres de bonnes*] so common in the Haussmannian buildings of Paris).

Research dedicated to the first appearance of this notion in literature should be carried out. An example of this can be found in Pierre Loti's *Vies des deux chattes* published in 1907. When he was not on board a ship, this adventurer and writer lived in Rochefort with his mother, his aunt, and his two cats. He recalls the moments spent in the evenings in "a small, warm living room … which was the most secret backstage of our family life". And he adds: "No other place has ever given me a more complete and sweet impression of a nest; nowhere have I warmed myself with more lulling melancholy than in front of the flames of this little fireplace." Family intimacy, warmth, sweetness of life.

Other novels have taken the opposite approach by evoking the nest, but entirely deprived of warmth. Let us refer to Daniel Odija's *Pusty Przelot* (2021), where the two brothers learn to live together in a house deserted by their father, and even by their mother lost in her dreams. The reference in Milos Forman's film *One Flew Over the Cuckoo's Nest* (1975), is even darker, as the insane asylum operates in a severe and authoritarian manner, depriving its patients of all warmth and also of their entire freedom. The notion of a nest is positive based on two conditions: the members of the given habitat must feel good, and they must have the possibility to fly away: not to escape from misfortune, but to become independent.

The Invention of the Notion of Empty Nest Syndrome

In the humanities, the use of the notion of the empty nest changes the perspective. These are the parents, or more specifically the mother, who observe their children's departure. Literature points to Dorothy Canfield Fisher who proposes the notion of "empty nest syndrome" in *Mothers and Children* (1914). This author believes that many women start experiencing problems when the house empties itself of children. Her work, consisting of essays and fiction (published either under her maiden name,

Canfield Fisher, under her married name, Fisher, or under her combined name) is critical of attributing parental roles based on gender (Wright, 2000).

Dorothy Canfield Fisher (1912) thus points to the confinement of women in family life by using the analogy of the "squirrel cage" to designate marriage. She advocates, on the one hand, a division of labour that depends on the history of the couple and not on stereotypes—notably in her best-selling novel *The Home Maker* (Canfield Fisher, 1924) where the spouses exchange roles (Bliss, 2020)—and, on the other hand, an education centred on the independence and autonomy of children in the perspective of the Montessori method that the author defends. So, originally, empty nest syndrome belongs to a wider critique of the fixed roles attributed to women.

A few decades later, in the 1960s and 1970s, this notion was taken up by psychologists to refer to symptoms such as depression, loneliness and low self-esteem that a mother suffers from when her last child leaves home. Numerous studies tested the hypothesis of the appearance of these symptoms, of this malaise, and initially confirmed it (Lowenthal & Chiriboga, 1972). Then new data showed either the appearance of these syndromes or, on the contrary, a kind of liberation, a satisfaction of reconnecting with the spouse, of taking better care of oneself (Bouchard, 2014). The effects associated with the empty nest are thus not unequivocal (Randhawa & Kaur, 2021). What is the reason for this ambiguity?

How Can Sociology Deal with the Notion of "Empty Nest Syndrome"?

When we read the sociological literature, in reference to the notion of the empty nest, it is the perspective on roles that predominates (even though others may coexist). This is because, in line with Dorothy Canfield Fisher's hypothesis, the empty nest should bring about a change in parental roles, especially for women. Other changes may also be associated with the departure of children, but the empty nest analogy has the effect of emphasising the way in which women recompose their roles when their maternal role diminishes. The roles perspective can be differentiated in at least three directions, which Lynn White and John N. Edwards (1990) clearly distinguish.

The first one, called role identity theory, considers the number of roles that the social actor plays is important for the social construction of their identity. One possible form of wealth would be the repertoire of roles: "the more roles the given person has at their disposal, the better". Peggy Thoits (1983) thus considers that "social identities provide actors with existential meaning and behavioural guidance" and improve their "psychological well-being". In relation to the empty nest, the question arises: whether or not the parental role is lost when the children leave.

The second one, called role change theory, says that any change of role is disruptive, destabilising in such a way that the effects are negative, at least in the short term during the transition period (Holmes & Rahe, 1967).

The third theoretical framework, outlined by Lynn White and John N. Edwards (1990), is called role stress (cf. Barnett & Baruch, 1985). The impact of the change in parenting role depends on the degree of stress or conflict associated with that role. If the role played is associated with stress, losing it may bring the given person satisfaction. Parenting is stressful (McLanahan & Adams, 1987), it often lowers marital satisfaction. So, the departure of the children does not cause empty nest syndrome, it rather loosens the constraints and leaves more room for other roles.

In summary, the sociological literature on the empty nest primarily explores the changes in parental roles, particularly for women, when their maternal role diminishes. Three key theoretical frameworks—role identity theory, role change theory, and role stress theory—shed light on the dynamics of this phenomenon.

A Link Between Empty Nest and Marital Happiness

If the departure of children resulted in empty nest syndrome, the effects would be negative for the parents concerned. However, taking into account the data collected by Lynn White and John N. Edwards (1990), we can observe, on the one hand, a positive relationship with the marital happiness indicator while, on the other, no particular effect on personal satisfaction. This distinction is interesting because it confirms the link between parenting and marital roles. At the beginning, when the child appears, marital satisfaction decreases, and here, at the end, manifested by the departure of the children, satisfaction increases. The existence of this tension was found in research on family life in Paris: "In the trade-offs, marital time often comes after parental time, family time and even personal time" (de Singly & Giraud, 2012: 161). The departure of the children seems to liberate time for the couple, which makes marital satisfaction increase. If this interpretation is correct, it means that the lack of effect on personal satisfaction would be evidence that the time freed up by a reduction in parenting burdens would not be converted into personal time.

Lack of a Link Between the Empty Nest and Personal Happiness

There are three results complementing this main observation.

First, Lynn White and John N. Edwards (1990) note that the absence of children altogether, not just older children or fewer children, is necessary for the departure to improve marital happiness. The decrease in the burden (with the departure of one of the children) is not enough to create the shock; there must also be a clearer marker of the change in the hierarchy of roles, with the parental role losing its priority. The adjective "empty nest" then takes on its full meaning.

Second, after the departure of the children, the role changes significantly without rupturing the relationship. However, according to Lynn White and John N. Edwards (1990), varying the frequency of visits or calls from children does not change the positive relationship between their leaving and the marital happiness results.

Third, the neutral relationship between departure and personal satisfaction changes with the frequency of contact. It becomes positive if contact is maintained with non-resident children and negative if the relationship becomes less frequent. This result proves that parents actually do not wish for the end of parenting that much, but rather a significant reduction in the workload associated with parenting when the child is in the same household as the parents.

The "empty nest" can have a positive effect on personal happiness only under certain conditions, probably also because the departure of the children also proves that parental work is accomplished. This by no means implies a desire to break with one's child or children. Parenthood—in the sense of parenting—continues to be important after the children have left. The "nest" may be "empty" but the relationship is not, it gets transformed.

For Lynn Whyte and John Edwards (1990), these effects provide at least some validation of the perspective discussed at the beginning of this paper, namely the stress associated with performing certain roles. At this level, the father and mother are relieved by the end of the cohabitation. By dissociating strong parenting from maintaining a relationship with the child, we observe the reduction of parenting constraints as positive for marital and personal happiness (however, only if contact with the child or children is maintained).

By analogy, we believe that maintaining links between parents and children without shared space can be likened to couples without shared accommodation, as in *Living Apart Together*. It is a way of maintaining ties while easing the constraints associated with sharing the same home. A comparison could be made with the situation of parents after divorcing when they opt for alternating custody. Some parents do not feel less of a parent despite the experience of disengagement from parenting (Hachet, 2021). Others, especially mothers, react in the opposite way, and refuse the very principle of alternating custody. Analysing the empty nest can help to shed light on the issue of raising younger children after divorce and vice versa.

A HISTORICAL REVERSAL OF THE SYNDROME?

When these results on the empty nest are found—which we will see, or not, in the pages that follow—we can question the initial notion by asking ourselves if the phenomenon in question, which can be observed at the level of the intergenerational relationship, should not be called *the syndrome of the full nest, from the second half of the twentieth century,* instead of the empty nest. This raises the question of whether White and Edwards are right in stating that "the impact of the empty nest is reduced by the close ties and frequent contact between parents and children", which are maintained despite the departure, suggesting that "separate residence is relatively minor for disengagement" (White & Edwards, 1990: 241).

Indeed, another interpretation can be made based on a theoretical condition, which is separating the parental dimension from personal identity and the workload associated with the parental role. Parental identity and parenting are not the same thing. With the end of the children residing under the same roof as their parents, these two factors separate: identity remains strong while parenting is less demanding.[2] It all depends then on what is implied by White and Edwards (1990) in the notion of disengagement. The criterion of the number of hours is undoubtedly a good indicator of commitment to the notion of a role, but this does not mean that this quantitative indicator is a good indicator of the place of this identity

---

[2] The return of the child home—the boomerang effect—is problematic as parents have to combine the two factors again.

dimension. Are working mothers less mothers in terms of identity than stay-at-home mothers? Many conservatives have thought so and still think this way, but it has never been proven. Moreover, it seems that based on what constructing the identity by the contemporary individuals concerns, the two factors, that is, the time spent and the place of the dimension in identity, are not dissociated either.

The empty nest can have a positive effect. To put it another way, you can feel like a mother and be happy to be one without devoting all your time to this role.

We must return to Dorothy Canfield Fisher (1914) who invented the notion of empty nest syndrome. This syndrome is the flip side of the assignment to women to be first and foremost mothers. The time spent and the place of identity of the maternal dimension were to merge (in the sense of social constraint). Today, with transformations of identity and, particularly, of women's identity, this confusion is criticised. The end of living together on a daily basis can be experienced as an opportunity to achieve this dissociation. If this is true, it is normal that empty nest syndrome will disappear to some extent.

THE SOCIO-HISTORICAL CONTEXTUALISATION OF PARENTAL ROLES

Reconciling Dorothy Canfield Fisher's (literary) hypothesis with its rather positive results associated with the current departure raises questions about the conditions under which empty nest syndrome has disappeared in many studies.[3] The answer can only come from the social and temporal contextualisation of observations. Indeed, sociology is not ruled by any law, as it is a historical discipline (Passeron, 1987). It is therefore necessary to place the surveys in their social and temporal environment. Thus, in the surveys presented in this book, the diversity of family forms is one of the possible variables of the comparison. Indeed, it can be assumed that women who are responsible for a "single parent family" experience a greater sense of emptiness than women who live with their partner. It was also observed in some research that the departure of children increases the marital happiness score. It is as if there were a communicating vessel between the two dimensions of the parental and the conjugal. Women

---

[3] If we assume more medical measures, there is no empty nest syndrome either (Dennerstein et al., 2002).

who are single parents cannot experience this principle, and are therefore more likely to experience empty nest syndrome, unless the departure of children gives them the freedom to enter into new relationships.

The comparison between Poland and France also makes it possible to examine the differences between these two European countries in terms not only of gender differences in parenting, but also the values at stake in child-rearing. The hypotheses put forward by Mandeep Randhawa and Jaismeen Kaur (2021) can be used as a basis. These authors believe that the variation in the importance of the place given to children's autonomy and independence in family socialisation must be taken into account. From their perspective, parents who value these two qualities will suffer less from the empty nest than others because the child's departure will be considered as a sign of educational success by them.[4] Mandeep Randhawa and Jaismeen Kaur (2021) claim that Western countries differ from Eastern countries in this educational dimension. This is true for example for the United States, where the value of "autonomy" became very important throughout the twentieth century, while the value of "obedience" continually declined (Alwin, 1988; de Singly, 2006).

The recent and numerous studies carried out in China show the existence of depressive symptoms in both elderly mothers and elderly fathers (Zhai et al., 2015). This is not just a temporary, transient effect. It is significantly higher among parents aged 70 and over, living in the empty nest. Other research in China adds a variable to the analysis, which was rarely measured before, namely the loneliness and feelings of loneliness (Cheng et al., 2015).[5] Empty nest symptoms will also depend on the lack of relationships, after the phase of living with the child or children is closed. Can the bonds of emotional closeness be maintained with geographical distance (cf. Tanis et al., 2017)?

CONCLUSION

The question of the transformation of maternal and paternal roles throughout life is central to the problem of the "empty nest". To what extent do new conditions for the exercise of these roles change them? Is this conversion difficult, and how much, for those who have to adapt? To what extent

---

[4] This also makes the return of the children, known as the boomerang effect, a possibly unpleasant phenomenon, not only because of the new burdens associated with resuming the parenting role, but also because of the fear of having failed as a parent.

[5] This feeling of loneliness is felt even by those who live in couples (cf. Cheng et al., 2015).

does this reconversion create the conditions for a reconversion of identity, leaving more room for other roles, particularly the marital role? To what extent does this conversion constitute a new phase of life, marking not only a form of liberation from the constraints of parental roles, but also a gradual entry into certain ageing? To what extent is the remote exercise of these roles (partly) possible? Which dimensions of the parenting "repertoire" (de Singly & Chaland, 2002) are maintained and which are set aside?

The problem of the empty nest is actually relevant in the social sciences insofar as it is linked to the more classic notion of the role.

References

Alwin, D. F. (1988). From obedience to autonomy: Changes in traits desired in children, 1924–1978. *Public Opinion Quarterly, 52*(1), 33–52. https://doi.org/10.1086/269081

Barnett, R. C., & Baruch, G. K. (1985). Women's involvement in multiple-roles and psychological distress. *Journal of Personality and Social Psychology, 49*(1), 135–145. https://doi.org/10.1037/0022-3514.49.1.135

Bliss, A. V. (2020). Home/bodies: Challenging gendered work roles in Dorothy Canfield Fisher's "The home-maker". *Women's Studies, 49*(5), 478–498. https://doi.org/10.1080/00497878.2020.1772793

Bouchard, G. (2014). How do parents react when their children leave home? An integrative review. *Journal of Adult Development, 21*(2), 69–79. https://doi.org/10.1007/s10804-013-9180-8

Canfield Fisher, D. (1912). *The squirrel-cage*. Holt & Company.

Canfield Fisher, D. (1914). *Mothers and children*. Holt & Company.

Canfield Fisher, D. (1924). *The home-maker*. Harcourt, Brace and Company.

Cheng, P., Jin, Y., Sun, H. M., Tang, Z. H., Zhang, C., Chen, Y. J., Zhang, Q., Zhang, Q. H., & Huang, F. (2015). Disparities in prevalence and risk indicators of loneliness between rural empty nest and non-empty nest older adults in Chizhou, China. *Geriatrics & Gerontology International, 15*, 356–364.

De Singly, F. (2006). *Les Adonaissants*. Colin.

De Singly, F., & Chaland, K. (2002). Avoir le second rôle dans une équipe conjugale. Le cas des femmes de préfet et de sous-préfet. *Revue Française de Sociologie, 43*(1), 127–158.

De Singly, F., & Giraud, C. (2012). *En famille à Paris*. Colin.

Dennerstein, L., Dudley, E., & Guthrie, J. R. (2002). Empty nest or revolving door? A prospective study of women's quality of life in mid-life during the phase of children leaving and re-entering the home. *Psychological Medicine, 32*, 545–550. https://doi.org/10.1017/S0033291701004810

Hachet, B. (2021). *Une semaine sur deux. Comment les parents séparés se réinventent.* Les Arènes.

Holmes, T. H., & Rahe, R. H. (1967). The social readjustment rating scale. *Journal of Psychosomatic Research, 11*(2), 213–218. https://doi.org/10.1016/0022-3999(67)90010-4

Kaufmann, J. C. (1988). *La chaleur du foyer. Analyse du repli domestique.* Méridiens Klinckseck.

Lowenthal, M. F., & Chiriboga, D. (1972). Transition to the empty nest: Crisis, challenge or relief? *Archives of General Psychiatry, 26*(1), 8–14. https://doi.org/10.1001/archpsyc.1972.01750190010003

McLanahan, S., & Adams, J. (1987). Parenthood and psychological well-being. *Annual Review of Sociology, 13*, 237–257.

Murard, L., & Zylberman, P. (1976). Le petit travailleur infatigable ou le prolétaire régénéré. *Recherches, 25.*

Odija, D. (2021). *Pusty Przelot.* Wydawnictwo Czarne.

Passeron, J.-C. (1987). *Le raisonnement sociologique: L'espace non-popperien du raisonnement naturel.* Nathan.

Perrot, M. (Ed.). (1987). *Histoire de la vie privée, tome 4, De la Révolution à la Grande Guerre.* Seuil.

Randhawa, M., & Kaur, J. (2021). Acknowledging empty Nest syndrome: Eastern and Western perspective. *Mind and Society, 10*(03–04), 38–42.

Tanis, M., van der Louw, M., & Buijzen, M. (2017). From empty nest to social networking site: What happens in cyberspace when children are launched from the parental home? *Computers in Human Behavior, 68*, 56–63. https://doi.org/10.1016/j.chb.2016.11.005

Thoits, P. A. (1983). Multiple-identities and psychological well-being: A reformulation and test of the social isolation hypothesis. *American Sociological Review, 48*(2), 174–187.

White, L., & Edwards, J. N. (1990). Empty the nest and parental well-being: An analysis of national panel data. *American Sociological Review, 55*(2), 235–242. https://doi.org/10.2307/2095629

Wright, E. (2000). Dorothy Canfield Fisher. In L. Champion (Ed.), *American women writers 1900-1945* (pp. 113–118). Greenwood Press.

Zhai, Y., Yi, H., Shen, W., Xiao, Y., Fan, H., He, F., Li, F., Wang, X., Shang, X., & Lin, J. (2015). Association of empty nest with depressive symptom in a Chinese elderly population: A cross-sectional study. *Journal of Affective Disorders, 187*, 218–223. https://doi.org/10.1016/j.jad.2015.08.031

PART I

The Family in 'The Empty Nest'

CHAPTER 3

Reconfiguration of the Mother's Role After the Departure of the Children

Magdalena Herzberg-Kurasz, Christophe Giraud,
Magdalena Anita Gajewska, Sophie David–Goretta,
and François de Singly

MOTHERHOOD IN THE EMPTY NEST

Motherhood is a phenomenon that occurs within a certain time frame; it does not happen suddenly. We notice that the significance and importance of the mother's role are particularly strongly visible at the beginning of the maternal journey, right after the birth of the child (Budrowska, 2000;

M. Herzberg-Kurasz (✉) • M. A. Gajewska
Social Sciences Department (Institute of Sociology), University of Gdańsk, Gdańsk, Poland
e-mail: magdalena.herzberg-kurasz@ug.edu.pl; magdalena.gajewska@ug.edu.pl

C. Giraud • S. David–Goretta • F. de Singly
Centre de recherche sur les liens sociaux (CERLIS, UMR 8070), Université Paris Cité, Paris, France
e-mail: christophe.giraud@parisdescartes.fr; sophie.david.goretta@gmail.com; francois@singly.org

Afflerback et al., 2014). According to classical perspectives, the mother stands at the top of the hierarchy of the young child's needs (Titkow, 1995; Budrowska, 2000). In this approach, the uniqueness of the mother–child duet is continually emphasised, and the role of the mother is seen as an essential part of feminine identity (Budrowska, 2000; O'Reilly, 2010; Sheriff & Weatherall, 2009; Titkow, 1995, 2007, 2012; Titkow et al., 2004). There is a tension between this traditional model and the emancipatory model in the associated attitude to the spectrum of women's roles (Hryciuk & Korolczuk, 2012; Imbierowicz, 2012). The possibility for women to realise roles other than the role of caring for offspring is due to the delay in taking on the maternal role among the younger generation (Titkow, 1995, 2007; Packalén Parkman, 2017). This is largely related to the existing tension between career and professional desires and the willingness to become a mother—which is a "carrier of femininity" functioning beyond time and territory (Gromkowska-Melosik, 2017). Such a strongly held, internalised cultural frame (that the role of the mother is one's primary life role) might have a significant impact on how mothers experience their children leaving the family home. In Poland and France, the mother–child relationship is subject to stronger social evaluation than the father–child relationship. Creating motherhood as a means of female fulfillment, idealising the person and the maternal quantity, and directing all responsibility for the multidimensional development of the child to the mother is perfect grounds for the emergence of crises within the role of the mother (Titkow, 1995, 2007, 2012; Badinter, 1998, 2013; Budrowska, 2000; Titkow et al., 2004; O'Reilly, 2010; Imbierowicz, 2012; Kaźmierczak-Kałużna, 2016; Packalén Parkman, 2017; Włodarczyk, 2017). Culturally ingrained beliefs about the inseparability of femininity from motherhood continue to have a significant impact on the experiences of those who become mothers and also of those who become mothers of adult children (Sheriff & Weatherall, 2009; Włodarczyk, 2017).

On the one hand, the independence and self-reliance of adult children can be seen as a parental success that can be celebrated and opens the door to living as a couple or pursuing the individual's needs and desires. It is adequate to the theoretical perspective of role strain (relief) where it states that there is a great release from stressful situations, time limitations and conflicts in the relationship with adult children. On the other hand, following the role loss approach where the departure marks the end of a long-standing project that gave life meaning—being a mother—a worsening in the mother's well-being might be witnessed (Umberson et al., 2005; Sheriff & Weatherall, 2009; Erickson et al., 2010; Bouchard, 2014).

Wojciechowska points to the possibility of a feeling of emptiness among mothers as a result of offspring, who used to make the home bustle with family life, leaving the nest. This phenomenon is mainly considered from the perspective of the mothers, not the fathers, which is justified by the importance of the parental role in the definition of women's identity. This does not mean that the parental role is less important for fathers. However, the set of roles performed by them is more diverse and balanced (Wojciechowska, 2008; Zalewska, 2012; Bouchard, 2014). The autonomy of the adult child and the moment of moving out is a strong stimulant to view the role of the mother "as her past and future, a future without the role of the mother" (Gajewska et al., 2023).

The transition to the empty nest phase implicates a change from the life of the "immediate motherhood role to whatever lies beyond" (Spence & Lonner, 1971; Mitchell & Lovegreen, 2009; Bouchard, 2014). Sometimes, it turns out that the departure of adult children from the nest does not necessarily lead to a release from the parental role. If a woman worries about her adult child and their future, she goes into a state of limbo or unfinished task, where she continues her mother's work, which corresponds to a liminal stage (Spence & Lonner, 1971; Gajewska et al., 2023) or the feeling of ambivalence (Wojciechowska, 2008; see Chap. 13). As Spence's study shows, the concern and worries for the adult child (associated with proper entry into adulthood, independent living) moving beyond the family nest, despite the desire to pursue new life goals, does not allow the mother to rid herself of a sense of uncertainty and ambiguity (see Chap. 13). For Spence, the difficulty of leaving maternal responsibilities may be due to the emotional bond created over time and of long-term expectations for adult children to be reaching into their future successfully. Some parents assume that the moment their children enter adulthood (through at least their departure from the family home) will represent a moment of new life opportunities. Meanwhile, only a confrontation with this experience (beyond previous imaginations) sometimes brings different experiences than expected (Mitchell & Lovegreen, 2009; Bouchard, 2014). Is it really the case, as Gullette claims, that "the benefits brought by postmaternity are taboo"? (Gullette, 2002).

Our question in this chapter is how the departure of the children implies modifications within the role of the mother (in its diverse dimensions). The starting point for our analyses was the question of what happens to motherhood and the experiences of mothers when children leave the family home. We wanted to see if women step out of their role as they once stepped into it, or is the parental role one of those social roles that cannot be extinguished. In our investigation we include two dimensions of the mother's role (material and relational) and the impact of different stages of departure of adult children.

MOTHER'S ROLE DIMENSIONS

In this chapter, the role of the mother is defined as a set of obligations within two main dimensions: material and relational. The first dimension is well-known in feminist research. In France and Poland, mothers have a major role at home in housekeeping, feeding the children, and washing the clothes (Kaufmann, 1992; Żadkowska, 2016). They have the responsibility of reproductive work (Delphy, 1984) and especially work on the children. If the mothers are employed, they experience even more of a mental load (Haicault, 1984). This overload comes from the fact that mothers, as home managers, have to think about the organisation of domestic tasks even during their professional time. In the upper class, they are the organiser of many activities for the children such as sports, and music classes, while in the working class, much free time is left to be devoted to the children (Lareau, 2021).

The second dimension of a mother's role concerns its relational aspect (de Singly, 1996). Mothers have to support their children psychologically and morally, and solve their children's daily problems. Mothers do not only provide material goods or services but also have to be cautious with the psychological well-being of their children. They feel they should nurture the desires and tastes of their children. With the spread of psychological norms (de Singly, 1996), they must ensure not only the academic skills development of children but also a good balance between school and leisure time. They try to ensure that children's peer relationships are not toxic or that their children are not isolated from other children. Finally, they feel they should help the child to develop self-confidence and skills for independent living (in the future). As Coll and others suggest: "A mother is assigned … to attend minutely (largely unassisted) to the emotional and psychological development of her children (far into adulthood)" (Coll et al., 1999).

This chapter is structured around three parts. First, we describe the extent of the role of mothers, right after the children leave (Budrowska, 2000; Nelson, 2006; Deręgowska & Majorczyk, 2012). Second, we look at how the maternal role reconfigures when the children are on their educational journey and have their own apartment (without full financial independence): mothers have to perform their parental practices remotely. Here, the household tasks are reduced but not necessarily absent, as the children may return at weekends (Mitchell & Lovegreen, 2009). Depending on the type of departure, psychological support is more or less present, and sharing is more or less possible. We analyse the maternal role from the moment the child is settled in a new home and financially independent from the parents. Finally, we see how the mother's role becomes latent when the children are living economically and residentially independently, and overall, when they live in their own new family (Gajewska et al., 2023). Our question is how dimensions of a mother's role evolve according to the different steps of departure. When the children are away at university but still economically dependent on their parents, how does the mother's role transform? Our hypothesis is that while some aspects of the first dimension (mental overload) are reduced, the second (relational) dimension remains strong even after the departure for university or for a first job (when children are still dependent).

METHODS AND RESPONDENTS

Within the framework of this chapter, (43) in-depth dyadic interviews (DDI) with couples in relationships of at least 20 years of marriage (Poland and France, Corpus A, both in urban and rural settings), as well as in-depth individual interviews with women in such relationships (after one year from the in-depth dyadic interviews with the same couples, which were a second interview in the project) were analysed. Additionally, we also analysed (41) individual in-depth interviews with women whose partners chose not to participate in the main study (only Poland, Corpus B). All of the women, aged 50–64, whose experiences were analysed in this chapter are married or in partnerships with the fathers of their children. Their children (numbering from one to four) were all adults and had moved out from the family home over the previous year or earlier. In many cases, the analysis concerned households in which the adult children had moved away to study.

RESULTS

With the continuation of a period of dependence linked to education process, where young people remain dependent on their parents, the housework dimension of the maternal role is reduced (1) (and concentrated on holidays or weekends, when young people return, see Chaps. 6 and 7). However, the material role is not completely abandoned, but rather partially continued from a distance (2). The maternal role is mostly sustained in its relational aspects. The transition from a close and continuous role to a remote and discontinuous role poses many challenges (3). Once the children have settled in independent housing (financially independent), often in couples, the maternal role becomes latent: the material dimension of the role does not exist anymore. At the same time, the relational dimension of the role continues in the form of a very loose watch carried out during visits or phone calls (4). The strength of attachment and interdependence between parents and children is much differentiated, as are its manifestations. Thise chapter focuses on general trends and typical experiences, leaving aside some differences and nuances between households on which some of the other chapters of the book focus more. Section "Reduction of Maternal Burdens", describing a reduction in maternal burdens, is about what changes within the mother role (role reduction) and Sect. "Continuation of the Maternal Role: Remote Tasks" is about role maintenance and its transformation.

Reduction of Maternal Burdens

The role of mother is made up of a wide range of tasks. This domestic work is carried out by women on a daily basis, on a continuous basis, and in physical proximity to the children. The departure of the children then leads to a reduction in continuous work in close proximity to the children.[1] In the analysed material, the reduction of maternal burdens manifests itself in two characteristics which will be described with examples in Sect. "Decrease in the Flow of Products and Number of Household Tasks".

Decrease in the Flow of Products and Number of Household Tasks

The first considerable effect of children leaving home is the reduction in spendings and everyday duties (like paternal household tasks, see Chap. 4). As explained by Agnieszka, mother of three boys who have left the family home one by one over the past five years, the biggest change for her as a mother is that she does not have to worry about providing food for her

---

[1] The emotions produced by this reduction in women's domestic work will be analysed in Chap. 13.

children. She is no longer worried about the need to be ready with a two-course meal every day, which brings a feeling of relief:

> Agnieszka: And when there were children at home, a person thought that there must be both a soup and a second course, that's how it was in our house. And so, you do not have to worry about it, because you can even say "eat something on your way back home". (A_PL_1G)

After the departure of the last child, major transformations in the maternal role can be seen in a reduction of all sorts of household tasks:

> Interviewer: And after your daughters left, were there fewer duties? (…)
> Maria: Less shopping, less cleaning, less cooking, less medication—that time is needed after all. (A_PL_2P)

What is more, a reduction in household chores is also followed by a reduction in planning and equipping the house and (e.g., the refrigerator) with the right products. A major challenge for Elżbieta at home with her adult children was to make decisions that would lead to meeting the culinary tastes of all household members:

> Elżbieta: Well, and it seems to me that such an advantage is also that when it comes to the refrigerator, yes? That a person doesn't have to think about who eats what and to provide for everyone what they like, now there are just the two of us and, for example, I know what I eat and how much my husband will eat, and there is no longer this kind of policing, that everything must be there, because you don't know who will eat what, just these purchases are smaller, no? Well, how to say it? Well, I just know that my husband likes this kind of sausage and I buy only this kind, yes? And my son, for example, would no longer eat it, well, and I would have to think about what to buy for my son. And this is already such a convenience here. (B_PL_25G)

At the same time, when children come home for the weekends or holidays, mothers might re-mobilise for all these tasks. When children return home regularly, a rhythm alternating between weekdays and weekends can be established. Then, very often, the "old order" returns or the children take on the role of guests and are relieved of certain household chores by their parents (see Chap. 6).

It is not just a matter of reducing household chores related to meal preparation, but also the amount of food prepared, the frequency of shopping and even the very expediency of visiting the shop (when going out of habit, without a clear need to do so):

> Agnieszka: (…) you don't have to cook for 5 people and you can go from XL size pots to S size pots, well these are such obvious ones, especially if you have adult boys. You don't have to do such huge shops, well these are the kind of things that come out (…) Well before that… when you have three boys who are 190 cm tall, well, they eat a lot. I used to go shopping every day. And now I see that I can go once a week, sometimes out of some kind of habit I go for something, but actually, I don't know what for (…). (A_PL_1G)

The quantities are reduced. Preparation is also simplified in cases where children have special diets such as for Valérie, who had to manipulate the kitchen menu because one of the children was on a vegetarian diet and the other refused to eat fish:

> Valérie: I had one who started to say that she was becoming a vegetarian, and the other one who didn't want to eat fish, so I had one who ate fish and the other who didn't… So you can see the dilemma, so it's true that it was very difficult, so it's much easier for two people, that's for sure. And it's true that when they're here now, I often find myself making four dishes. (A_FR_6)

The reduction in working time also affects the very female sector of laundry. Men are present in the laundry entering it through the technical channel (loading and unloading the washing machine), but remaining rather in the position of their wives' students (Kaufmann, 1992; Żadkowska, 2016).

> Angèle: I take care of the whole family's laundry and frankly I see the difference. As a result, I have started to buy much less washing powder. (A_FR_19)

> Agnieszka: Before I washed every day, therefore there was also a lot of ironing, and now I can wash once a week and iron once a week, for example. This are so evident. And this is what I somehow missed at the beginning. There's no "what am I going to put in the washing machine, there's nothing", also it's the kind of thing you notice. (A_PL_1G)

The quotations above demonstrate that the reduction in domestic work results in both relief and loss. As Agnieszka admits, everyday laundry was something she missed at first. While housework is commonly seen as burden, it also strongly relates to the maternal role and it is an expression of care.

Reduction in Time Pressure and in "Mental Load"
The departure of the children makes people aware of the rhythm of the various activities in everyday life, especially in families from affluent backgrounds who function by accumulating leisure activities for the children. The reduction in time pressure and in "mental load" is another dimension in reducing maternal burdens. Valérie is a teacher. She has two daughters, who study in big cities. She has been living with her husband Eric, also a teacher, for three years.

> Valérie: We have more time to do our work, professionally, because sometimes you say to yourself "how could you manage to do everything, to manage four people at home, the girls", Well, preparation for classes had to be the last thing you did when you could free up some time. Yeah, it seems crazy to think that at some point you had to fit it all in, so maybe now you spend more time doing something, or you take the time to do it, whereas before it was all a bit of a rush, or you did it when you could. (A_FR_6)

What also changes considerably is the 'mental workload', that is, the work taken on primarily by women linking professional and domestic activities, which manifests itself in the preparation of family activities during professional work.

> Véronique: At one point, it was like .... over. Because it was always very demanding. I was commuting to work in Paris. I was stressed, what am I going to do for dinner tonight? (...) We knew that a good balance was also needed for them to work well. I know that there has to be a good meal. (A_FR_18)

Véronique, 62 years old, a mother of three, all moved out, two of whom are still students, expresses this feeling of the liberation of her mind:

> Véronique: (...) What am I going to make for dinner? It's all there (...) Have I done the laundry and that thing? Etc. There are always these little things. And now, the fact that she's no longer at home (...). Well, I feel that it frees my head. (A_FR_18)

But also, freedom from planning and forward-looking, like Agnieszka, mother of three boys:

Agnieszka: (...) indeed, you have more freedom, you do not have to worry. You do not have to think, to have all this in your head, what to make for dinner, because even if this dinner will not be, well, the husband will eat that fried egg or something. (A_PL_1G)

The departure of adult children from the family home, and the reduction of maternal burdens that follows it, is often a moment of intensified reflection, as well as a trigger for mothers to take certain actions (change and/ or modify some practices).

Agnieszka: Because as long as there are these children, a person doesn't see it, I guess, and when they suddenly move out, you have such an awareness of.... well I don't want to say passing away, because I still feel 20 years younger than I am, that's how I feel inside, but suddenly a person notices such things, that this is a different stage of life. (A_PL_1G)

This is the moment to physically realise the entry into a different stage of (family) life. It is directly related to changes in various practices within the family home, which have always been associated with the role of the mother.

Continuation of the Maternal Role: Remote Tasks

Although the children's departure reduces the mother's role, it often does not completely eliminate it, but rather leads to its redefinition. Usually, the departure of children to university or their first job implies a continuation of the maternal role. However, this role takes on new forms: whereas they used to act in proximity and every day, mothers must now work at a distance and in a discontinuous manner. The maternal role continues by adapting the implementation of its material dimension to living away from the children (the mother ensures the circulation of objects and individuals) and above all a relational dimension (monitoring the emotional well-being of their now adult children). Mothers thus reconvert part of their maternal skills, from physical ones to remote ones. What one can see is that mothers balance between distance and involvement, which is not an easy task.

Remote Material Tasks

Using examples of the material aspects of the maternal role, the reduction in the mother's role was shown one by one in Sect. "Reduction of Maternal Burdens". It will now be presented that in other aspects, the role of the mother does not always cease when the children leave, contrary to what one might expect from Sect."Reduction of Maternal Burdens".

Mothers continue to supply the children's accommodation. Laurence (A_FR_32), for example, continued to do the shopping for her eldest son for two years after he had left [she has three children anyway]. As the children's apartments are small, the parental house remains a storage space for objects (see Chap. 5). The parents must then ensure the circulation of objects between the house and the child's apartment (by mail or by travelling with those objects). A more or less continuous flow of resources but also objects and services circulate between the two residences. As the mother of Léa and Emanuelle, who have gone off to study, explains:

> Valérie: Afterwards, there are still a lot of activities that are still geared towards them. Oh yes, going to see Léa, taking this to her, taking that to her, going to pick her up, or even going to see Emanuelle. (A_FR_6)

Among the objects that circulate, food is central for this mother, who organises herself so that her daughters can cook for themselves:

> Basia: No, then we had to go shopping, take provisions, and plan meals. Well, I'm quite focused on meals, but it's still really important. To manage to structure a life where not everything depends on your parents, where you can take responsibility for yourself. (A_PL_4G)

Sometimes remote tasks involve having to commute to the adult child's place of residence, and sometimes they are expressed in the presence of objects (in the form of jars of food) given to the children by the mother. Basia accurately called this "such a partial extension of maternal tentacles":

> Basia: That's something we didn't say—it's **such a partial extension of my maternal tentacles,** because once in a while when they come home, they always take something from home.
> Rysiek: They serve a menu to order.
> Basia: Some kind of jars, containers, some kind of salad. This is partly an extension of those home-cooked meals because I prepare them here. (A_PL_4G)

Other mothers prepare meals themselves. Sandra, a mother of two, prepared meals for her sons herself when they came home. This mother teased them by assuming out loud that he was coming home for the services more than for his parents [one sense that the service is not enough for this mother: officially one comes home to see one's parents, not for the service].

> Sandra: And then, in fact, after a month, he came back every weekend and I told him "Hey, shouldn't you come back only once in a while?" Then I told him "You're coming home for my lunch" because I was making him meals and he was leaving with food for the whole week, so he was leaving with good things to last all week, so it wasn't unpleasant for him. But he managed his laundry, fortunately in Aix. But he left with his lunch because they all ate together but each of them had to make their own dinner, but they shared these moments. (A_FR_15)

Finally, the parents assist in transferring their adult children from one place to another. For some young people who study far away and do not yet have a driving license, this activity is central.

> Valérie: There was just the inconvenience of the journey. And so it's true that she came home almost all year, every weekend, it took her 3 hours. It was stressful because she had to get the train… she had to go to Bordeaux to catch her train from Toulouse, so it had to go smoothly, so it was important not to miss the train that she took in Gujan to be in Bordeaux. To shorten the journey, we often took her to Biganos because there were more trains to Bordeaux. So on Sunday evening, it was always a bit of a race. Around 4-5 pm, she would leave, but she wouldn't arrive until 9 pm, yeah, for her it was hard. (A_FR_6)

Valérie, who accompanies her daughter to the train, is a perfect example of this common phenomenon.

Remote Relational Work

The mother's role encompasses not only work related to the material security of the child but also involves psychological tasks. One of the tasks of modern mothers is to build and care for the relationship with their adult children. The second dimension of the remote maternal role is the relational work of listening to and supporting the child. It also continues after the child has left. They are supposed to answer the questions about daily life that the young person has to deal with on their way. The first moments of independence in a new home can be very complicated for young people who have always been looked after by their parents:

Marie-Dominique: How to kill gnats?

Jean-Luc: Yes, yes.

Marie-Dominique: Can you eat a three-day-old steak?

Jean-Luc: For the gnats, you just told him "Well, you can't, you just have to clean your house" (laughs). Afterwards, he asked you about cleaning products too.

Marie-Dominique: Yes, how do you clean your washbasin? He took pictures of the household products at Auchan to find out.

Jean-Luc: Oh yes, but that was a long time ago.

Marie-Dominique: Yes, but that's when he was at the beginning, but yes, that counts. Yes, we give him help.

Jean-Luc: And he asks his father, he asks questions about DIY.

Interviewer: Did Gaël himself ask for this support or not?

Marie-Dominique: Yes.

Jean-Luc: Yes, every time, every time it's him, he's crying on the phone "yes, I don't know what to do anymore". (A_FR_44)

This part of relational work lies in practical advice. Parents like Marie-Claire, mother of two children, both students, and Jean-Luc, her husband, are still supporting their children in solving practical problems. Another part of this relationship work is emotional support. Parents have to "cheer up" the children. Another example is Carole, 53 years old, the mother of two children, still students:

Carole: So it's a psychological hotline already. It's just as soon as they need, um, when there's a slump, or when they're not in good spirits, which may have happened, we're here all the time, um, available 24 hours a day, 7 days a week, it's a premium service, it has to be said, so we're available for them. (A_FR_40)

She sees her role as a hotline for her children, available around the clock to support them when they need consultation, advice, or support.

Continuity of Daily Moral Support

Even if, in theory, there is a reduction in daily moral support, it happens that adult children invite their parents into solving their private and personal problems. Both Irena and Elżbieta have similar experiences with their adult daughters, who either involve them in some issues which are quite emotionally burdensome:

Elżbieta: In terms of this empty nest, she is present with me all the time. So emotionally, because she also does not give… does not allow such a departure, which I, for example, need, because I would already like to have a little… This sphere of just, problems, life decisions (…) I would like to be consulted either what I would do in her place, or if I had such a situation, but not in the way she does it (…) This is difficult for me because I'm very concerned about everything. I would like to get it over with, but I don't think it will ever be like that. I don't know if it's going to happen and if there's a chance for it to happen. (B_PL_11P)

Or as in Irena's case, her adult daughter, who moved out 7 years ago, interferes with her free time, when she is supposed to rest and spend time either alone or with their partners/friends, like in the example below:

Irena: She's on the phone and I've noticed that you know… I think I've actually let her out of the nest… and still, she calls me, we're on a walk, we're climbing (…), she calls us, and we're on our bikes, for example, and I have to interrupt what we are doing (…) and talk to her. So, it's like we're having a good time (…) and then my daughter calls and interrupts our fun. Of course, it's not a problem, it's just a fact, isn't it? (…). (B_PL_60G)

Interestingly, these examples differed in the amount of time that had passed since the two children moved out and the nature of the departure itself. Elżbieta's daughter, Paula, moved abroad 10 years ago. It was a definite move out, with no regular returns to the family home, despite the young age at which the move occurred (19 years old). While Irena's daughter, who also moved out at a young age to study (19) to another city in Poland, 6 years ago, returned regularly to the family home on weekends for a long time.

Tools and Pitfalls of the Remote Role

The transition from a close role to a remote role is delicate because the mother feels like she should protect the child who has left (by intervening with him or her) but at the same time encourage the child's autonomy (thus not interfering too much). Remote maternal work is therefore always a challenging balancing act between these two constraints. The intensity of maternal work will depend on the child's personality as perceived by the parents, and on their reaction to independent life and being on their own. It implies a particular organisation of contact between children and parents to find the appropriate distance.

Difficulty in Finding Balance Between Proximity and Distance

The first key issue to be addressed is contact between parents and their children. Some parents opt for very regular phone calls or even organise regular 'compulsory' calls with their child who has left for school. Other parents opt for less control. For example, they decide to contact their children through short messages that allow the children to call or answer when they are free. In doing so, parents try to preserve the autonomy of the children: this is the case of Delphine, mother of two student children aged 20 and 19.

> Delphine: I very often use short messages on the phone. With messages, little jokes or things like that, like "Hi, I haven't heard from you in a while, are you all right?". It depends because Colin doesn't want me to disturb him too much, otherwise I'll quickly be seen as the annoying mother, so I accept the fact that they don't reply. If they don't answer me, it's because I shouldn't insist. With Sofia it's going to be very different. But most of the time it's going to be texting. I use their way of working because it's a bit more practical, you can answer when you want, with work it's better, I answer between two patients. But yes, contact is important. I used to do it a lot with Sofia when she was in Italy, we had WhatsApp videos too, and with Sofia, it worked well. With Colin, seeing each other is not his thing, he will answer precisely to something, and he will move on. (A_FR_26)

Delphine is the one who expects the children to respond to her requests and forces them to exchange information. She is also the one who constantly contacts the children without waiting for them to contact her first. For Delphine, being intrusive is the counter-model to the maternal role, which is to let the children breathe. However, the freedom not to answer is not a lack of interest. Delphine is particularly attentive to the signs that might be a sign of problems appearing in her children's lives. Their return is an opportunity to continue her work as a mother.

Some parents take a while to find the right rhythm of communication with their children, as this mother of two, who have gone abroad explains:

> Sandra: when they don't need anything, they don't call, and uh, I call to get news when I feel the need, but I admit that I don't call much because I don't want to intrude. On the other hand, I send text messages, yes, I send text messages a lot in our group of 4, in the family group. So I used to send a lot, and a little bit, and then I got the impression that it bothered every-

one, so I understood that no one needed to communicate as much as I did, so I did it less, I waited for it to come from them too, so when they write to me to know if I'm okay I'm happy. (A_FR_15)

But Sandra accepts that the moments of conversation are irregular in time, adapting to the needs of the children. For some mothers, this means accepting the silence of busy children. Like in the case of Zofia and her son Kuba who studies in a different city. It is difficult for her to accept the lack of contact with her son. This causes her to feel anxious and worry about his safety. It does not suit her that her son only contacts her when he needs something:

Zofia: That's the problem—Kuba doesn't call or write to us. I told him to send at least an emoticon, a smile so that I know he is alive. I already called once, because I said Jesus, maybe something has happened to him these first weeks, because for a whole week nothing. No, no, everything is fine—it didn't occur to him that someone was worried. And now, practically always when he calls, it's to say that he needs something, for example, or to ask if I can arrange something, or if the scouts can come to you and pick up something from my room or something like that—on that principle. But for him to ask if we are alive and well, no. (A_PL_3P)

Often, parent–child contact only occurs when mothers initiate it. The child turns to their parents mainly when they need support. Without the role of mothers in this regard, the number of accounts would decrease. It shows how difficult the search for a good distance between parents and children is at this particular stage:

Teresa: Maybe it would also be different if they were in a relationship, but they are still together [brothers living together], and it seems to me that this parental contact with them is also different. We keep getting more into what they do, how they do it and why. I keep explaining to myself that it's out of concern for them, that I'm worried—**that's the truth, although maybe sometimes we exaggerate, but let's not kid ourselves, sometimes it's hard to centre where the line is that it's a concern and where it's exaggeration or hyperactivity on our side.** (A_PL_5G)

However, not every mother looks forward to daily contact. It also happens that contacts undertaken by adult children are overwhelming in their quantity (and quality) for mothers. They get a report on virtually every activity of the day. Ultimately, it seems very difficult and not obvious to find the right and satisfying way (for each side) in family communication.

> Elżbieta: (…) she hangs on by a single hair, this umbilical cord, that if there are problems she comes forward and wants to talk, which is good, although I would like most of all not to have to deal with her problems. But if she has them—I wouldn't want to know about everything either, and she still burdens me with such problems all the time. And then, for example, she forgets to tell me that she doesn't have this problem anymore. This is what we need to work on. It's difficult for me—she had a terrible problem last spring, she burdened me with it—I couldn't sleep for a week and after a week I finally dared to ask her how the matter was—and she said it had been solved the following day. I just spent a week thinking I was going to die, I was afraid to ask her (…). (B_PL_11P)

As Ela mentioned, even though her daughter Paula moved out almost 10 years ago, the "umbilical cord" still hangs by a thread and she, as a mother, is burdened with problems she would rather not disvover.

The Difficulty of Letting Go of One's Role

Some mothers are forced to "let go", that is, to give up close control of the child and intervene in their problems. Valérie, whose two daughters have moved to two different French provincial towns, is bitterly disappointed. She is disappointed that she could not physically intervene when her child needed it. The disappointment also comes from the perception of their powerlessness, the child now evolving in an environment that the mothers no longer control.

> Valérie: One of the first evenings she phoned crying, she couldn't find her way home, she was lost in the streets of Bordeaux, she didn't know how to get home. So you say "well yes, that's it", you've let go of your child, they're now in an area which is not hostile but where everything is more complicated for them and you're no longer there, you can't do anything to make things easier, so we're hyper-formatted parents now. We're always looking after them, always feeling guilty about "whether we are doing enough", and "whether we are being good parents", so being good parents, or maybe it's a mistake, is just taking on a lot. And um, when the child doesn't need you, well, they can't rely on you any more, they're going to have to take responsibility for themself, it's difficult to think that they're going to manage like that so easily. (A_FR_6)

Other mothers spoke of their anxiety at not being present to deal with their child's problems, of their difficulty in 'letting go' of the demands of their role.

> Fabienne: When they phone when there's a problem and they're far away, you feel, um... you have to be there, you have to reassure them, but you feel... It generates a lot more anxiety. Well, for me, because they're far away and I can't see them and... I always get the impression that if I were there, I would solve everything at once and that's it. It's a protective instinct and I make myself, and often it happens that I make films in my head: what if this happens and then if it's this and then well. But in the end, it's nothing at all. (A_FR_2)

Fabienne is on disability following a burn-out in 2017 after a long career as a training manager. That was the same year that her two children left home for university. Since then, she has devoted herself fully to her role as a mother and does not want to give it up. Her son has been back for two years. But she is still very concerned about her youngest daughter, at the risk of having her over-investment in her role as a mother mocked by her friends.

> Fabienne: My colleagues always found that I was a mother hen, that I was too nurturing. Not that I was covering for them, that I didn't let them manage on their own, but that I was too much like a mother hen with her chicks under her wings. I have the impression that when I'm with them nothing can happen to them, which is completely stupid. So uh... So now, is it true or not? I don't know. It's the feeling I have. (A_FR_2)

Zofia puts in a lot of effort and is very careful not to be intrusive towards her adult child:

> Zofia: Because I kept it locked inside me that I missed her a lot, because I knew that it was more important that she didn't feel that (...) because I'm not her child, she's my child. And I wanted to give her so much freedom, but it was hard for me to give her, because I wanted to know everything about her at the beginning, but I held back because I knew it would hurt our relationship a lot and I preferred to be colder, not to be so interested. (B_PL_9P)

Although it is difficult to relinquish control, Zofia now recognises it is essential to preserve her daughter's autonomy.

Latency of the Maternal Role When Children Are Settled

Children's access to secure employment allows them to have access to stable housing, either alone or as a couple. The economic independence of young people opens a new stage in the process of leaving, a stage marked by greater autonomy in relation to the parents. Children return to the parental home less often. As we saw (see the Chap. 1), they have less recourse to parental assistance because they have to show that they are now independent. On the mothers' side, the maternal role in its material dimension (preparation of meals for the children, circulation of objects, food) almost completely stops. The moral support dimension, on the other hand, continues, but in the form of very loose supervision of the children's psychological well-being and the search for any problems that need to be solved. But at this stage, the norm of independence of the children (who must manage themselves) prevails.

This mothballing of the mothering role is never better seen than in families where siblings are at different stages of the departure process, for example where some are in employment (and in cohabiting couples) while others are still students. This is the case in couple 13, a family from a higher education background with four children, two of whom are 28 and 24 years old and two students aged 21 and 19.

> Interviewer: Okay, and do you still provide them with assistance, financial assistance, or buy them food or material assistance...
>
> Eric: Yes, of course. For the two older children, less so. The two older ones, they manage. But for Théo and Alina, yes, of course, we help them a little bit, for food, for everyday life, we give them pocket money to live. (A_FR_13)

The rooms rented for the younger children were like an annexe to the family home (even if access was not always easy), whereas the new independent homes of the settled children are not as a rule a new home for the parents. In some families, mothers emphasised that it does not work both ways. Even though the adult children rent apartments, the family home is still willingly and frequently "used" by them, they feel like homemakers. In the situation where they live in their final "adult" home, being financially independent—their new nest does not become a family nest for their parents. Nour, who is very involved in her role of mother, because she is a housewife, does not like going to her children's houses [two of them already have families], because she does not feel at home:

Nour: I'm always a bit uncomfortable because [hesitation] well, it's not my house. I know that when they come to my house, they know it's their house because they lived there, but when I go to their house, I've never lived there, I don't sleep there, so sometimes I feel a bit uncomfortable. I don't feel that I can go into the kitchen and help myself or wander from room to room. I prefer it when they come because I feel more comfortable, I can do more things. I take care of them in fact, and the opposite bothers me because when I go to their houses they will take care of me, serve me and I'm not used to it so... I don't like it very much. (A_FR_39)

This takes away her ability to surround her children with care, which happens when they visit her at the family home.

The relational register of the maternal role may persist in the form of very loose monitoring of the children's psychological well-being. Mothers show concern for their well-being after children have settled down, like Clarisse, whose son is 24 years old and works in the army.

Clarisse: There is a question of trust: who they come across, you never know. They may be swindled, so I keep a close eye on them. For me, the most important thing is that my children are happy, they're not just for me, I didn't make them for me. (A_FR_12)

This concern for children persists in the minds of mothers. Some are ready to reactivate this maternal role at any time in case of trouble, despite the norm of independence that children should take care of themselves. The following statement also reflects the attitude towards social norms and expectations and the clear need to compare oneself with others in one's maternal actions:

Interviewer: So you continue to help them?
Béatrice: I will take responsibility for my children until the end, even if they have left home... **I'm not like some parents** (...) who... you're 18, you can get out of the house and that's it... you can be in trouble... I'll pretend you don't exist... No, I'll take it for my whole life. (A_FR_14)

Some mothers also feel that a secret bond persists even after the separation between them and their children. Thinking about their children silently is a mental trace of this maternal role. This is the case of Clarisse who has three children (two of whom are already parents) and compares her feelings with those of her husband.

Clarisse: They [the fathers] don't have the same connection with their children as the mother has with her children. (...) I have the impression that I haven't yet cut the cord. Well, it's still there, it's invisible. (...) But it's still there, whereas the father may have it differently. But uh they don't, they don't have that stuff anyway, they can't have it. It was, it's unique to the mother. (A_FR_4)

"Not cutting the cord" means seeing the child, and being connected to the child at all times, even when the child is gone. We can see here a form of expression of this latent role of the mother, a role that no longer exists because the children are independent and do not need the parent's help, but a role that persists nonetheless through the mother's silent concern and worry (through an invisible link).

The maternal role is latent but can be reactivated at any time in the event of a problem. Children can return to live at home, something that happened especially during the COVID-19 pandemic, or at any time in the case of professional or marital problems (Gaviria, 2020; Żadkowska & Herzberg-Kurasz, 2022) (see Chap. 7). Some parents may also feel that they will reactivate this part of their role when they become grandparents. However, in the French corpus, only one couple mentioned this grandparental perspective.

Fabienne: And that's why I say we're ready to be grandparents. Why? Because we're going to start again with the grandchildren, and it's great just to think that we're going to accompany (...) these little ones again in life, explaining the world to them, deciphering things, we're ready, we're on the ball. We've been doing it for a long time with Charlotte, now we have to get on with it, so we're ready! (A_FR_20)

Among Polish couples, we found far more examples of grandmothers and mothers looking forward to becoming one. Some interviewees are very much waiting to become one. Like Zofia (B_PL_9P) who bought her daughter baby clothes even though she was not even pregnant yet, nor planning to be in the near future. However, we cannot speak of a smooth transition of the role of mother into the role of grandmother as a pattern noticeable in the material on Polish mothers, because many of them set the boundaries of their new/potential role, approaching it more reflexively, with a ready-made plan. As in the case of Krystyna, who has two sons who already have children of their own, where she underlines referring to the need to preserve her time and space. Moreover, as a couple, they appreciate the time they spend together:

> Interviewer: But also, as a couple, that you prefer to be on your own...
> Krystyna: Also—**as a couple, that we are as a couple.** We've become so separate—us and Roman (son) with his family have completely different arrangements, are different families. They have different customs, and Roman, especially with this family, have a completely different way of life. And we respect that, but to put up with it long term would be difficult for us. (…) That kind of contact is great, I love them in general (grandchildren), you know I want to—I like to—and with the older ones and the younger ones to talk and be in contact, great, **but I also like to have my time and space.** (A_PL_12P)

For Magdalena, whose daughter comes from abroad and stays more often than not for an extended stay, it is obvious she is both happy when they visit and when they leave again:

> Magdalena: **we are happy twice: when they come and when they are gone** (…) this is already our family joke, everyone knows it! The daughter too, doesn't get angry, she even says it herself. As I say, "We are waiting impatiently for them to come to see the grandchildren", as it is usually for 3 weeks, once they leave after 3 weeks, oh my, we are back to our lives! (A_PL_26G)

Elżbieta, mother of Patryk and Marysia, whose nest has been empty for eight years now, does not yet have grandchildren but her attitude is very definite:

> Elżbieta: Sometimes, when there is a situation, then yes. And so permanently, then no. I don't know, well I also raised my children myself and I worked, so I think one can manage. But there are situations when, of course, I would help… Because it's not just the parents, right? Sometimes you drop off the children, and grandchildren, like a child is sick, and cannot go to kindergarten. Well, someone must stay with this child. But to take care of the grandchildren all the time, then no! (B_PL_25G)

Thus, she acknowledges the possibility of providing occasional care support, but she cannot envision taking on the role of a daily grandmother.

CONCLUSION AND DISCUSSION

Mother Role: The Role that Never Ends but Fades?

This chapter described the gradual process of reconfiguration and with examples showed that this process continues all the time, because the practices that sustain the role are constantly changing. When an external factor appears—the departure of adult children from the family home— the reconfiguration process acquires intensity. The reconfiguration of the mother's role is not only managed by mothers, but also happens in collaboration with their adult children and with their partner (fathers of their children), depending on how relationships with one another are shaped when they lived together in the full nest.

A mother's role has dimensions attached to material tasks (feeding, tidying, supplying, transporting) and relational work (listening, talking, advising, supporting). The second aspect of the role, relational work, has become more important while going remote (when the children moved out). The transition from a close role to a remote role is subtle. Remote maternal work is therefore a balancing act between the need to protect the child who has left and not to interfere with adequate autonomy.

The analysis of the interviews collected showed the diversity of solutions and experiences that mothers have. They also showed that the reconfiguration of the mother's role is a process staggered over time. The reduction of the mother's role is understood as a reduction in everyday tasks in a woman's life and is the reverse of the process of entering the mother's role (where the responsibilities are gradually increasing). The daily household chores are removed from her in favour of caring for the relationship with her child. Moreover, the reduction in maternal tasks may only be temporary. The children may return regularly at a rate that depends on the proximity of the place where they are studying. Every weekend, once a month, or for every short holiday, young people may systematically return home (see Chaps. 6 and 7). Studying has become an expected and normal situation for young adults. Compared to the traditional model of entry into adulthood, studying implies young people's prolonged dependence on their families and a de-cohabitation for reasons of studying (Galland, 1997).

The mother's role is a subject of social evaluation. Mothers (mainly in Polish project cases) have a strong maternal identity: they feel relief after their children leave—because of the reduction of maternal burdens. At the same time, they feel guilty about being relieved (see Chap. 13 for more about the ambivalence of emotions). This comes out clearly from the statements of Polish mothers, who, presenting their experiences and reflections, often compare themselves with "other" mothers. Rather than referring to the patterns of behaviour of their own mothers, they more often compare themselves to other mothers of adult children "from their environment" (without specifying who they are).

Based on the example of Poland and France, what could be explored further is how the relationship with the children differs by gender, as well as how it affects the reconfiguration within the mother's role itself. Our analysis showed that the reconfiguration of the mother's role is a staggered process over time, but what would also be very interesting to investigate further is how the different socio-cultural contexts in which the family lives affect the process. Moreover, the reconfiguration of the maternal role seems to happen earlier for families from affluent backgrounds concerning their children's biography, because they more often attend university through which independence and a sense of autonomy are achieved more quickly. As a result, the remoteness of the maternal role might be shorter among families from the working class because the educational path takes less time, and young adults traditionally enter adulthood. It would be very intriguing to verify this thread and elaborate on it in further quantitative research, as it is only a hypothesis.

Contrary to the idea that the maternal role withdraws after the children leave, our research showed that the maternal role is prolonged and adapted to the new family circumstances and settings, and might be expressed in new practices.

References

Afflerback, K., Anthony, A. K., Shannon, C., & Grauerholz, L. (2014). Consumption rituals in the transition to motherhood. *Gender Issues, 31*(1), 1–20. https://doi.org/10.1007/s12147-014-9115-0

Badinter, É. (1998). *Historia miłości macierzyńskiej* (K. Choiński, Trans). Oficyna Wydawnicza. (Original Work Published 1980).

Badinter, É. (2013). *Konflikt: kobieta i matka.* (J. Jedliński, Trans.). Wydawnictwo Naukowe PWN. (Original Work Published 2006).

Bouchard, G. (2014). How do parents react when their children leave home? An integrative review. *Journal of Adult Development, 21*, 69–79. https://doi.org/10.1007/s10804-013-9180-8

Budrowska, B. (2000). *Macierzyństwo jako punkt zwrotny w życiu kobiety.* Monografie FNP Seria Humanistyczna.

Coll, C. G., Surrey, J. L., & Weingarten, K. (1999). Mothering against the odds: Diverse voices of contemporary mothers. *Infant Observation, 2*(2), 118–121. https://doi.org/10.1080/13698039908400553

de Singly, F. (1996). Le soi, le couple et la famille, Essais et recherches. *Sociologie du travail, 39*(1), 123–125.

Delphy, C. (1984). *Close to home: A materialist analysis of women's oppression.* The University of Massachusetts Press.

Deręgowska, J., & Majorczyk, M. (2012). Poglądy młodych kobiet na rolę matki we współczesnym świecie. Komunikat z badań. In J. Deręgowska & M. Majorczyk (Eds.), *Konteksty współczesnego macierzyństwa. Perspektywa młodych naukowców* (pp. 11–52). Wydawnictwo UAM.

Erickson, J. J., Martinengo, G., & Hill, E. J. (2010). Putting work and family experiences in context: Differences by family life stage. *Human Relations, 63*(7), 955–979. https://doi.org/10.1177/0018726709353138

Gajewska, M., Herzberg-Kurasz, M., Żadkowska, M., Kostecka, M., & Dowgiałło, B. (2023). Room of her own: Remaking empty nest and creating herspaces in practices of Polish mothers whose children left home. *European Journal of Women's Studies, 30*(1), 7–21. https://doi.org/10.1177/13505068221110336

Galland, O. (1997). *Sociologie de la jeunesse.* Colin.

Gaviria, S. (2020). *Revenir vivre en famille. Devenir adulte autrement.* Le bord de l'eau.

Gromkowska-Melosik, A. (2017). Rekonstrukcje tożsamości współczesnych kobiet. Paradoksy emancypacji. *Pedagogika Społeczna, 2*(64), 95–116.

Gullette, M. M. (2002). Valuing 'postmaternity' as a revolutionary feminist concept. *Feminist Studies, 28*(3), 553–572.

Haicault, M. (1984). La gestion ordinaire de la vie en deux. *Sociologie du travail, 26*(3), 268–277.

Hryciuk, R., & Korolczuk, E. (Eds.). (2012). *Pożegnanie z Matką Polką? Dyskursy, praktyki i reprezentacje macierzyństwa we współczesnej Polsce.* Wydawnictwo Uniwersytetu Warszawskiego.

Imbierowicz, A. (2012). The Polish mother on the defensive? The transformation of the myth and its impact on the motherhood of Polish women. *Journal of Education Culture and Society, 1,* 140–153.

Kaufmann, J. C. (1992). *La trame conjugale. Analyse du couple par son linge.* Nathan.

Kaźmierczak-Kałużna, I. (2016). Matka w tradycji i kulturze polskiej. Rola kobiety-matki i jej przemiany w na przestrzeni wieków. In I. Przybył & A. Żurek (Eds.), *Role rodzinne. Między przystosowaniem a kreacją* (pp. 139–151). Wydawnictwo Naukowe Wydziału Nauk Społecznych UAM.

Lareau, A. (2021). Les inégalités invisibles. Classe sociale et «élevage» des enfants dans des familles noires et des familles blanches. In S. Octobre & R. Sirota (Eds.), *Inégalités cuturelles, retour à l'enfance* (pp. 39–101). Ministère de la culture-DEPS.

Mitchell, B. A., & Lovegreen, L. D. (2009). The empty Nest syndrome in midlife families: A multimethod exploration of parental gender differences and cultural dynamics. *Journal of Family Issues, 30*(12), 1651–1670. https://doi.org/1 0.1177/0192513X09339020

Nelson, M. K. (2006). Single mothers "do" family. *Journal of Marriage and Family, 68*(4), 781–795.

O'Reilly, A. (Ed.). (2010). *Twenty-first century motherhood: Experience, identity, policy, agency.* Columbia University Press.

Packalén Parkman, M. A. (2017). Macierzyństwo bez lukru i retuszu. Wizerunek Matki Polki w literaturze polskiej po roku 2000 i blogach. *Postscriptum Polonistyczne, 2*(20), 63–83.

Sheriff, M., & Weatherall, A. (2009). A feminist discourse analysis of popular-press accounts of post-maternity. *Feminist and Psychology, 19*, 89–108.

Spence, D., & Lonner, T. (1971). The "empty nest": A transition within mother-hood. *The Family Coordinator, 20*(4), 369–375. https://doi. org/10.2307/582168

Titkow A. (1995). Kobiety pod presją? Proces kształtowania się tożsamości. In A. Titkow, & Domański H. (Eds.), Co to znaczy być kobietą w Polsce (pp. 9–39). Instytut Filozofii i Socjologii PAN.

Titkow, A. (2007). *Tożsamość polskich kobiet. Ciągłość, zmiana, konteksty.* Wydawnictwo IFiS PAN.

Titkow, A. (2012). Figura Matki Polki. Próba demitologizacji. In R. Hryciuk & E. Korolczuk (Eds.), *Pożegnanie z Matką Polką? Dyskursy, praktyki i reprezentacje macierzyństwa we współczesnej Polsce* (pp. 27–48). Wydawnictwo Uniwersytetu Warszawskiego.

Titkow, A., Duch-Krzystoszek, D., & Budrowska, B. (2004). *Nieodpłatna praca kobiet: Mity, realia, perspektywy.* Wydawnictwo IFiS PAN.

Umberson, D., Williams, K., Powers, D. A., Chen, M. D., & Campbell, A. M. (2005). As good as it gets? A life course perspective on marital quality. *Social Forces, 84*, 493–511.

Włodarczyk, E. (2017). Misja mama. Wyzwania i trudności. In E. Włodarczyk (Ed.), *W trosce o macierzyństwo* (pp. 53–68). Wydawnictwo Naukowe UAM.

Wojciechowska, L. (2008). *Syndrom pustego gniazda. Dobrostan matek usamodzielniających się dzieci.* Wydawnictwo Instytutu Psychologii PAN.

Żadkowska, M. (2016). *Para w praniu. Codzienność, partnerstwo, obowiązki domowe.* Wydawnictwo Uniwersytetu Gdańskiego.

Żadkowska, M., & Herzberg-Kurasz, M. (2022). "Boomeranging covidowy" – o powrotach dorosłych dzieci do domów. Perspektywa rodziców. *Przegląd Socjologii Jakościowej, 18*(1), 40–61. https://doi.org/10.18778/1733-8069.18.1.03

Zalewska, S. (2012). *Syndrom pustego gniazda.* Wydawnictwo UKSW.

CHAPTER 4

The Empty Nest as a Phase of Fatherhood

Christophe Giraud, Radosław Kossakowski,
Magdalena Żadkowska, and Bogna Dowgiałło

INTRODUCTION

Understanding of fatherhood and father involvement has changed over time. Fatherhood has always been a multifaceted concept, although over time the defining theme has shifted sequentially from moral guidance to breadwinning, to gender role modelling, marital support and finally nurturing (Lamb, 2000).

The male breadwinner/female homemaker family model, a famous analytical construct, dominated family research during the second half of the twentieth century. In Western societies, after the Second Demographic

C. Giraud (✉)
Centre de recherche sur les liens sociaux (CERLIS, UMR 8070),
Université Paris Cité, Paris, France
e-mail: christophe.giraud@parisdescartes.fr

R. Kossakowski • B. Dowgiałło
Social Sciences Department (Institute of Sociology), University of Gdańsk,
Gdańsk, Poland
e-mail: radoslaw.kossakowski@ug.edu.pl; bogna.dowgiallo@ug.edu.pl

© The Author(s), under exclusive license to Springer Nature Switzerland AG 2024
M. Żadkowska et al. (eds.), *Reconfiguring Relations in the Empty Nest*, Palgrave Macmillan Studies in Family and Intimate Life, https://doi.org/10.1007/978-3-031-50403-7_4

Transition, the collapse of the housewife figure as a life career, and the collapse of the Parsonian family initiated the vanishing of the long-standing hegemony of the male breadwinner family model (Esping-Andersen, 2009).

Nowadays, fathers spend more time with their children than at any time for which there is comparable data. In the second half of the twentieth century, they doubled the time dedicated to housework and childcare (Bianchi et al., 2006; Smith, 2010; Marsiglio & Roy, 2012). Along with mothers' emancipation, fathers are less likely to be the sole or even primary financial providers in their families (Raley et al., 2012). Changes in family policies (cf. paid paternity leave) influence the number of stay-at-home-fathers (Suwada, 2021). Fathers obtain greater sociocultural pressure to be more involved in caregiving than they used to receive in the past (de Singly, 1996; Henwood & Procter, 2003). They are even viewed as acquiring maternal traits and losing paternal traits (Banchefsky & Park, 2016). They organise significant moments with their children and are generally satisfied with the time spent together (Chatot, 2020). Similar practices of "New father" can be noticed in Poland (Sikorska, 2009; Suwada, 2021; Włodarczyk, 2022) and worldwide (Doucet, 2006; Banchefsky & Park, 2016). Correlatively, in France, authority is now shared more with the mother since the laws on joint parental authority (1970 and 1993) reduced the father's monopoly (Castelain-Meunier, 2005). However, as Eurostat data show (2020) 65% of Poles believe that the main role of a man is to earn money (French express less traditional believes with the result of 31%). Women devote more work to household and caring, and men work longer hours and have more free time—the gender gap in time spent on domestic duties can be observed in different European countries, including Italy (Gallo & Scrinzi, 2016), the United Kingdom, Poland, Germany, Austria (Crespi & Ruspini, 2016) or Sweden (Suwada, 2017) and in European comparative perspective studies (Fahlén, 2014).

M. Żadkowska
Social Sciences Department (Institute of Sociology), University of Gdańsk, Gdańsk, Poland

Centre de recherche sur les liens sociaux (CERLIS, UMR 8070), Université Paris Cité, Paris, France
e-mail: magdalena.zadkowska@ug.edu.pl

The biological differences between mothers and fathers still serve as an explanation for the diversification of maternal and paternal obligations of being a parent (Suwada, 2015, 2017). Women remain the primary caregivers, and men are perceived in terms of a secondary caregiver or a helper (Kaufmann, 1992), whose role is to support the mother in everyday life (Thevenin, 1993). The father's primary obligation is to provide economically for his family. This differentiation of a mother's or father's obligation has consequences for the organisation of work within the family (Suwada, 2021). Traditional conceptions of fathering are seen, in contrast to mothering, in relation to his achievements in the public sphere and being a good provider and supporter for the family (Finn & Henwood, 2009). In this perspective, paternal authority is still associated with the potential to exercise power and control in a gender-differentiated home (Tannen, 1990).

While taking gender dimension into account, we can also see differences between men and women in different stages of life. Fathers still contribute far less time to childcare and household chores than mothers do (Schoppe-Sullivan & Mangelsdorf, 2013), and they often face a workplace backlash for trying to do so (Rudman & Mescher, 2013). The "rush hour of life" (30–49 years old) strongly influences what happens in the "third age" (Phillipson, 2015; Bonvalet et al., 2021) and the "late working life stage" (50–65 years old) when men still spend fewer hours on unpaid work than women (around 5–6 hours a week for the French and Poles) (Coelho et al., 2021).

In contemporary times, even though sociologists observe that the male breadwinner model has been replaced by an involved caring father (Engster & Stensöta, 2011; Fransson et al., 2016), gender biases very strongly influence both fathering and mothering. As Maume concludes in her study devoted to sleep within gendered work–family responsibilities: "women subjugated their own sleep needs to those of their husbands, who needed sleep to be their best at work." (Maume et al., 2010: 764).

Fathers in the Empty Nest

Existing research on the empty nest phase rarely focuses exclusively on the perspective of fathers. This is related to women's traditionally understood role in raising children as primary caregivers.

What we do know from early 1970s studies is that for men, the departure of their children makes them more dependent on the work role and that the transition to an empty nest might be difficult for some of them

(Bart, 1972). Especially for those, who, due to the role of primary economic provider, failed to build relationships with their children when they were still at home and in the empty nest phase, feel guilty and have difficulties coping with it (Barber, 1989). The empty nest transition is stressful, especially for fathers with fewer children, and a higher caring and loving involvement (Barber, 1989). The emotional distress is more difficult for them to express due to the perceived gender roles (Lowenthal & Chiriboga, 1972). In an empty nest situation, fathers become less authoritarian and directive, and relationships with their children, which were previously forced by coresidence, become more voluntary (Bozett, 1985).

There is still a notable gap in studying the empty nest phase from the fathers' perspective. A study in the British popular press indicates that men may also find the experience of children leaving hard, but one of the reasons for this is the regret associated with their absence from their children's lives at earlier stages (Sheriff & Weatherall, 2009). The same study also suggests that, unlike women, men are not at risk of being judged as bad parents if they experience the empty nest period as joyful. Other researchers report that fathers, contrary to mothers, regarded the children leaving as a step toward encouraging child maturity, and having matured and well-raised children was positively related to low-stress levels (Lomranz et al., 1996; Bouchard, 2018).

Although recent studies emphasise the contemporary transformations of the father's role (Coles et al., 2018; Bosoni Mazzucchelli, 2019), little is known about how men respond to this change in the empty nest phase (Randhawa & Kaur, 2020). Randhawa and Kaur (2020) argue that the lack of research might suggest that men are unaffected by the departure of their children, or that they are not affected in the same way as their wives in regard to mental health, for example. As Lewis, Freneau and Roberts noticed more than 40 years ago: this dearth of scientific outcomes is unfortunate since more fathers appear to be investing time and concern into childcare (Lewis et al., 1979) and his observations still seem very up to date.

While analysing changes in fathering, it is difficult to believe that such an event as the departure of adult children would not influence fathers, especially since we also know that parents (both mothers and fathers) act as "scaffolding" and "safety nets" to aid their children's successful transition to adulthood (Swartz et al., 2011). The study by Swartz et al. (2011) shows that good relations between fathers and children trigger independent leaving, not prolonged cohabitation. The findings also suggest that relationship quality between mothers and fathers may be based on different criteria, with distinct implications for intergenerational support.

The chapter focuses on (1) the life course perspective of the empty nest phase, showing how fathers perceived the new phase of the family life course, (2) the changes in the breadwinner role and (3) on the new fathering practices that appeared in this phase. As empirical data demonstrate, the roles of fathers are not disappearing but, in many cases, they are transformed in a particular way. The findings are based on the analysis of interviews with fathers from France and Poland. The thematic analysis was carried out on Polish corpus A and B and French corpus A.

RESULTS

The End of the Full Nest Phase

In the stories of fathers in an empty nest, there are strong signals indicating the end of a certain phase of the family life course.

For Jan, 62 years old, a doctor, the departure of his two sons (34 and 30) and their economic and housing independence suggest that now he can live his own life in "peace and quiet".

> Jan: And now we live alone we have peace and quiet. Well, we live very well. (...) Such a big mental shortcut happened after the children moved out, I would say, peace and quiet. Elegant peace and quiet, oh! Which I value terribly, by the way. Elegant peace. We sometimes turn off our mobile phones, you know, to have peace and quiet. That's how I would characterise it. You know, the kind of peace of mind that the kids are doing as well as they can, that they're rather healthy, that everything is somehow going ok there, and they have something to live on. Well, I also guess that it would be possible for a person to actually leave, to die, and at the same time, the kids are no longer naked, poor, yes? Well. (B_PL_8P)

Many men described the transition to the "empty nest" as a "natural process", the "natural order of things". For Mieczysław, 53 years old, a University professor, father of two daughters (25 and 23 years old), the slow dynamics of the transition softened the end of the full nest phase. Mieczysław confirms he was prepared for it:

> Mieczysław: The point is that in the case of both daughters, this departure from home was so, I would say, gentle. It wasn't on the principle that you

come home and there's your daughter standing in the doorway with her bags, saying she's moving out. It was all done on the principle that, she'd stay the night somewhere... especially since this house has stayed like this, that these things of theirs are here. So it kind of seems like they're gone for a while, it's like a family member came and said something to her... then she didn't move out at all. Like I remember the layout of the room, in terms of books lying around or some stuff. So it's like this—usually a person more easily accepts things that come so gradually, it just happens. Someone was gone for a day, then two days, then disappeared for a week, and so on. And it came so naturally. (...) And when it happens in such a smooth way, it just happens. A person accepts it with much greater ease, just—when I look at these books, it seems to me that in a moment the door will open and she will come back, back. And ok—it will come... it's kind of an illusion because that's probably not going to happen, but that's kind of the way it works out, on that principle. (...) But **I was internally prepared for the fact that this is how the world is arranged.** (B_PL_4P)

As fathers seem to possess certain beliefs about the "natural order of things" it makes them first feel prepared for the "empty nest phase", especially regarding the absence of children. They also find themselves less worried and less terrified in comparison to their wives. Wiesiek, 51 years old, a maritime engineer, admits that he does not worry about his 22-year-old son. He also knows that the family situation has changed but he has activities he can devote his free time to instead of performing paternal duties.

Wiesiek: That's what I think, I wasn't worried about it at all—like I didn't have any fears, whether something would happen to him or not, whether he would cope or not. It can happen anywhere, whether here or there—you can choke on a sip of tea and die. But no, I wasn't afraid, Elka certainly had some greater concerns about this lonely life of his. I always said, well gee, he may be very young, but he's an adult, he wants to, so he has to manage. (...) Well... well, that's just it. Yes—this is certainly ... this aspect of a full and empty nest, it certainly affects the functioning of everyone in the nest, no? So yes... Certainly, something will change somehow. I for one have an easy escape, so to speak, into sports. It's easy for me to just escape into it—I add one more workout or an hour more on the bike or in the pool or whatever, it's easy for me. I think Elka will have more of a problem with that (...) And it will be the same in the future—she will certainly have more problems with filling this kind of free time, because somehow the absence of this duty of parenting makes you have a little more time, you know, so you will have to fill it with something. To me it seems that it will be easier for me, at least for now, for her it may be more difficult. (B_PL_1P)

Eric, 54 years old, father of two daughters (23 and 21 years old), also demonstrates a processual attitude towards their departure, even though he worries about his younger daughter:

> Eric: But afterwards, deep down, I have always considered (I inherited this from my own family) that the fact of reaching student age is great to finally be free. So, I've always thought that this is a chance for my daughters, and I'm quite optimistic about it, I'm not apprehensive, which doesn't mean that as soon as they need it I don't go. I always go and I've always been confident. (A_FR_6)

As Eric is aware that his two daughters will manage once they have left, he confirms the empty nest phase is a new beginning for him:

> Eric: For me, it is a form of freedom, as if I was the one who was becoming a student (laughs), free again. (...) I don't need to have a permanent link, the permanent presence of my daughters. It doesn't make me sad. I'm happy for them to go and do things, I don't care, I'm not worried. It never makes me cry, I trust them, it's normal... (A_FR_6)

Grzegorz and Robert name the transition straightforwardly, that it has finished:

> Grzegorz: I don't know if it can be called a closed topic anymore, that they will never come back, because you never know what will happen in life. But this stage has closed—they live in a new place, moved out, gone out on their own, **and that stage is behind us. Now we are in the middle of the next one.** (B_PL_7P)

> Robert: Of course, they can always count on us, **but it's no longer that stage,** as they say, that a person is just waiting when there will be a phone call that "Dad, mum, rescue me," no? (B_PL_13G)

We have noticed that the fathers' narrative about the "natural order of things" might be related to certain behaviours encouraging the children's departure. Adam even uses a comparison to the animal world:

Adam: Especially since we knew that he had wings to fly—because he worked and she worked [the girlfriend]. So from the point of view of the child's welfare, **it's like birds—they push it out, throw it out of the nest.** There, somehow, there are no great dilemmas—bird-mom sees that it has wings, so if she pushes it out, it's sure to fly away. And so maybe even with a little premeditation, we did it for the sake of our child, knowing that sooner or later it had to happen. (B_PL_2G)

In interviews with French and Polish fathers, the sense of the certain rhythm of life was strongly connected with children moving out and this understanding influenced the attitude towards the empty nest phase.

The End of Domestic Tasks Overload in the Full Nest

For many fathers, as for most women, the departure of the children is linked to a reduction of material tasks (housework). For example, Claude echoed Angèle, who has seen her daily workload lightened since their three children left home for school.

Angèle: I do all the family's laundry, and frankly, I can see the difference. As a result, I've started to buy a lot less washing powder.
Claude: It's the same for me. I cook for everyone most of the time. I buy much less food, and I spend much less time in the kitchen. (A_FR_19)

Even when fathers didn't do many household chores, they would still often notice fewer of them as a result of their children moving out. Jérémy, a manager, was a father who was "very present for his children". He asked for part-time work when his first child was born (80%) and took parental leave for 8 months for the second. However, he is not very involved in household tasks (the couple pays a household helper). For example, he helps with the washing up and notes that this small task has lightened since his two children left for school:

Sabrina: The only thing for me is that I have less laundry and less ironing …
Jérémy: I'd say that they must have left if I have the impression of having less housework.
Sabrina: But what kind of housework did you have?
Jérémy: No, but I have the impression that since they're no longer here, it's just the two of us eating, so there are fewer dishes. (A_FR_29)

Not all fathers invest time in housework. So relief in this matter is only for the fathers who get involved in domestic tasks. Didier and Delphine (A_FR_26), both independent workers (osteopathy), reduced their professional activity (80%) when the children were at home. Now they still share the housework: Delphine does the cleaning and Didier does the cooking.

In contrast, men who were not involved in domestic chores don't speak about a reduction in domestic work. Some men feel little change since the children left. Fabrice, 64 years old, a father of two, said this.

> Interviewer: And for you, Fabrice, has anything changed?
> Fabrice: Well, um, for me it's like... They left, it was for a good professional level, for professional training. I didn't miss much, because my work took up a lot of my time, um... It was not, how can I put it, the discussions were less and the worry was less. The problem was more for Fabienne than me. So if you're not... The absence didn't weigh on me. (A_FR_2)

Fathers who were focused on their professional activities and absent from home, have established limited intimacy with their children, and for them, the end of domestic chores overload is not "their story".

The End of the Breadwinner Role?

For men, the breadwinner husband norm is less strong after the children become independent. Housing independence for children means a reduction of major financial efforts. Fathers feel less of a need for a massive financial contribution and can disengage themselves relatively. This can lead to a reduction in investment in professional work (with a reduction in working hours and sometimes dual activities or working on the side to earn more). The career cycle makes working more than one job less conducive as opportunities for upward mobility are fewer. One may decelerate professionally (fewer opportunities offered, less investment in new positions, more routine with a job that one has done). With the departure of the children men enter the last phase of their professional life and they are on their way to retirement. As the household is smaller and the financial needs are less demanding (children finally become residentially and economically independent), many men seem to decelerate professionally. On the other hand, the freed-up resources let accelerate one's career and self-development. There are fathers who use the time they gain after children' departure to work more.

For many men, the departure of their children coincides with a particular moment in their career. Around the age of 50, professional opportunities become scarcer. This can lead to a form of distancing from work. For Claude, a senior executive in a large company, his involvement in work has reached its limits, and this end of his career takes the form of a deceleration.

> Claude: At the point where we are in our careers, that is to say in the last part, opportunities for evolution are gradually disappearing. So it wasn't at all driven by the logic of "well, I have more time, so I'm going to take on more responsibility". (A_FR_19)

For men with a lower income, a reduction in working hours, and sometimes even additional jobs they take on is also a sign of change. Grzegorz, 49 years old, a middle education clerk, two daughters (25 and 22 years old) admits gaining free time after his daughters' departure.

> Grzegorz: Yes, I mean, before that, I was coddling, I was doing the so-called "second jobs", and now I don't—I was practically never at home, only at night, and at the moment I don't do it anymore or very rarely. So generally there is time now. (B_PL_7P)

There are men who admit that they "are slowing down" and have stopped working over weekends. Mieczysław is 53 years old, a University professor, and has reduced the amount of work he used to have; he does not work on weekends. He wants to decelerate professionally.

> Mieczysław: You know, there is no denying that a person is already reaching **a certain age**, and more so in the professional sphere, in an industry such as I work in, I would say, one could say that despite **the fact that I am not too far from retirement age, it is just the way the world is arranged that I have already reached my maximum in a certain way**. Now, you could say that I am slowly reaping the benefits… I am trying to give the field to younger people. Possibly even slowly give some advice or whatever I can, but again—**this is the order of things and at some point, you have to give way.** This, among other things, makes it possible for me not to read an email for a day and a half, in the sense of what 3–4 years ago was virtually unimaginable. (B_PL_4P)

There are also fathers who continue to accelerate their professional careers. The phase of the "third age" gives them the opportunity to consider their professional careers to be very important and they focus on earning money and saving for retirement. Jan, 62 years old, who is a doctor, was stressed about being a breadwinner and also had many tasks related to parental duties. Now he mainly focuses on work and is even more overworked:

> Jan: We do not really have that time, relatively for ourselves, yes. Despite the children moving out. Since... well, you know, there are simply very few doctors in Poland in terms of numbers, on top of that we have these specialisations and that makes... Well, you probably understand me, yes? That I stress the importance of work, right? (...) well, I like my work, it is literally for me like being a little medical detective for me sometimes, so... Well, it's so nice for me and so I try to continue it, no? But that means less free time. But that's out of the question! (B_PL_8P)

There are fathers who had a strong investment in childcare, the empty nest is also an opportunity to work more. For Vincent, Sandra's husband, the children's departure is an opportunity to work more and spend less time with the family than he used to. He can focus more on his work, which is the central part of his life. Sandra does not even force him to have dinner with her when he comes back from work, whereas she used to do so when the children were still at home.

> Sandra: The fact that the kids were around a lot, it didn't change the fact that you were extending your work hours anyway.
> Vincent: Not at all.
> Sandra: Well, it just reinforced the fact that he could work even later. So, he had more to do. I made him more... well, no, the exact term is that I put more pressure on him, on the fact that he wasn't there in the evening. Because as long as the children were there, I made it a point of honour that we at least had dinner together. Now they do not see it. (A_FR_15)

Eric is a teacher and while his two daughters were at home he used to be very involved in parental tasks, mainly related to his younger daughter's education. The departure of the children allowed Eric to devote more time to his teaching activity. It can be realised though, more for his personal career purposes than to fulfil the breadwinner's vocation.

> Eric: We are both teachers. When you're a teacher, you have a limited amount of time in front of the students, but then you're a teacher a bit all the time. You have to read, you have to correct papers and that takes up a

lot of space. So we probably do it less quickly than before, we have a little more time to do it, but we don't gain so many extra hours that could be leisure time. It's a little bit of the job that tends to eat up the space that's been recovered, I think. But not completely either. There is a small margin. But it's not a net gain either.

Valérie: We saved time because when they were here, we often had to drive them around. There were activities... That was a bit of a hassle, so it freed us up, yes.

Eric: It's not a total revolution in our way of life. It's simply more space, more freedom in the head. But not necessarily a lot more possibility. (A_FR_6)

The transformation of the work domain for men after the departure of the children is quite ambiguous. The two tendencies (reinforcement and deceleration) are visible but the strain to be a family provider has weakened.

New Roles for Fathers in the Empty Nest

The reduction of parental burdens does not mean that paternal work disappears altogether. Work changes in nature and frequency. Many mothers have a practice of remote monitoring that fathers do not do directly. Fathers, in contrast, are available to help but wait to be asked explicitly to intervene. Their position is to trust the child. They have an on-demand role. They may also continue to care for (or maintain specific links with) a child to whom they were particularly close before the departure.

In Chap. 3 we saw that mothers did loose monitoring work to see if the children who had left were coping or needed support. Interestingly, fathers can continue to perform or take over the monitoring work. Tomasz admits his anxiety whenever his daughter was travelling for work:

Tomasz: But I still have such a thing in the back of my mind that yes, well, if anything happens, how can I help her? Well, because here we are ok and ok, but you would like your children to be safe. Nothing more! Safe simply, yes? And those things were mentally overwhelming me, no? This distance. I say, I laugh, that her first flights, listen, it was tragic for me, because I really did, she was taking off, and I sat down at the computer on flightradar right away. And until she had landed somewhere out there, on the other side of the world, I followed the flight. (A_PL_22P)

The father's role is more or less important depending on the degree of autonomy of the children who have left home. This autonomy is a representation constructed by the parents, but it can be confirmed by how often the children ask for help. There are relatively large differences between Poland and France. Several Polish fathers seem to intervene a lot, leaving their children little autonomy. Robert is the father of two children, aged 30 and 25. He has an intellectual job. The eldest, a boy, left two and a half years ago. Robert allowed himself to go to his son's house without warning, after his son had left (he was 27), to maintain contact but also to check that everything was OK.

> Robert: There came a time when I started to miss him and then, when I had a bit more time, well, then I would go to his place, for example, when I was going somewhere to do some big shopping, I would do some shopping for him, I would drop it off, to help him on the one hand, and on the other, to keep in touch, right? And at the moment it looks like we can already see and have it confirmed that he's coping, right? [...] (B_PL_13G)

It should be noted, however, that the children's autonomy varies according to the time that has elapsed since the moment the nest became empty. Over time, Robert gains confidence and no longer expects his child to ask for help or have a problem. He recognises that his child is becoming more independent.

Some fathers show a need for control that leads them to be particularly controlling from a distance. Ryszard, a father of two, whose eldest child left at 17, expresses this need to avoid risks for them:

> Ryszard: I'm one of those people who likes to be in control of everything— instead of taking risks, I do everything to avoid those risks. I neutralise certain situations more than simply reacting later so that there's no need to react, I try to do certain things earlier so that there's no trouble. (B_PL_4G)

The following excerpt shows how closely this father monitors the movements of his children who live in a nearby town. This leads him to accompany them regularly (even after they have left) to avoid any problems. Ryszard, a man from a wealthy background (he is a lawyer and his wife is a teacher), makes himself available for the evening of the trip, rather than living independently of the children. He continues to provide an escort service even though his (young) son is settled elsewhere.

> Ryszard: When they were going somewhere for some event in the city, I thought about it intensely and even asked them if they had transport, what time they would be coming back, etc., so that I would know—if I needed to go out in the evening, so that I would know—if I could have a beer in the evening or if I had to wait in the starting blocks and wait for a signal to drive somewhere in [a town near Poznań] to pick them up because after midnight the public transport in [a town near Poznań] is, to put it mildly, average. (...) we are here in the starting blocks, my starting blocks, so to speak. (B_PL_4G)

For Leszek, father of two children, and an entrepreneur, giving life advice and moral support is inscribed in his role as a father. He gives advice to his eldest daughter and her boyfriend.

> Leszek: I tell them that simply, well it should be done in such a way, and then they either accept it or they don't accept it. Mostly they accept it and then put it into practice. (B_PL_3P)

It is worth mentioning that Leszek's primary aim is to make his children believe that they will manage. In that sense, he is fundamental moral support for them. But this involves his daughter and son-in-law interfering in the household.

On the part of French parents, the appreciation of children's autonomy modifies the participation of parents (and the father in particular). This autonomy is assessed on the basis of several signs: the fact that they know how to manage themselves and ask little of their parents (from a material, economic or administrative point of view), and the fact that the child knows what they want for themself ('decision' criterion). According to these criteria, fathers can be "confident" or "worried". It is mainly these criteria that are used to qualify the relationship with their children. Mothers can say they are worried or not, but also sad, which fathers say less.

Francis, an administrative employee (whose wife is an account manager), is the father of a 23-year-old daughter, enrolled in a master's degree programme, who chose to spend a year in Mauritius. He is proud of his daughter's ability to make good decisions for herself.

Francis: It doesn't matter what she chooses to study. That she decides it, not that (...) that we decide for her what she will do later on. And we've always explained it to her and I think we've done pretty well, she's always been very independent and she knows exactly where she wants to go. (A_FR_20)

Both parents accept this temporary departure of their daughter, who has since returned home during the pandemic. Vincent, a father of two and a senior executive in a large company, values the energy that his eldest daughter put into her choice of higher education:

Vincent: No, but above all the motivation Sophie had and the energy she put into taking charge of herself, how can I put it, managing herself.
    Sandra: Yes, yes, to take care of everything...
    Vincent: Exactly and so we intervened very little, I would say except for administrative things because sometimes they asked her, well we had certain things to do but it was, I would say, the energy and autonomy that she had, that she had, to organise herself, to take all these steps which resulted in the fact that she was selected by 2–3 schools and that she had the choice. (A_FR_15)

This autonomy leads Vincent to trust his children and not monitor them. He expresses this freedom in a way that is very different from that of Ryszard above: he refuses to anticipate problems.

Vincent: At a certain point, there is no point in trying to anticipate too much. If you start to get ideas and then maybe you go in the wrong direction. It's done, it's done and then, well I'm speaking for myself, we might be better off doing it like that, as we go along, than trying to tell ourselves a whole bunch of thoughts we might have, ideas we might have. (A_FR_15)

This trusting attitude leads to a form of distance from the fathers in relation to the supervision of the children. They adopt a rather passive attitude, less based on controlling the children. These fathers wait to be called upon by the children, unlike the mothers (see Chap. 3).

The Exercise of an "On-Demand" Role

For many fathers who give a large amount of autonomy to their children, the father's role after the departure of the children depends on the demands of the children. It's an "on-demand" role. As we have seen (see

Chap. 3), mothers usually monitor the psychological state of children who live further away. Fathers do not initiate many calls or personal meetings: they are "passively available". They have a sense of solidarity, but they are waiting to be asked. In contrast, most women are available but are also active in ensuring that the children do not have any problems or lack anything. Their availability is "active".

Father's telephone exchanges are often short and focused on a more or less practical problem. For example, Fabienne and Fabrice show this difference between long conversations for no reason other than to check on the children and conversations focused on a problem. Fabienne likes to receive calls from her daughter at regular intervals and asks her for news for no other reason than to maintain the relationship.

> Interviewer: Do you call each other? Do you write messages to each other?
> Fabienne: Well, I don't really write messages, I have to be on the phone, so... I like it when she calls me. Because when I call her, I often get her answering machine on her mobile. And I don't like to leave a message, but I like it when she calls me.
> Interviewer: And does she call you often?
> Fabienne: Oh, once a week. And sometimes when I think I haven't heard from her for too long... And when I feel the need to call her because I think I haven't heard from her for a long time, I send her a message like "Hello, how are you?". And then she contacts me at that moment. (A_FR_2)

For Fabrice, on the other hand, the exchanges are linked to requests for services. Here, for example, he fulfils the role of taxi driver.

> Interviewer: Ok. And you, Fabrice?
> Fabrice: By SMS [Short Mini Messages]. Yes, usually by text message.
> Interviewer: And how often is that?
> Fabrice: No, not too much, it's when I need it. Yes, it's true, it's when I need a little knock, knock, knock: a little text message. Especially an SMS when she is coming home for the train timetable. (A_FR_2)

In the same way, we see another example of the same division between the regular small-talk conversations Laurence (a housewife) has with the children and the rarer conversations about a particular problem with the father Mounir (on disability leave, a working-class family).

Laurence: It's rare that they'll call their father.

Mounir: But yes, he calls me to ask me questions about specific things too, that's all. He'll call, he'll talk to his mother and then half an hour later, he'll call me and say "Dad, I need to know", and then he'll ask me questions.

Interviewer: Questions about what?

Mounir: Many things! It could be, so it depends...

Laurence: ...the car.

Mounir: It's his job, his car, he has to make an estimate, he has to do that. Or if he has a problem with a colleague or how he should react and what he should do. You have to advise him because even if he always has the right idea more or less, so he needs an adult to explain to him... and so that reassures him in the end, what to do and what not to do.

Laurence: If you like, he's just starting his professional life now. And he did a sandwich course but it's not the same. It's not the same as entering professional life now. In his adult life after all. (A_FR_32)

Polish fathers, especially in the first months following the departure, may also feel that children always address them "when there is a problem". Leszek, an entrepreneur, and father of two children, explains his relationship with his younger son who is on his way to move out and live separately:

Leszek: Well, and when he calls, he will call and say, "does that sofa from Ikea have to be tightened up properly, or can it be a bit loose?", well I say, "it has to be tightened up properly", then he says "oh fuck, then we'll have to fix it again". He always calls me when there's a problem. If he can't do something, something even mechanical, or if there's a bigger problem. He calls about specific issues, right? He doesn't call to chat; he calls to deal with a specific issue. Like I call to find out what's going on there. (B_PL_3P)

The dynamics of contact between fathers and their children are changing. The conversations differ from dialogues between children and mothers and very often have specific goals.

The Performance of the Masculine Domain: Father as a 'Handyman' and as 'Particular Advisor'

Occasionally helping the children is another important dimension of the paternal bond after the children have left. In working-class areas, this help is usually in the form of male domestic tasks such as car maintenance and DIY work. Men remain fathers through their masculine skills.

Carrying out small repairs (being a 'Handyman' for a child) is not only about helping to solve technical problems: it is also a way of maintaining a bond with the child. Wiktor (49 years old), the father of two sons (25 and 22 years old), a foreman in a shop, admits that he and his wife (a saleswoman, 49 years old) differ as far as building a connection with the children is concerned.

> Interviewer: Do you have, for example, a different way of talking with the children?
> Wiktor: Well, I think yes. But do I know how? It's known that my wife would want to just talk with them... when they talk with me it is: help me with this, help me with that, we talk about some bullshit, and it's about the car or what they need me to do. The younger one was, he did catering let's say, he brought some hams to be smoked, I used to do that for him—that's the kind of different relationship we have. (B_PL_11G)

Doing DIY jobs results, for Wiesław, 62 years old, owner of a guesthouse, in reducing the distance between himself and his children (a son who is 35 years old and a daughter who is 32 years old) and their spouses. He feels almost at home at both his son's and his daughter's places. He feels even more at ease there than his wife, a 56-year-old nurse, who is not engaged in such activities.

> Wiesław: I feel at home. For example, I know how to switch on the coffee machine, although we have a different one, to make myself, let's say, a latte there. But my daughter always gets up and knows that I like it, so she even prepares breakfast for me straight away. I feel at home. And my son-in-law absolutely accepts it... By the way, we also sit at their place for a long time when we arrive. Just as they feel at home at our place, so do we at theirs. I feel is even a bit more than my wife. Well, as I say, well I helped a bit, painting, you know how it is when finishing a house. (A_PL_33G)

Sometimes a father not only helps but takes control of the whole technical part of installing children in a new place, showing gendered skills in the family. When Delfina, the daughter of Leszek, a 45-year-old entrepreneur, was moving to another city, her father felt responsible for preparing the new flat for her:

> Leszek: When Delfina was leaving, well there were preparations, I was going, there I was preparing her flat. When she came by car, we packed it, it was literally like in American films and the car was full. (B_PL_3P)

It is worth mentioning that parental support also continues when a certain period of time has passed after the children have moved out. For example, material support (e.g. in the form of renovation work, DIY) continues even after the children are stable in their marriage. Melanie, the first daughter of Gérald, lives with her boyfriend, but he isn't interested in DIY work. So she asks her father to help them.

> Gérald: Now, Melanie, she needs me, it bothers me... not because she needs me, it's because she actually needs me, because her boyfriend doesn't want to do it. It bothers me because they're actually living as a couple but no, um, she's managing her business, she calls me to do things when I'm not doing them at home... to do things, that's what's terrible. Don't tinker because I don't like to, but I'll do it for her because she's my daughter. And... she knows it, she knows she can count on me. It bothers her to call me for some things, for others she should call me because he can't do it or doesn't want to do it. I think it's more like, there are things where you don't want to piss him off. And then I say to him, "I'm willing to do it for you, I don't see why I should bother with it when I don't do it at home, but you've got a guy who doesn't want to do it". (A_FR_14)

In this case, the father, a truck driver by profession, takes action on behalf of his daughter, even though he does not like the work. But he also has to carry out work in his own house at the request of his wife. In this family, gendered skills are strong.

Father as a Pal

In the statements of the respondents, a change in the relationship with the children from a typically protective, even authoritarian one to a more partner-like, even pal-like one is sometimes apparent. This is particularly noticeable in the case of father–son bonds.

Here we have Wiesiek, 50 years old, a maritime engineer, father of a 22-year-old son. His son is back home after three years of living independently.

> Wiesiek: The relationship is still super, I think it's as it should be, but it's on such a... he's a grown man, it's more like with a pal than a child. (B_PL_1P)

One father described the common journey he has with his son, some kind of 'men's adventure', 'men's belonging', which is something wives (or generally women) are absent from. Jan is the father of three sons, whose last left home six months ago.

> Jan: So I went with my middle son [25 years old], we went on a holiday together, a great one. One that, because of the low standard of accommodation, my wife would never go on in her life. And we liked it very much. (B_PL_1G)

These 'being together' moments seem to be significantly important for fathers. Here is Marcin, a retired police officer, and father of one 28-year-old son, who left home three years ago and is now married.

> Marcin: Because here the relationship with my son is really cool and fine and (...) as he's like willing and all the time on his own, every year he wants to go with me, for years we've had it like that, up in the mountains somewhere for 4–5 days or something, some kind of trip together, no? We did a nice one half a year ago to [a country in the Mediterranean] up north, the two of us, and so on. So it kind of proves that it's ok, right? That it's not like I'm snatching his time away from him, taking it away from his wife, because now she has to go with her father. It's just based on sheer will and desire (...). (B_PL_12G)

The relationship with the son is also pal-oriented in that the son has become an equal partner in conversation and sometimes even an expert on a particular topic. Thus, there might be an exchange of services between fathers and sons or even a reversal of these roles, with the son helping his father with minor repairs or technological problems. Ksawery, a watchmaker, father of a 35-year-old son, agrees that it is his son who gives him assistance in dealing with new technologies.

> Ksawery: Yes. The TV has been working weirdly lately because it's this internet app, all this stuff that sometimes gets lost. So I called him the day before yesterday and he was here yesterday and he wanted to help us here, no? And that's it, isn't it? (A_PL_30G)

In France, for fathers whose authority was strong, having their child move into an independent home and, above all, acquire economic independence improved their relationship with time. This is the case of Gérald, a truck driver and father of two daughters, who acknowledges having a certain authority over them.

Gérald: Alicia [the youngest], she left to go away Alicia. She needed independence, she needed to be alone. I think she also needed to detach herself from my authority because I had authority... and instead of doing like her sister and talking with me, she shut herself off, so my authority was even more constraining for her. Because for her, there was no way to discuss it with me. Now [Alicia has a career and an independent home] we talk much better, we are much freer, we joke, we... Well, you see my sense of humour... So we talk to each other now. (A_FR_14)

For many fathers, their children moving out is still an important symbol of their transition into adulthood. Often, this step has an impact on their relationship, transforming it into an adult–adult dynamic.

CONCLUSIONS

The analysis of the interviews with fathers who were experiencing the empty nest phase shows that, in the dimension of their relationship with their children, the following patterns are constituted. First, although the fathers confirm the end of a long-lasting phase of the family life course, the full nest phase, their role is not over, it is reconstructed. Their role changes into a more advisory, supportive one, and new practices of fathering appear. They become the person the children call about unplanned problems but are no longer a daily assistant. Fathers accept that they have 'on-demand' status and that their support should be more technical, pragmatic and, to a lesser extent, emotional, although they do not shy away from moral support. This shows that despite the less authoritarian nature of the relationship they have built with their children, their role and status still have a certain traditional trait—they are seen as 'technical' rather than strictly caring parents. If they are authorities, it is in those matters that are associated with traditionally male responsibilities.

Second, both social and personal expectations (probably also family expectations) for fulfilling the role of the provider are waning. How much time men devote to work begins to depend primarily on what individual goals they have set for themselves, how passionate they are about work, and their physical strength and health, which are related to ageing. For some, the time of the empty nest is associated with an increase in personal time and with redundancy, for others this time will only occur after retirement.

In some cases, fathers have no problem crossing over into partnership or even pal status with their children. The fact that being a 'mate' for one's child primarily concerns the relationship between father and son still has a certain symbolic, to some extent traditional dimension. It is still the construction of a kind of male belonging, although already on somewhat different terms than when the child was younger.

Men's perspective on their children's departure from home does not necessarily indicate a significant milestone in their own life course. Rather, they tend to view it as "something will change somehow", with vague expectations about the process and its outcomes. Men adapt to this new situation by engaging in new fathering practices such as being available when needed, offering practical support, and being a friend and advisors to their children. This approach should not be mistaken as a withdrawal from paternal responsibilities, but rather as a means of assisting their children in achieving independence and building or sustaining their father–child relationship in a new way.

REFERENCES

Banchefsky, S., & Park, B. (2016). The "new father": Dynamic stereotypes of fathers. *Psychology of Men & Masculinity, 17*(1), 103–107. https://doi.org/10.1037/a0038945

Barber, C. E. (1989). Transition to the empty Nest. In S. J. Bahr & E. T. Peterson (Eds.), *Aging and the family* (pp. 15–32). Lexington Books.

Bart, P. B. (1972). Depression in middle-aged women. In V. Gornick & B. K. Moran (Eds.), *Women in sexist society* (pp. 163–168). The New American Library Inc.

Bianchi, S. M., Robinson, J. P., & Milkie, M. A. (2006). *Changing rhythms of American family life*. Russell Sage Foundation.

Bonvalet, C., Gallou, R., & Ogg, J. (2021). Transitions in later life and the reconfiguration of family relationships in the third age: The case of the baby boomers. In A.-M. Castrén, V. Česnuitytė, I. Crespi, J.-A. Gauthier, R. Gouveia, C. Martin, A. M. Mínguez, & K. Suwada (Eds.), *The Palgrave handbook of family sociology in Europe* (pp. 591–609). Palgrave Macmillan.

Bosoni, M.-L., & Mazzucchelli, S. (2019). Generations comparison: Father role representations in the 1980s and the new millennium. *Genealogy, 3*(2), 17. https://doi.org/10.3390/genealogy3020017

Bouchard, G. (2018). A dyadic examination of marital quality at the empty-Nest phase. *The International Journal of Aging and Human Development, 86*(1), 34–50. https://doi.org/10.1177/0091415017691285

Bozett, F. (1985). Male development and fathering throughout the life cycle. *American Behavioral Scientist, 29*, 41–54.

Castelain-Meunier, C. (2005). *Les métamorphoses du masculine*. PUF.

Chatot, M. (2020). L'articulation travail-famille «au masculin». Des pères empêchés de paternité? *Les Politiques Sociales, 2*(3–4), 30–44.

Coelho, B., Maciel, D., & Torres, A. (2021). Gender, social class, and family relations in different life stages in Europe. In A.-M. Castrén, V. Česnuitytė, I. Crespi, J.-A. Gauthier, R. Gouveia, C. Martin, A. M. Mínguez, & K. Suwada (Eds.), *The Palgrave handbook of family sociology in Europe* (pp. 45–67). Palgrave Macmillan.

Coles, L., Hewitt, B., & Martin, B. (2018). Contemporary fatherhood: Social, demographic and attitudinal factors associated with involved fathering and long work hours. *Journal of Sociology, 54*(4), 591–608. https://doi.org/10.1177/1440783317739695

Crespi, I., & Ruspini, E. (Eds.). (2016). *Balancing work and family in a changing society. The fathers' perspective*. Palgrave Macmillan.

de Singly, F. (1996). *Le soi, le couple et la famille*. Nathan.

Doucet, A. (2006). *Do men mother? Fathering, care, and domestic responsibilities*. University of Toronto Press.

Engster, D., & Stensöta, H. O. (2011). Do family policy regimes matter for children's well-being? *Social Politics, 18*(1), 82–124. https://doi.org/10.1093/sp/jxr006

Esping-Andersen, G. (2009). *The incomplete revolution: Adapting welfare states to women's new roles*. Polity Press.

Fahlén, S. (2014). Does gender matter? Policies, norms and the gender gap in work-to-home and home-to-work conflict across Europe. *Community, Work & Family, 17*(4), 371–391. https://doi.org/10.1080/13668803.2014.899486

Finn, M., & Henwood, K. (2009). Exploring masculinities within men's identificatory imaginings of first-time fatherhood. *British Journal of Social Psychology, 48*(3), 547–562.

Fransson, E., Sarkadi, A., Hjern, A., & Bergström, M. (2016). Why should they live more with one of us when they are children to us both? Parents' motives for practicing equal joint physical custody for children aged 0–4. *Children and Youth Services Review, 66*, 154–160.

Gallo, E., & Scrinzi, F. (2016). *Migration, masculinities and reproductive labour: Men of the home*. Springer.

Henwood, K., & Procter, J. (2003). The 'good father': Reading men's accounts of paternal involvement during the transition to first-time fatherhood. *The British Journal of Social Psychology, 42*(3), 337–355. https://doi.org/10.1348/014466603322438198

Kaufmann, J. C. (1992). *La trame conjugale. Analyse du couple par son linge*. Nathan.

Lamb, M. (2000). The history of research on father involvement. *Marriage and Family Review, 29*, 23–42. https://doi.org/10.1300/J002v29n02_03

Lewis, R. A., Freneau, P. J., & Roberts, C. L. (1979). Fathers and the postparental transition. *Family Coordinator, 28*(4), 5140–5517.

Lomranz, J., Shmotkin, D., Eyal, N., & Zohar, Y. (1996). Launching themes in Israeli fathers and mothers. *Journal of Adult Development, 3*, 159–170.

Lowenthal, M. F., & Chiriboga, D. A. (1972). Transition to the empty nest. Crisis, challenge, or relief? *Archives of General Psychiatry, 26*(1), 8–14.

Marsiglio, W., & Roy, K. (2012). *Nurturing dads: Social initiatives for contemporary fatherhood*. Russell Sage Foundation.

Maume, D., Sebastian, R., & Bardo, A. (2010). Gender, work-family responsibilities, and sleep. *Gender & Society, 24*, 746–768. https://doi.org/10.1177/0891243210386949

Phillipson, C. (2015). The political economy of longevity: Developing new forms of solidarity for later life. *The Sociological Quarterly, 56*, 80–100.

Raley, S. B., Bianchi, S. M., & Wang, W. (2012). When do fathers care? Mothers' economic contribution and fathers' involvement in child care. *American Journal of Sociology, 117*, 1422–1459.

Randhawa, M., & Kaur, J. (2020). Acknowledging empty Nest syndrome: Easternand Western perspective. *Mind and Society, 10*(03–04), 38–42. https://doi.org/10.56011/mind-mri-103-420214

Rudman, L. A., & Mescher, K. (2013). Penalizing men who request a family leave: Is flexibility stigma a femininity stigma? *Journal of Social Issues, 69*, 322–340. https://doi.org/10.1111/josi.12017

Schoppe-Sullivan, S. J., & Mangelsdorf, S. C. (2013). Parent characteristics and coparenting. *Social Development, 22*, 363–383. https://doi.org/10.1111/sode.12014

Sheriff, M., & Weatherall, A. (2009). A feminist discourse analysis of popular-press accounts of post-maternity. *Feminist and Psychology, 19*, 89–108.

Sikorska, M. (2009). *Nowa matka, nowy ojciec, nowe dziecko*. Wydawnictwa Akademickie i Profesjonalne.

Smith, R. (2010). Total parenting. *Educational Theory, 60*(3), 357–369. https://doi.org/10.1111/j.1741-5446.2010.00363.x

Suwada, K. (2015). Being a traditional dad or being more like a mum? Clashing models of fatherhood according to Swedish and Polish fathers. *Journal of Comparative Family Studies, 46*(4), 467–481. https://doi.org/10.3138/jcfs.46.4.467

Suwada, K. (2017). *Men, fathering and the gender trap: Sweden and Poland compared*. Springer.

Suwada, K. (2021). *Parenting and work in Poland: A gender studies perspective*. Springer.

Swartz, T. T., Kim, M., Uno, M., Mortimer, J., & O'Brien, K. B. (2011). Safety nets and scaffolds: Parental support in the transition to adulthood. *Journal of Marriage and the Family, 73*(2), 414–429. https://doi.org/10.1111/j.1741-3737.2010.00815.x

Tannen, D. (1990). *You just don't understand: Women and men in conversation.* William Morrow and Company.

Thevenin, T. (1993). *Mothering and fathering.* Avery Publishing Group.

Włodarczyk, J. (2022). *Tata 2022. Raport z badania polskich ojców.* Fundacja Dajemy Dzieciom Siłę.

CHAPTER 5

Adult Children's Bedrooms and the Emptying Nest: Mechanisms of Transition

Marta Skowrońska, Filip Schmidt, Emmanuelle Maunaye, Marianna Kostecka, and Cyrano Andre–Vieille

INTRODUCTION

In this chapter, we examine the processes of transition from the full nest to the empty nest phase of the family life cycle by studying changes in the domestic space and domestic objects. While much attention has been paid to family home space, there has been little interest in the dynamics introduced by adult children leaving it (Maunaye, 2001; Hachet, 2014). To fill this gap, in this chapter we investigate parents' narratives about what happened to their children's old bedrooms. By analysing the process of transforming the materiality of children's bedrooms, their use and decoration, we look at the accompanying changes in the parents' agency and identity.

M. Skowrońska (✉) • F. Schmidt • M. Kostecka
Faculty of Sociology, Adam Mickiewicz University, Poznań, Poland
e-mail: marta.skowronska@amu.edu.pl; fschmidt@amu.edu.pl;
markos10@amu.edu.pl

© The Author(s), under exclusive license to Springer Nature
Switzerland AG 2024
M. Żadkowska et al. (eds.), *Reconfiguring Relations in the Empty Nest*, Palgrave Macmillan Studies in Family and Intimate Life, https://doi.org/10.1007/978-3-031-50403-7_5

We also highlight the importance of external factors in managing the room, such as housing conditions and the degree of confidence that the child has gained autonomy and will not return to the family home. The analysis distinguished room transformation scenarios in the narratives of Polish and French parents whose children had recently moved out.

MATERIALITY AND SOCIETY

While sociological and anthropological interest in material objects and space is not new, increased attention to materiality has been observed within social sciences for several decades (Dant, 1999, 2004; Preda, 1999; Woodward, 2007). Numerous aspects of the relationship between humans and objects have been studied. Ethnographic interest in the material culture of everyday life (Douglas & Isherwood, 1982; Mauss, 2002), analysis of the social status, lifestyle and consumption (Miller, 1987; Shove & Warde, 2002; Warde, 2005) have been complemented with a more recent focus on materiality as actors involved in the production of social order. Objects have also been studied in the context of embodiment, habits and practice in general (Law & Mol, 1995; Schatzki, 2010) and the imposing power and beliefs connected with objects and related rituals (Julien & Rosselin, 2005). For at least several decades, researchers have studied the role things play in developing and expressing identity and self-definition (Belk, 1988; Low & Altman, 1992; Lincoln, 2014; Ramos, 2016). The composition of objects in space sets the stage for everyday life (Chevalier, 1992; Segalen & Le Wita, 1993). Studies on materiality let us follow how individuals appropriate space using objects, adapt them to themselves and transform them into a medium for self-expression (Lefebvre, 1986; Serfaty-Garzon, 2003). These analyses make it possible to measure and

E. Maunaye
Département Carrières Sociales (UMR 6051), Université de Rennes, Rennes, France
e-mail: emmanuelle.maunaye@univ-rennes1.fr

C. Andre–Vieille
Centre de recherche sur les liens sociaux (CERLIS, UMR 8070), Université Paris Cité, Paris, France
e-mail: cyrano.andre–vieille@etu.parisdescartes.fr

understand the self's evolution and the ego's reflexive work mediated through material objects (Ramos, 2016).

Materiality, Home and Housing. The Evolution of a Bedroom

Sociological attention given to materiality is mirrored in the studies of home and housing. Although the main focus in studying the home has long been housing conditions and housing policy (Moore, 2000), a growing amount of work has also touched upon the home as the site of consumption and social differentiation (Amaturo et al., 1987; Madigan & Munro, 1996; Woodward, 2001), self-expression (Csikszentmihalyi & Halton, 1981; Duncan, 1981; Ramos & de Singly, 2000; Ramos, 2002; Reimer & Leslie, 2004), privacy and comfort (Shove, 2003; Cieraad, 2006; Newell et al., 2015; Skowrońska, 2015), and agency, power and gender relations (Madigan et al., 1990; Allen & Mack, 1991; Madigan & Munro, 1991; Allen, 1996; Baydar, 2005).

A significant stream of research on the history of home space emerged as part of the history of private life developed by the third generation of the Annales School. Michelle Perrot (2008) demonstrates that the evolution of the bedroom reflects the gradual appropriation of the body and the intimacy of the individual. As she observes, the history of the child's bedroom helps understand the evolution of the child's place in the family (Perrot, 2018). In our chapter, we also observe the evolution of the child's status, but in the biographical context of a family life course rather than from a historical perspective.

CHILDREN'S BEDROOMS AND IDENTITY, AGENCY AND APPROPRIATION

Nowadays, psychological research reinforces the rising importance of children's space. The significance of a child's room is placed in the context of psychological well-being, sleeping habits, sense of security, privacy and independence, access to leisure time and media use, and the possibility to develop and express the self (Lincoln, 2014). As Ramos (2016, 2018) observes, adolescents' bedrooms provide intimacy, autonomy, and separation from other family members, which are crucial elements of gaining independence. Especially the psychological and sociological studies on privacy referred to the importance of having one's own room as a chance for self-development, a sense of safety and agency (Altman, 1977; Pedersen, 1997; Zaleski, 1998; Jędruszczak, 2005; Decup-Pannier, 2016; de Singly, 2016; Ramos, 2018). Moreover, according to the commonly accepted European norms, a flat or house should consist of a shared space (living room, dining room), a bedroom for the parents, a room for each adult, a room for two children under the age of 12, a room for two children of the same sex aged between 12 and 17, a room for each person aged between 12 and 17 not included in the categories above (cf. Eurostat).

The bedroom space constantly evolves during adolescence (Glevarec, 2010a, b). The bedroom expresses the culture and identity of the child, then of the adolescent and finally of the teenager. The changes in the material expression of the bedroom are strongly influenced by the evolution of child culture. They express belonging to a youth group and distancing from the culture inherited from the parents (ibid.). The room's personalisation also shows the child's autonomy in their tastes and practices. However, this autonomy is relative, as parents are still involved in decisions concerning the bedroom. Children's freedom may be even more restricted today because their parents are more present and concerned (ibid.). A right to one's room is thus related to the question of power—an individual bedroom is a "power base" (Ratecka, 2011; Krzaklewska & Ratecka, 2014), a vital resource which is often negotiated between the family members during the family life cycle (Munro & Madigan, 1999). Appropriation of home space (Lefebvre, 1986) is a continuous process rather than a constant arrangement (Ramos, 2002). Therefore, the child's bedroom is a place of appropriation practices, such as decoration, which conflict with parental practices of control. A bedroom is a place where parental tastes, habits and beliefs are confronted with children's attempts to express their agency while remaining within the family framework. As Glevarec (2010a, b) observes, this process varies according to social class.

Children's Bedrooms and the Transition to the Empty Nest

The children's departure introduces significant changes to the family network of relations and the material space of the home. We mentioned earlier the transition of children's bedrooms that follows as children gradually gain independence and separate from their parents. In the case of children's departure, the bedrooms' transformation may also reflect the process of distancing and separation, and a split between the child self, attached to the family of origin and inscribed in the materiality of the parental home, as well as the self of an independent "young adult" (Maunaye, 2000). As Gajewska et al. (2023) demonstrate, the transition to the empty nest is also a chance for women to acquire a separate, private space and to inscribe it with their new identity, in which the mother's role recedes into the background (cf. Chap. 13). While not devoted to the empty nest period, Hachet's (2014) study on children moving between two homes in divorced families indicates important dilemmas over children's rooms that arise when the child is at the other parent's place. These dilemmas concern the questions of privacy and agency. The parents cannot entirely appropriate the room; they sometimes use it but protect the intimate space of their children from intrusion by not letting strangers in.

Although numerous studies have analysed the role of materiality in everyday life, life course transitions have rarely been investigated in the context of material objects. To fill this gap, we are analysing the process of transition to the empty nest through the lens of material objects and home space. In this chapter, we analyse the transformation of adult children's rooms to examine the question of agency, identity in the transition to the empty nest stage of the family life course. As in other chapters, our analysis focuses on the parents' perspectives. We examine their narratives regarding their children's former bedrooms, which reveal how parents view their parental roles and adjust their identities during this transition.

METHODS

This chapter is based on an empirical study undertaken in Poland and France. The research material comprises 62 qualitative, in-depth dyadic interviews conducted in 2018–2020 (corpus A). The couples, aged 50–64, whose children (ranging from 1 to 4) were all adults and had moved out within the past year, were interviewed. We included an exception of one couple whose child was still at home, which helped us see interesting elements of the transition process. The analysis was a multi-staged process. While it resembled grounded theory to some extent (the coding process was iterative and quite open), it should best be described as a reflexive thematic analysis (Braun & Clarke, 2021). First, we identified and analysed the excerpts related to changes in the children's bedrooms after their departure. We distinguished several recurring ways of transforming or preserving the function and appearance of these places, collated into three types: continuity, partial transformation, and change. Second, we used these excerpts and other parts of the interviews to examine the role of:

1. Agency (or the power of decision-making): Who decided on the room's décor and function?
2. Identity (or the family roles): How is the role of being a parent experienced in the process of the empty nest transition? How much does the parental role define the self and the children–parent relationship? These two problems can also be analysed in terms of continuity and change. In addition, the analysis identified two other factors relevant to the transition process: housing conditions and the degree of certainty that the departure was definite.

RESULTS

The study shows significant differences in the degree and shape of the children's bedroom transition. The type and pace of room transformation relate, on the one hand, to the agency and identity of the children and parents and, on the other hand, to contextual factors (housing conditions and un/certainty of departure). Transition is slowed or hindered if the children can still decide about their (former) room and accelerated if the parents take control over its function or aesthetics. Change is also hindered when parents stick to their role and believe children must be cared for. Housing conditions may also hamper or accelerate the transformation. A strong need for additional space is a stimulus for change. In contrast, spacious homes allow for keeping children's bedrooms untouched. Finally, it is essential whether a child's departure is defined as definite.

As we demonstrate, all these factors interact with each other in the process of room transition. We present three possible scenarios of what may happen to adult children's bedrooms after their departure—from continuity (1) through partial transformation (2) to complete transformation (3). Some families move from one scenario to another over time, but this is not a rule. The eventual shape of the analysed rooms may change in the future, and we only focus on the moment of the interview and the months and years that preceded it.

Continuity

The first scenario refers to the cases of continuity, which means that the children's bedrooms have stayed the same since their departure.

The narrative of Monika and Józef combines all aspects of continuity. First, parents continue to be attached to their parental roles. In their view, the unchanged bedrooms signalise "a refuge" to which their daughters may always return. They assume that their daughters are in potential need of their care and support, which they declare to provide no matter what ("a relationship may break up, and they can always come back"). Second, children continue to own their rooms, and their power over them remains absolute. Without the daughters' permission, parents would never decide to change anything. "We would decide together, with them", they claim, stating that the agency over the bedroom space has not shifted. "We'll always say: this is Werka's room and this Małgorzata's room", they emphasise. The daughters additionally force the continuity of their agency over their bedrooms. They disallow even the slightest violations of their power. When the father tidied up the room, he threw away an object that the daughter cared for, which caused a conflict and reassured the parents of their decision to keep the bedrooms intact.

> Józef: Everything stayed the same.
> Monika: Yes—and they didn't like it when we went inside and changed something.
> Józef: When they were gone.
> Monika: They disliked it terribly—it happened several times that my husband... Because I know about it and I don't throw anything away. But my husband did—he thought it was something unimportant, but it turned out to be very important for her [the daughter]. And now we don't throw anything away. (A_PL_23G)

Material conditions of this household also support the decision to leave the children's bedrooms unchanged. The couple has a spacious house, and they do not need any additional rooms. Finally, the daughters are still studying, and the parents feel their departure is not definite.

Delphine and Eric as well as Fabienne and Francis are also clear examples of continuity. The two youngest children (21 and 19 years old) of Delphine and Eric are still students and regularly come home at weekends. Similarly to some Polish parents, the father or mother "cannot imagine" changing their two youngest children's rooms. "When [our daughters] come back, they have their things", they say. The father insists on the daughters' agency of these rooms: "they keep their room", and "they have their things". Fabienne and Francis also keep only daughter's room untouched. She is still a student who went to Spain for several months to develop a humanitarian project as part of her studies and join her boyfriend. Her departure is not perceived as definitive, partly explaining why the room has been kept unchanged. The father and mother agree on this point:

> Francis: (…) She still has her room; she can return whenever she wants (…). it wasn't a definitive departure. (…) I think that played a role, too.
> Fabienne: Well, no, because we knew she would come back, so (…) we left the room as it was; we didn't touch it. (A_FR_20)

The three examined cases are clear examples of continuity, which is not questioned or conflicted by any other factors. The departure is not perceived to be definite. The family houses are spacious, so the parents do not need an additional room. The children's status as requiring care is dominant and eliminates any potential thoughts of reclaiming the room or making small changes. Children also stick to their roles and define the room as theirs. The room reflects the care and is a tool to manifest it. For Francis and Fabienne, keeping the daughter's bedroom is a way of telling their child that she still belongs in their home, which underlines the importance of their identities and roles as parents and caregivers.

> Francis: She must feel that she still has a place at home and that (…) and that she is always welcome. That's it! (…)
> Fabienne: Yes, family is important! (A_FR_20)

However, a room may remain unchanged, even if not all the factors support continuity. One or two powerful brakes on change may prevent it if the pushing factors are not strong enough. For example, Magdalena and Stanisław demonstrate that even when housing conditions would support room transformation, the uncertainty of departure, strengthening the caring role of the parents, prevents this process. The younger daughter of Magdalena and Stanisław goes to a secondary school in a town 50 kilometres away and stays in a rented flat with her older sister and nephew. The transition to the empty nest is incomplete; the younger daughter is underage and may return to the family home if she does not get to college. Leaving her bedroom unchanged seems unquestionable for the parents, who assume their daughter still lives in the family home, as she returns every weekend. The returns are also obvious for the daughter, who still needs parental support. In addition, the departure at a young age gives rise to parents' fears about fulfilling caring roles. Declaring to keep their daughters' bedrooms in the distant future, the parents reduce dissonance, which resulted from remorse for 'pushing' the child out of the nest so early, and reassure themselves and their children of the continuity of their care. They want their children to have "their place on Earth".

> Stanisław: Exactly. I said so, and I'll always repeat it; my parents also repeated it: they can always come back. (...) their bedroom remains here. (A_PL_26G)
>
> Asked if they need additional room, the interviewees say they do because their flat is not big, and they would happily accommodate more space. But they immediately rule out the possibility of room transformation, which would contradict their caring role.
>
> Interviewer: So you don't need them [the rooms] for any other purpose?
>
> Magdalena: Well, we do, obviously. But no, no! Absolutely not! They have their space, their rooms, the same as before. (A_PL_26G)

In this case, the younger daughter's age and her early departure, forced by poor educational offers in her hometown, strengthen the parental identity and weaken the impact of housing conditions.

However, even when children live independently and the departure is definitive, the strength of other factors may successfully hamper the room's transformation. Honorata and Mirek are strongly focused on their parental role. They continue to be very worried about their daughter's future. Although she has completed her education and has a full-time job, they still send her money every month and give expensive presents, notwithstanding their modest financial resources. They want to support her as long as possible, believing it is their duty. In one moment of the interview, they say parents have an obligation to provide for their adult children: "[parents] should do it. (...) Not even should, they must!". Their strong orientation towards caring for their daughter is reflected in the narrative about her bedroom. Nothing has changed since her departure because they want her to feel comfortable when she visits:

> Interviewer: I just wanted to ask about it—is her bedroom still hers?
>
> Honorata: Yes, it has stayed exactly in the same state; even her clothes still hang there, so no, nothing has changed. We have not redesigned or moved anything—she has everything as she left it. And when she visits, she sleeps there, and I think she feels good there. (A_PL_24G)

While in the case of Honorata and Mirek, the continuity mainly resulted from the parents' attachment to their caring role, in the case of Laurence and Mounir, the most vital impulse comes from the daughter's need to leave her room intact. Her claim to retain control over the room and, perhaps, sustain "a place on Earth" in her parents' house is supported by a suitable housing situation—her parents do not need any additional space. The parents do not consider her return because the daughter moved a while ago and has a full-time job, a stable relationship, and her own house. Their relationship has changed—they no longer worry about her and treat her as an adult. Still, a part of her needs the symbolic place in the family house that stays untouched. Her request to leave the room made a few years back is still respected.

> Laurence: Ambre told me the day she left: "leave the room as it is". (laughs) "You mustn't touch it; she said" (laughs). (A_FR_32)

It is worth noticing that the continuity may sometimes result from inertia rather than efforts to keep the parental identity. Children's bedrooms sometimes stay unchanged because no one has the time, energy or need to care about them. In such cases, the continuity results only from good housing conditions rather than any other factors. For example, one of the interviewed couples, Irmina and Ksawery, whose house is much bigger than they need, hardly ever goes upstairs where the son's old bedroom is. They once thought their son and his wife might want to live with them (they decided not to), so the upper floor may serve as a separate flat. Ksawery reflects on their situation, saying that while some people lack personal space, he has the luxury of leaving the entire floor unused just because "he doesn't need to use it".

> Ksawery: Other people have poor housing conditions, and they squeeze (..) children don't have their own rooms, they can't study, they can't develop! And I haven't been in a room in my house for a year... Because I don't have such a... [need] (A_PL_30G)

The narratives of the first scenario, in which the room is kept untouched, are very similar in Polish and French interviews and underline the importance of the child's place in the parents' home, even after the departure. The room symbolises preserving the child–parent relationship, particularly the parent's caring role and the child's agency. The scenario is supported by good housing conditions and the incomplete character of the child's departure.

Partial Transformation

In the second scenario, partial transformation, rooms have changed since the children's departure but have not entirely transformed. We deliberately use the term "partial" rather than "incomplete" to avoid suggesting that the room must eventually change completely or that it is only a stage of an inevitable process. Partial transformation may be a phase, but it may also remain permanent. The partial ownership of the room illustrates the processual, nuanced and ambivalent character of the transition to the empty nest. The room may belong to parents and children simultaneously, and the sense of ownership may shift and gradually change. Sometimes, change is hampered by children who still mark their possession over a space or a need for parents' care and attention. Sometimes parents stick to their roles and fear letting their children move out for good. Finally, materiality and uncertainty of departure may slow down the process of a room transformation.

Anchors: Remaining Objects as Barriers to Change

In the quotation below, the son who moved out took his sofa bed to his new flat and has no intention of returning to his parents' place. He relinquished power over his room and is no longer interested in its décor or function. The departure is definite. Wiktor and Małgorzata, the parents, accept their son's independence and do not plan to keep his bedroom "just in case" he returns. While the room's transformation seems inevitable, it has changed only a bit. Without a bed or a sofa, it is no longer a bedroom, but it serves as a storage place.

> Małgorzata: Yes. Arek's room has changed because he took his couch—he took the furniture he had. It's more of a stash now. There are some hangers, some jackets—they [Arek and his brother] still have their stuff in there that they didn't take (...).
> Wiktor: Maybe they don't even know it's there. (A_PL_11G)

Similarly, the daughter of Béatrice and Gérald uses her bedroom for storage:

Béatrice: Aurelie's room, well, apart from the bookcase which I've taken out, otherwise there's all the furniture that was there when she was here... There are just the boxes which are hers. (A_FR_14)

In both cases, family roles and identities have transformed—the children are now independent and their parents accept this. The parental role has moved to the background. There has also been a shift of agency over the space. However, the overwhelming number of items that would need to be sorted sustains the temporal character of the room as "no man's land". When parents' housing conditions allow them to have an additional, unused room, temporality may change into a permanent state. A problem appears when children refuse to empty their rooms even when parents ask them to. In the case of Julia and Zenon, the room still stores their son's stuff, but Julia is gradually taking over the wardrobe and shelves to store her things. She is so discreet that even her husband has not realised that the room is transitioning.

Zenon: In their rooms, they have their private things (...)
Interviewer: No one uses their rooms in the meantime? When your children are gone, don't you use their rooms?
Julia: Nah, I started to take them over. My husband doesn't even know that I started taking them over.
Zenon: I don't know what my wife is up to! (A_PL_32G)

The son bought his own house and has no claim on his room. He doesn't even spend time there when he visits. The only obstacle to his mother taking over his bedroom is the piles of objects that need someone's attention. All the family members are hoarders—they gather plenty of things, and even their spacious house can hardly accommodate them. The reason the objects stay is that there is space to store them. The partial solution Julia worked out is using the remaining shelves and racks to pack her things. Throwing everything away is not an option—even if frustrated or impatient, parents usually wait until the child symbolically hands power over the room to them: "I want him to decide", Julia says.

Interviewer: So he wouldn't mind, would he? He doesn't come and say: "What have you changed here, mom?" (....), does he?
Julia: Nah, we don't have that. Just the opposite, I'd like him to remove these things; I don't want to throw them away; I want him to decide.
Interviewer: Do you think he wouldn't want to throw them away yet?

Julia: No, he can't find time to do that. (…)
Zenon: As there is space and these things don't have to disappear (immediately), they stay. (A_PL_32G)

Similarly, in the home of Dorota and Franciszek, boxes remain and are waiting. In this case, however, the son seems attached to his old magazines and video games and wants them to remain in the family home, even if he never intends to use them. While the son's perspective is only narrated by the parents (the study did not include interviews with the children), we may assume that the old objects symbolise a part of the son's identity he does not want to abandon.

> Franciszek: A lot of things are left, a lot. You don't know what to do with them; cos Jerzy collected some IT magazines, some video games, CDs with old games, you don't know what to do with them (…) There are many things you don't know what to do with. He doesn't need them, but he says: dad, leave them. I would prefer to…
> Dorota: And he won't allow us to throw them away. (A_PL_9G)

Children's rooms may sometimes retain their temporary status due to lingering clutter. In certain cases, parents quietly assume control of the room as they await their children's decisions regarding its future. However, the sentimental attachment to old possessions, which symbolize identity, can hinder the room's transformation.

Update: Same Function, New Decor

Another case of partial transformation is when the room's function stays the same, but the parents or the children change the décor. The room is defined as a child's room, but "adult" décor is introduced instead of teenage furniture and colours. Parents may want to make their own decisions, marking their agency and power over the space, but in some cases, children's agency over the room continues.

One of the typical first signs of the parents "reclaiming" the child's room is tidying it up. Couples Carole and Erwan and Basia and Ryszard belong to many of those in which the question of cleanliness and tidiness used to be an agency struggle between parents and children. When the children moved out, the parents reclaimed at least some rights to the bedroom—they cleaned it and enjoyed the cleanliness at least until the next visit of their children. The parents' role as caregivers continues, strengthened by the possibility of the children's return after graduation. There are no plans for the room's appropriation—the only shift is the parents' control over the room's aesthetics.

> Carole: Yes, we tidied Robin's room because he's so messy. So when his back was turned, we took the opportunity to tidy up his room a bit. (A_FR_40)

> Basia: We took these bags and filled 7 of them, really, taking out all sorts of rubbish, crisp wrappers, chocolate wrappers—there was everything. And [at times] when I felt bad [that our son had moved out], my husband said: look at the old pictures of his room, you'll get better; because we literally decluttered that room. We cleaned it very well, and even painted a part of the wall, and it was perfect. The mess in his room was a big sticking point in our relationship because there was no way you could get him to clean it up (…). And I thought to myself when I felt bad; I'll look at the mess in the room and remember the problem we had at home. (A_PL_4G)

Parents' efforts to set their own aesthetic and cleaning standards may meet resistance. Konrad and Iwona, who could not stand the look of their son's bedroom, cleaned and painted it right after his departure. Although their son initially said he had no colour preferences, he was finally very dissatisfied with the grey shade the parents had chosen. To his parents' relief, he did not mind that they were using half of his wardrobe—as the son's bedroom is the biggest room in the house, the parents decided to use some space to store their things. The wall colour, however, turned out to be an essential means of the son's identity expression—greyness did not reflect his personality.

> Iwona: He got the biggest room (…) enormous, really. And we cut out a bit and made our wardrobe—a bit of the wardrobe is ours, and a bit is his (…). And he doesn't mind that, but he does mind this terrible greyness that it does not reflect him; it is not his, and he did not choose it. (A_PL_7G)

A further step typical for an *update* is redecoration. In addition to the partial agency shift, redecoration signals the child's transition into an independent adult. Desks that served to study are now replaced with coffee tables, single beds with sofas or double beds for children as adult visitors. Rooms are defined as belonging to children but reflect and reinforce their new role and status as independent adults.

Agnieszka: (we plan to) arrange one bedroom into a room with a double bed for them when they visit. One is not married but lives with his girlfriend, and she's his partner; they often come together so... I want them to have a guest room. (A_PL_1G)

Basia: (...) we rearranged his room regarding his new life situation. His desk was still there, his LEGO collections, as he had left them in high school. And I recently decided to change it. We threw the desk away because he visits us with his girlfriend, his fiancée, and they need a corner to sit in, an adult room. (A_PL_4G)

Sometimes, an update is done under the watchful eye of a child controlling the process. Zdzisława and Gracjan, whose daughter could always decide about her room's décor, continues to leave most room-related decisions to her. While they initiated the process of change, their daughter managed it. In other words, the parents and daughter agreed that the room should reflect the girl's status as an adult, but there was no shift of agency.

Gracjan: She was free (to decorate her room) because parents cannot always furnish their children's lives!
Zdzisława: Even when we redecorated her room lately, we bought a bed, but she had to accept it first.
Gracjan: She had to see it in the photos.
Zdzisława: She decided. And the old furniture, it was also her idea how to renovate them, Paints, tapestries for furniture [renovation]—she chose them as well. (A_PL_31G)

As we can see, redecoration signifies the child's transition to independent adulthood, with rooms reflecting their new roles. Parents may aim to assert their agency and power over the space by introducing more adult-oriented décor, but children's agency in the room can persist.

Shifts: Temporal Ownership
In the case of shifts, parents use their children's rooms, but remove all signs of use for their visit. The agency is thus a bit unclear, but it seems stronger on the children's side as parents do not make any permanent changes and try to remove the signs of their activity in the room. Housing conditions (a need for additional space) usually push parents towards

change, while other factors (attachment to role, children's claim on agency, unclear status of the departure) hamper this process.

> Interviewer: What's the function of this room?
> Zdzisława: I mean, when she's away, I take all the dry laundry there, I fold it. (...) But when she's visiting, we hide everything; we hoover the floors so she won't notice.
> Interviewer: That it was used?
> Zdzisława: Yes. (...) the room is empty; for example, if guests are brave enough to visit, despite our dog, they have a place to sleep. (A_PL_31G)

For some parents, the temporary occupation of the child's room fills the emotional void and the need to get closer to the child.

> Carole: We put a shelf in the corridor with all the work files but didn't annex her room. I just put my computer there when she wasn't there. I felt close to my daughter, and at the same time, I was working at home, you know? (A_FR_40)

However, sometimes using the child's room does not bring the expected joy or sense of closeness but instead reinforces the feeling of emptiness.

> Delphine: When she went to Italy, I painted. And I indeed missed her terribly, so I said, "I'll put my painting stuff there, my easel, and when I get bored... I'll go upstairs to her room". Except it was even worse to have the feeling of emptiness. I never managed to do a painting up there. (A_FR_26)

In all cases of partial transformation, parents are still in the transition process and are attached to their parental identity. They also believe the room belongs to their children. Temporal use of the room is usually explained in terms of the need for additional space. However, it may also even serve to increase the parental identity and emotional closeness with the child.

Complete Transformation

This scenario concerns completely transformed rooms that officially no longer belong to the children. The room may become a personal, individual space of one of the parents, an intimate space for the couple (bedroom) or a room without one specific owner: a guest room, a laundry room or a storage room.

Magdalena and Stanisław illustrate an explicit parent–children agreement that their rooms should be transformed. Almost all factors push towards change. The children's departure was an opportunity for the parents to finally gain a bedroom or a study after years of sacrificing space for the sake of their children (it is not uncommon in Poland that a couple is deprived of a separate bedroom, which does not serve other functions). Children are independent: they have jobs and stable partners and do not intend to return. The parents regain agency over the children's bedrooms, and the children are happy to give them up. While this family also experienced the previously discussed problem of boxes with the children's old possessions, a strong need for additional space made parents force their son to remove his stuff.

> Magdalena: And so we said we were making this room our bedroom. How long can a room stay cluttered like this?
> Interviewer: So… it was irritating that it wasn't used?
> Magdalena: It was a useless room. Even now, when they visit, it's better they stay in this room, cos it's arranged so one can sleep there, than in a cluttered room, full of various computers and cables! (…) And so we redecorated, and we moved in…
> Interviewer: Did he [your son] have anything against it?
> Magdalena: No, no, no.
> Stanisław: No, our children had nothing against it.
> Magdalena: They even encouraged us to use these rooms. (A_PL_26G)

When the children visit, they sleep in the living room, or their parents give them their bedroom. Living in a very small flat, they cannot afford to keep the children's bedrooms. While Magdalena and Stanisław are still attached to their parental identity and practices of care, housing conditions are the reason for the appropriation of the room.

> Magdalena: I don't understand it. Must the bedroom be kept so the children feel they have their place?
> Stanisław: They can always come back!
> Magdalena: They can always come back. This is how it will always be.
> Stanisław: [But to] leave the room unchanged? My brother can afford it because he has a big house and can have such a room. (A_PL_26G)

Another couple's narrative demonstrates the importance of a definite character of departure, which allows parents to think of room transformation and supports the transition of the parent–child relationship. The eldest daughter of Gérald and Béatrice, who is married, has a good job, lives in a 100-square-metre flat, and no longer needs parental help. Her room has been rearranged according to Béatrice's needs and taste: "the way I want it", she says. The furniture was given away as a sign that the transition was complete.

> Béatrice: Yeah, and then all the furniture in Melanie's room went to my sister's (…). So now I can furnish Melanie's room as I want… (…) here we are in Melanie's room, it's become Béatrice's teleworking office and an ironing room… it's… we've taken it over, we are reorganising the space.. (…). So now Melanie's room can be rearranged the way I want it. (A_FR_14)
>
> In contrast, the younger daughter's life and financial situation are less stable, and her unchanged room reflects that.
>
> Gérald: Melanie and Alicia don't have the same space. Melanie has a house of 100 square metres with garages (…). Aurelie has 29 square metres. (A_FR_14)

An interesting test of whether the transformation is complete comes when the child returns home, as in the case of Juliette and Claude. The daughter, who moved back into the family home for a few months after a marital break-up, no longer had a room and had to sleep on the sofa. Her father had adapted her room into his study—he used to work in the garage before her departure.

> Claude: Oh well, when she returned, we told her: no problem. But you're going to do what your brother did, you're going to sleep on the sofa. (A_FR_5)

Similarly, in the case of Valerie and Sylvain, the father's rapid reappropriation of the only daughter's room communicates the emphasis put on parts of his identity other than parental ones. The daughter's departure made room for him to expand his interests. The departure seemed definite, as she had finished her studies and was looking for a teaching post near her partner's home. Even so, the room's transformation was unusually rapid. Shortly after the daughter moved out, Sylvain "needed to reclaim the space", explains Valerie. He likes music and cinema, so he set up a home studio. But he describes the suddenness of the transformation:

Sylvain: Here we are, changing everything. It's not about erasing our daughter. But [we need] to reappropriate the space, so it's not a sanctuary but a living room. So that's it. That's why I started the work relatively quickly. (A_FR_17)

Sylvain's needs were not the only push factor. We soon learn that Valerie was sad when her daughter left and had great difficulty returning to the daughter's room. "It took me a long time to get back upstairs", she confessed. "It was a bit of a no-go area for Valerie", explains Sylvain. The complete transformation of the room helped Valerie use all the space in the house, spared her from confronting emotionally charged areas and accelerated the role transition process. Today, their daughter's former room is used as a home studio and winter bedroom.

Valerie: In winter, we sleep in Léonie's old room.
    Sylvain: So there's a sofa, so there's the heat from the stove (...). It's all about the comfort of warmth (A_FR_17)

The room's transformation facilitated the transition to the empty nest phase. Without traces of the daughter's identity in the room, it is easier for the mother to use this space. Nevertheless, as her father admitted, this rapid transformation was a bit shocking to the young woman. She interpreted the change as a signal that her parents had abandoned their caring role, which hurt her.

Sylvain: At first, when I moved in and started to transform the room, she said, "ah, well, you didn't wait long before transforming my room, did you...?". (...) we felt that we were erasing traces of her very quickly. (A_FR_17)

As we have demonstrated, in some cases, children's rooms are completely transformed and no longer officially belong to the children. These rooms can become personal spaces for one of the parents, a couple's intimate space (bedroom), or serve various functions like a guest room, laundry room or storage room. Room transformation can result from agreements between parents and children, the children's definite departure, or the need for additional space. While such changes may facilitate the transition to the empty nest phase, they can also be emotionally challenging for the children.

Discussion

In this chapter, we investigated how several factors (agency, identity, materiality and biographical stage) may explain different stages of the transition of children's rooms after their departure. The fact that the child's bedroom has remained unchanged even after a definite departure may relate to the continuity of the general parental identity and parental role. The child may also manifest their agency by forcing the parents to leave the room as it is. The uncertain character of the child's departure significantly reinforces parental roles and hampers the process of change. The need for additional space may push for room transformation, but if it is not strong enough, other factors overcome it. In a scenario of complete change, push factors win over hampering factors. Children's independence and definite departure, their surrender of agency over the space, parents' need for additional room and the weakening of their caring role accelerate the transition. If all the discussed factors push towards either continuity or change, the process is clear and smooth. However, there are often tensions between different factors, when some of them favour room change, while others tend to inhibit it. They may result in conflicts between parents and children; for example, the room's transition can be experienced as too rapid or forceful. They may also lead to cognitive dissonances. For example, parents may feel the need for extra room but also that taking it over would conflict with their idea of a good, caring parent. Tensions reflected in materiality are best observed in the partial transformation scenarios and are worthy of further analysis.

This study illustrates how materiality is involved in producing and reconfiguring family relations. First, it reflects the shifts or continuity in the relationship between children and parents, their agency and identity. Second, it is an actor in shaping family relationships by encouraging or preventing change. Material objects reflect transitions but also have an impact on them. For example, erasing material traces of the child can accelerate and facilitate the change or loss of the parental role. Additionally, adequate housing conditions are necessary to even engage in the dilemmas regarding the future of the children's bedrooms. More studies that consider materiality in these three roles as an indicator, facilitator and condition of family development and change would be fruitful in exploring the potential of this approach.

The complexity of the process of transforming a child's room shows that the transition to the empty nest is a process that may take a significant amount of time, switch directions and pace, and result in tensions. Similar results are found in the analyses described in other chapters. In this sense, studying the materiality of a child's bedroom is a useful way of observing the complexity of the transition to the empty nest, which is a process rather than a distinct stage of life. It would be helpful to study other stages in the family's life, including the transformation of the living interior over a more extended period.

Another potential line of research would be to compare changes over time and between generations. Several factors that hinder the transition of the children's rooms have increased. They include the increasing number of children who have their own room, and the strengthening idea of a child's privacy, which allows the child to develop a strong attachment to this particular type of space. The prolonged period of education, combined with the economic crisis and neoliberal housing policies, and the young people's difficulties in achieving economic independence reinforce the parental role and slow down the transition of the children's bedrooms.

References

Allen, A. L. (1996). Privacy at home. The twofold problem. In N. J. Hirschmann & C. Di Stefano (Eds.), *Revisioning the political: Feminist reconstructions of traditional concepts in Western political theory* (1st ed., pp. 193–212). Westview Press.

Allen, A. L., & Mack, E. (1991). How privacy got its gender. *Northern Illinois University Law Review, 10*(3), 441–478.

Altman, I. (1977). Privacy regulation: Culturally universal or culturally specific? *Journal of Social Issues, 33*(3), 66–84. https://doi.org/10.1111/j.1540-4560.1977.tb01883.x

Amaturo, E., Costagliola, S., & Ragone, G. (1987). Furnishing and status attributes: A sociological study of the living room. *Environment and Behavior, 19*(2), 228–249. https://doi.org/10.1177/0013916587192008

Baydar, G. (2005). Figures of wo/man in contemporary architectural discourse. In H. Heynen & G. Baydar (Eds.), *Negotiating domesticity. Spatial productions of gender in modern architecture* (1st ed., pp. 30–46). Routledge.

Belk, R. W. (1988). Possessions and the extended self. *Journal of Consumer Research, 15*(2), 139–168. https://doi.org/10.1086/209154

Braun, V., & Clarke, V. (2021). One size fits all? What counts as quality practice in (reflexive) thematic analysis? *Qualitative Research in Psychology, 18*(3), 328–352. https://doi.org/10.1080/14780887.2020.1769238

Chevalier, S. (1992). *L'ameublement et le décor intérieur dans un milieu populaire urbain: approche ethnographique d'une vraie-fausse banalité* [Doctoral dissertation, Université de Paris X-Nanterre]. Université de Paris.

Cieraad, I. (2006). *At home: An anthropology of domestic space.* Syracuse University Press.

Csikszentmihalyi, M., & Halton, E. (1981). The meaning of things: Domestic symbols and the self. *Cambridge University Press.* https://doi.org/10.1017/CBO9781139167611

Dant, T. (1999). *Material culture in the social world.* McGraw-Hill Education.

Dant, T. (2004). *Materiality and society* (1st ed.). Open University Press.

de Singly, F. (Ed.). (2016). *Libres ensembles. L'individualisme dans la vie commune.* Armand Colin.

Decup-Pannier, B. (2016). Avoir une chambre chez chacun de ses parents séparés. In F. de Singly (Ed.), *Libres ensembles. L'individualisme dans la vie commune* (pp. 275–296). Armand Colin.

Douglas, M., & Isherwood, B. C. (1982). *The world of goods.* Norton.

Duncan, J. S. (1981). *Housing and identity: Cross-cultural perspectives.* Croom Helm.

Gajewska, M., Herzberg-Kurasz, M., Żadkowska, M., Kostecka, M., & Dowgiałło, B. (2023). Room of her own: Remaking empty nest and creating herspaces in practices of Polish mothers whose children left home. *European Journal of Women's Studies, 30*(1), 7–21. https://doi.org/10.1177/13505068221110336

Glevarec, H. (2010a). Les trois âges de la «culture de la chambre». *Ethnologie Française, 40*(1), 19–30. https://doi.org/10.3917/ethn.101.0019

Glevarec, H. (2010b). *La culture de la chambre. Préadolescence et culture contemporaine dans l'espace familial.* Ministère de la Culture – DEPS. https://doi.org/10.3917/deps.gleva.2010.01

Hachet, B. (2014). La chambre des enfants en résidence alternée: Un sanctuaire? *Strenae: La chambre d'enfant, un microcosme culturel. Espace, consommation, pédagogie, 7.* https://doi.org/10.4000/strenae.1187

Jędruszczak, K. (2005). Prywatność jako potrzeba w ramach koncepcji siebie. *Roczniki Psychologiczne, 8*(2), 111–135.

Julien, M.-P., & Rosselin, C. (2005). *La culture matérielle* (7th ed.). La Découverte.

Krzaklewska, E., & Ratecka, A. (2014). Władza w intymnych związkach heteroseksualnych refleksja nad badaniem władzy w kontekście równości płci. *Acta Universitatis Lodziensis. Folia Sociologica, 51*, 149–167.

Law, J., & Mol, A. (1995). Notes on materiality and sociality. *The Sociological Review, 43*(2), 274–294. https://doi.org/10.1111/j.1467-954X.1995.tb00604.x

Lefebvre, H. (1986). *La Production de l'espace* (3rd ed.). Anthropos.

Lincoln, S. (2014). "I've stamped my personality all over it": The meaning of objects in teenage bedroom space. *Space and Culture, 17*(3), 266–279. https://doi.org/10.1177/1206331212451677

Low, S. M., & Altman, I. (1992). Place attachment. In I. Altman & S. M. Low (Eds.), *Place attachment* (pp. 1–12). Springer US. https://doi.org/10.1007/978-1-4684-8753-4_1

Madigan, R., & Munro, M. (1991). Gender, house and 'home': Social meanings and domestic architecture in Britain. *Journal of Architectural and Planning Research, 8*(2), 116–132.

Madigan, R., & Munro, M. (1996). 'House beautiful': Style and consumption in the home. *Sociology, 30*(1), 41–57. https://doi.org/10.1177/0038038596030001004

Madigan, R., Munro, M., & Smith, S. J. (1990). Gender and the meaning of the home. *International Journal of Urban and Regional Research, 14*(4), 625–647. https://doi.org/10.1111/j.1468-2427.1990.tb00160.x

Maunaye, E. (2000). Passer de chez ses parents à chez soi: Entre attachement et détachement. *Lien social et Politiques, 43*, 59–66. https://doi.org/10.7202/005186ar

Maunaye, E. (2001). Quitter ses parents. Terrain. *Anthropologie & sciences humaines, 36*, 33–44. https://doi.org/10.4000/terrain.1168

Mauss, M. (2002). *The gift: The form and reason for exchange in archaic societies.* Routledge Classics.

Miller, D. (1987). *Material culture and mass consumption.* Basil Blackwell.

Moore, J. (2000). Placing home in context. *Journal of Environmental Psychology, 20*(3), 207–217. https://doi.org/10.1006/jevp.2000.0178

Munro, M., & Madigan, R. (1999). Negotiating space in the family home. In I. Cieraad (Ed.), *At home. An anthropology of domestic space* (pp. 107–117). Syracuse University Press.

Newell, B. C., Metoyer, C. A., & Moore, A. D. (2015). Privacy in the family. In B. Roessler & D. Mokrosinska (Eds.), *Social dimensions of privacy* (pp. 104–121). Cambridge University Press. https://doi.org/10.1017/CBO9781107280557.007

Pedersen, D. M. (1997). Psychological functions of privacy. *Journal of Environmental Psychology, 17*(2), 147–156. https://doi.org/10.1006/jevp.1997.0049

Perrot, M. (Ed.). (2008). *Historia życia prywatnego. Od rewolucji francuskiej do I wojny światowej* (Vol. 4, 2nd ed.). Ossolineum.

Perrot, M. (2018). *The bedroom: An intimate history.* Yale University Press.

Preda, A. (1999). The turn to things: Arguments for a sociological theory of things. *The Sociological Quarterly, 40*(2), 347–366. https://doi.org/10.1111/j.1533-8525.1999.tb00552.x

Ramos, E. (2002). *Rester enfant, devenir adulte: La cohabitation des étudiants chez leurs parents.* L'Harmattan.

Ramos, E. (2016). *L'expérience individuelle et les "chez-soi".* Sciences de l'Homme et Société. Université Paris Descartes.

Ramos, E. (2018). La chambre à l'adolescence à l'ère des écrans connectés. Ancrage spatial et mobilité numérique. *Cerlis.* Retrieved January 4, 2023, from https://www.cerlis.eu/portfolio-view/la-chambre-a-ladolescence-a-lere-des-ecrans-connectes-ancrage-spatial-et-mobilite-numerique/

Ramos, E., & de Singly, F. (2000). La défense d'un petit monde pour un jeune adulte vivant chez ses parents. In F. de Singly (Ed.), *Libres ensemble. L'individualisme dans la vie commune* (pp. 155–176). Armand Colin.

Ratecka, A. (2011). Niedokończona egalitaryzacja: O władzy w polskich małżeństwach. In K. Slany, B. Kowalska, & M. Ślusarczyk (Eds.), *Kalejdoskop genderowy: W drodze do poznania płci społeczno-kulturowej w Polsce* (pp. 255–270). Wydawnictwo Uniwersytetu Jagiellońskiego.

Reimer, S., & Leslie, D. (2004). Identity, consumption, and the home. *Home Cultures, 1*(2), 187–210. https://doi.org/10.2752/174063104778053536

Schatzki, T. (2010). Materiality and social life. *Nature and Culture, 5*(2), 123–149. https://doi.org/10.3167/nc.2010.050202

Segalen, M., & Le Wita, B. (1993). Chez-soi: Objets et décors, des créations familiales? *Autrement: série «Mutations», 137,* 11–23.

Serfaty-Garzon, P. (2003). *Chez-soi, les territoires de l'intimité.* Armand Colin.

Shove, E. (2003). *Comfort, cleanliness and convenience: The social organization of normality.* Berg Publishers.

Shove, E., & Warde, A. (2002). Inconspicuous consumption: The sociology of consumption, lifestyles, and the environment. In R. E. Dunlap, F. H. Buttel, P. Dickens, & A. Gijswijt (Eds.), *Sociological theory and the environment: Classical foundations, contemporary insights* (pp. 230–251). Rownan & Littlefield.

Skowrońska, M. (2015). *Jak u siebie. Zamieszkiwanie i komfort.* Zakład Wydawniczy Nomos.

Warde, A. (2005). Consumption and theories of practice. *Journal of Consumer Culture, 5*(2), 131–153. https://doi.org/10.1177/1469540505053090

Woodward, I. (2001). Domestic objects and the taste epiphany: A resource for consumption methodology. *Journal of Material Culture, 6*(2), 115–136. https://doi.org/10.1177/135918350100600201

Woodward, I. (2007). *Understanding material culture.* Sage. https://doi.org/10.4135/9781446278987

Zaleski, Z. (1998). Prawo do prywatności. Spojrzenie psychologiczne. *Czasopismo Psychologiczne, 4*(3–4), 218–238.

CHAPTER 6

Adult Children's Visits to Their Parents: Recomposition and Renegotiation of Family Roles and Responsibilities

Marta Skowrońska, Emmanuelle Maunaye, Dorota Rancew-Sikora, and Cyrano Andre–Vieille

M. Skowrońska (✉)
Faculty of Sociology, Adam Mickiewicz University, Poznań, Poland
e-mail: marta.skowronska@amu.edu.pl

E. Maunaye
Département Carrières Sociales (UMR 6051), Université de Rennes,
Rennes, France
e-mail: emmanuelle.maunaye@univ-rennes1.fr

D. Rancew-Sikora
Social Sciences Department (Institute of Sociology), University of Gdańsk,
Gdańsk, Poland
e-mail: dorota.rancew-sikora@ug.edu.pl

C. Andre–Vieille
Centre de recherche sur les liens sociaux (CERLIS, UMR 8070),
Université Paris Cité, Paris, France
e-mail: cyrano.andre–vieille@etu.parisdescartes.fr

INTRODUCTION

This chapter investigates how family roles and interaction patterns are recomposed during adult children's visits to parental homes in Poland and France. We aim to show the empty nest as a stage for domestic hospitality, a trigger for family roles, and a display of a family ideology (Finch, 2007; James & Curtis, 2010). Our analysis focuses on the transition from adult–children to new, adult–adult relationships (Scabini & Cigoli, 1997; Maunaye, 2006), which are reflected and re-established during family gatherings. We examine adult children's visits in detail to observe how different families interpret this new situation, which is an intersection of a family setting and a staged, hosted event. Do parents believe their children should be invited and received like other guests? Or do they expect them to behave like household members? How do these practices differ among Polish and French families and change over time?

The Context of Intergenerational Relations in the Family

Although the departure of adult children may seem like a rupture in children–parent relations, "involved parenting" (Sørensen & Nielsen, 2021) may include frequent and intense intergenerational contact. In France, 43% of adult children see their father or mother every week (Régnier-Loilier, 2006). This study also shows that the frequency of visits after the children's departure relates to several factors, of which geographical distance is the most prominent. The Generations and Gender Survey (Kotowska, 2019; Régnier-Loilier, 2019) demonstrates that Polish adult children live closer to their parents than their French counterparts (87% of Polish adults can reach their parents in an hour or less compared to 76% of French adults). In addition, 22.6% of adult children in France live six or more hours away from their family home, while only 4.6% of adult Polish children live so far. Further distance results in limited face-to-face contact. Polish adult children are slightly more satisfied with their relations with their parents than the French. Generally, parents' satisfaction is greater than that of the children in both countries.

A considerable amount of literature has been published on the relationship between parents and underage children during everyday life. Many aspects of everyday family life have been analysed, such as shared meals as part of domestic life (Ochs & Shohet, 2006; Aronsson & Gottzén, 2011; Cappellini & Parsons, 2012a; Brannen et al., 2013) and leisure and shared family time (de Singly & Ramos, 2010; Brunet & Kertudo, 2013; Céroux & Crépin, 2013). However, less attention has been given to family meetings in the empty nest phase (Maunaye, 2001, 2002; Hogg et al., 2004; Gram et al., 2015; Rancew-Sikora & Skowrońska, 2022).

In the context of intergenerational family relations, visiting family members can be experienced as a return to being a close family again. However, it is an experience limited to a short period together, having quality time and celebrating special, festive occasions (Cappellini & Parsons, 2012a, b). Maunaye (2001) has demonstrated that adult children strongly associate the idea of 'home' with their family home. Young adults, particularly single students, use the expression 'I'm going home' to describe visits to their parents' places (Ibidem). Although they have moved out, adult children are not yet fully independent of their parents for economic, material, and emotional support (Portela & Raynaud, 2019). Maunaye (2006) details the evolution of the meaning of encounters between parents and children while the young person is gaining independence. She highlights that they move from the status of a child to an adult by becoming a couple.

Visiting parents strengthens bonds and provides real help to those who need it; thus, these visits can be an essential element of intergenerational solidarity (Silverstein & Bengtson, 1997). It is worth noting, however, that the expected models of maintaining parents–adult children relationships and the degree of individual autonomy of family members or intergenerational connectedness vary among cultures (Trommsdorff, 2006). Western models are more based on the independence and individuality of family members than Eastern ones, and this trend can be observed even within Europe. Within one culture, families also differ. Members of the same family may disagree in this respect due to their relational strategies and interests associated with their age, gender, status, life situation, and individual preferences. Family meetings help observe the "family in a nutshell" signs of its change and continuity (Ochs & Shohet, 2006). By expressing their mutual expectations and negotiating modes of engagement, participants create new routines for being together and respecting the new roles of other family members (DeVault, 1994; Ochs et al., 1996; Cappellini & Parsons, 2012a, b; Fiese et al., 2006).

In this chapter, we explore the transformation of family roles and interaction patterns as adult children revisit their parental homes in Poland and France. Our main goal is to find regular transition patterns among different families and in different national contexts. Specifically, we aim to examine adult children's visits in their parents' narratives and observe how they interpret this new situation, which is an intersection of a family setting and a staged event. To do this, we use the notions of host and guest and see how they relate to the exchange between adult children and their parents.

On Receiving Guests and Hospitality

The terms "hosts" and "guests" are usually used in the context of hospitality. For Anne Gotman (2001), "hospitality is literally the space made for the Other (…) different and therefore disturbing (…) wherever he or she comes from—from afar or from the vicinity (…)—and whoever he or she may be, a stranger or a family member". The best-known works on hospitality are those published by anthropologists who conducted their field research in cross-cultural contexts, such as Boas (1888), Stefánsson (1913) in the far North, Pitt-Rivers (1972) in Spain, Herzfeld (1988) in Greece, and Shryock (2008, 2009) in Yemen and Jordan. For this reason, anthropological accounts of hospitality emphasize cultural distances (Lashley & Morrison, 2001; Lashley et al., 2006) and are generally dominated by a male perspective (Rancew-Sikora, 2021). A second important strand of research in this area is philosophical considerations of the ethical meaning of openness towards strangers. Recently, a lot of research into hospitality has been conducted in the context of tourism, and slowly a less romanticized, more realistic, and gender- and class-balanced approach to hospitality is being developed (Bachórz, 2013; Horolets, 2014; Skowrońska, 2014, 2019, 2020; Bloch, 2021). Still, there are few studies on hospitality among long-term friends and family circles, perhaps because in the West the traditional function of receiving guests in private homes has largely been taken over by gatherings held in public and commercial settings (Habermas, 1991; Selwyn, 1996; Cohen, 1988; Duval, 2003; Candea & Da Col, 2012; Simoni, 2017).

From a comparative perspective, the "traditional" type of generous and self-sacrificing hospitality persists, especially where commercial infrastructure and the public service sector are underdeveloped or where their availability is limited. There is a tendency to attribute generous hospitality to cultures defined as more peripheral or archaic and to poorer populations and lower classes, which has been criticized in literature as paternalization (Doja, 2011, 2014; Bachórz, 2013; Horolets, 2014). Domestic hospitality, relatively less prevalent in the West, remains essential in organizing and sustaining closer friendships and family relationships. There are subtle national, regional, class, generational, and gender differences, as well as individual/family variations of beliefs about the degree of preparation and care related to domestic hospitality and about sharing the responsibility for it (Matyska, 2013; Rancew-Sikora & Żadkowska, 2017; Skowrońska, 2020). Notably, women are still burdened with a greater involvement in hospitality, even in more egalitarian societies (Blichfeldt & Gram, 2017).

From a sociological perspective, hospitality in modern societies counteracts the isolation of families and reduces risks in their relationships with the outside world (Znaniecki, 1938). The principle of reciprocating hospitality creates stable solidarity circles that link different households together. These circles can also facilitate connections among individuals of a similar age and gender, supporting them and promoting status shifts within groups (Mauss, 1992). Temporary coalitions between members of different families can reinforce and neutralize asymmetries arising from taking host and guest roles or in-group hierarchies (Rancew-Sikora, 2015). As Allerton (2012) demonstrated, referring to the Indonesian context, even close friends and family tend to be nervous about playing the role of guests, even if it allows them to eat and be served better than usual. The tension may result from believing that a wrong course of events may harm their relationship. The festive formality, occasionally intruding into an intimate personal relationship, emphasizes social distance. Formal celebrations make the guest an outsider with the right to make observations and judgements from the position of a stranger. According to Herzfeld (2012), the formalization of hospitality inevitably produces ambivalence and tension. It lacks a sense of casual intimacy, which returns after the guest leaves or stays in the house for longer.

From this perspective, and in the context of children's visits during the empty nest period, are children "disturbing guests", as Anne Gotman (2001) would suggest, who take up space that the parents have reappropriated? Do they become guests? Do the parents consider themselves hosts? Of what type? Do parents believe their children should be invited and received like other guests? Or do they expect them to behave like household members? How do these practices change over time?

To answer these questions, we will present four parents–children encounters demonstrating the (un)changing relationships, expectations, conflicts, and ambiguities. First, we examine cases of returning to old patterns, when children and parents behave as if the children still lived in the family home, and there is hardly any change in intergenerational relations.

Oftentimes, the asymmetry of exchange combined with children's disengagement in the interaction results in parents' dissatisfaction. Second, we analyse visits, which modify how parents anticipate, organize, and live the meeting according to hospitality patterns. Here, the asymmetry of exchange is compensated by the children's involvement and their role of grateful guests. Third, we present a balanced and more symmetrical encounter during which children take more responsibility for the meetings with their parents. Finally, we observe situations where visits are rare or without real intergenerational exchanges.

The chapter is based on an empirical study undertaken in Poland and France. The research material consisted of 87 (42 Polish and 45 French) qualitative, in-depth dyadic interviews conducted in 2018–2020 (corpus A). The couples, aged 50–64, whose children (one to four) were all adults and had moved out within the previous five years, were interviewed. The analysis focused on the interview part devoted to the question of adult children's visits—their frequency and character and how they were experienced. However, the remaining parts of the interviews were also read to provide context and to find other mentions of visits and family meals.

RESULTS

Particularly in the first years after their departure, children's visits to their family homes are processes of renegotiation and reconfiguration of family roles and practices. They are influenced by several factors, such as the model of family bonds and relations (hierarchical or democratic, distanced or close, harmonious or conflictual), the attitude to hosting others (as something formal or informal, tiring or relaxing, symmetrical or asymmetrical), the occasion (birthday, Christmas, or a regular visit), and the susceptibility of the family system to modification. Seeing an adult child may be a return to an almost-intact relationship pattern and a chance for a new role and perspective.

In general, the way in which children are received varies according to the occasion, the structure of the household, the distance of their residence, the frequency of the visits and also the stage of departure, understood as a long process of gaining independence by adult children who have moved out of the family home. In this chapter, we analysed generalized descriptions of children's visits provided by their parents. We focused on regular visits rather than special occasions. Instead of differentiating various factors that might influence the shape of the visit, we decided to observe the evolution (or lack thereof) of the parent/child relationship after the departure mirrored in their encounters. We were also interested in how these visits relate to the general understanding of hospitality and receiving guests. While the exchange between parents and children is almost always asymmetrical (parents give and children receive), the meaning of this asymmetry changes with the evolution of the parent/child relationships towards more balanced and adult-to-adult relationships.

Return to Home and Old Patterns of an Asymmetrical Children– Parents Relationship

This type of encounter involves adult children "returning" home rather than "visiting". Parent–child interaction patterns have not changed or only changed slightly. They involve more work and effort from the parents, who tend to give their children much more than they receive. Continuing asymmetry of intergenerational relationships is a source of possible parental frustration.

Valérie and Eric quoted below emphasize that their daughters return home as if they never left. They lead the lives of teenagers who hide in their rooms, derive comfort from familiar surroundings and parental care, and remain uninvolved in household duties:

> Eric: She keeps us company from time to time, but otherwise, she comes to visit her "brother", our rabbit (laughs) (…) Here there is a form of comfort (…) the meal is ready; the house is warm, and two grumbling oddballs will do the housework. (A_FR_6)

> Valérie: And Emanuelle, she hides in her room (…) she's looked after as if she were a child, she doesn't do much in the way of material things, you know, preparing a dish, vacuuming, ironing her clothes, nothing. So you see, it's a bit uncomfortable. (A_FR_6)

The parental narrative includes frustration or irritation at the daughters' behaviour. Parents expected that their daughters' departure would begin a role transition process and the relationship between them would be more partner-like and balanced. The daughters, however, stick to the small child's role. Another part of the interview demonstrates another aspect of this problem: since the daughters still haven't got a driving license, their parents have to pick them up and drop them off:

> Valérie: Well, it indeed creates a burden when they're here because, in the end, they want an urban life, but here there's no possibility of having it, so it makes them dependent on us, which is not good. (A_FR_6)

The Polish interview below demonstrates another source of family disagreement. Julia and Zenon were disappointed by their children's insufficient involvement in family life. However, contrary to the previous example, the parents did not iron their children's clothes or drive them anywhere when they asked—they employed a distancing strategy instead:

> Zenon: We don't dance attendance around them. If they want to lock themselves in their rooms, they can do it (…). When they're hungry, they come downstairs and prepare something. So it's not absorbing. (A_PL_32G)

Krzysztof and Magdalena expected more intense interactions and involvement. To them, their son Kuba was neither an adult household member who would perform his housework duties nor a guest who would offer his attention. Instead, to his parents' discontentment, he resembles a hotel guest with no obligations towards his hosts:

> Krzysztof: There's one problem with Kuba—I complained about it [to my colleagues] at work. He visits us, and he's away all day (…), so he's kind of here, but in fact, he's not because he goes out, here and there. (A_PL_3G)

Kuba's parents expected their son to take up the new role of an engaged guest while he continued to perform the child's part, only receiving care and attention but not obliged to give anything. In this sense, both families share a similar problem—parents expect their children to take up the new role of an adult visitor, who knows the obligations of a guest, and children need to continue the old patterns. Similarly, Gérald said that he had to explain to his youngest daughter that he expected to spend some time together. Otherwise, the visit would resemble a hotel stay rather than domestic hospitality:

> Gérald: There was a moment when I got a little bit angry with her and her first boyfriend… because it was (…) "well, we're sleeping here tonight… but we're not eating here tonight". After a while, I said to her: "Wait, Melanie, (…) this is not a hotel; it's not a guesthouse where you can do what you want. (…) if you come home, but we don't see you, then don't come home". (A_FR_14)

Parents who refrain from taking action to reduce their frustration signify their desire to avoid open conflict:

> Fabienne: We don't want to clash. Well, it's true that she doesn't live here anymore, and we don't know what she's going through; sometimes, we're not on the same wavelength. And we do our utmost so that... we understand each other. (A_FR_2)

Many teenagers living in their family homes are accused of "treating home as a hotel"—use of parental care and help without involvement in family life. Parents' narratives reveal their hope that their children's departure might be an opportunity for a more balanced relationship. However, in some cases the old pattern of imbalance continues unchanged. The continuity of old patterns may relate more to families where children still study and do not have a permanent place of residence (Maunaye, 2001, 2006). Some parents assume that children will return to the "real" (family) home every weekend and holiday. In these cases, the process of departure has only begun, so there is little space for role transition. For Marie-Dominique and Jean-Luc, quoted below, the return of their eldest son, a student, to the family home every holiday was self-evident:

> Interviewer: How did you decide that he would come back every school holiday?
> Marie-Dominique: Well, we didn't give him a choice (laughs).
> Jean-Luc: No, but we still wanted to see him, and during the holidays, his school is closed, so he comes back. (A_FR_44)

To conclude, this scenario involves adult children "returning" to their parental homes, maintaining parent–child interaction patterns with little change. Parents often provide more care and effort than they receive, leading to potential parental frustration. Some adult children continue to act like teenagers, seeking comfort and parental care while avoiding household responsibilities. The continuity of these patterns may relate to children who still study and maintain a connection to their family home.

Parent-Hosts and Children-Guests in an Asymmetrical but Mutually Aligned Relationship

The other type of visit refers to situations of clear asymmetry in exchange of work and effort, balanced by the children's involvement in the encounter. The children are treated as "special guests" whose presence activates great parental efforts. Satisfaction is derived from the greater attention that children pay to their parents, marking a desire for a relationship of equals.

In the Polish families, the interviewees' stories of meetings often included the image of tables overflowing with an abundance of food and mentioned intense preparations for visits:

> Interviewer: Does one need to prepare for their visit? How does it usually look when you know they're going to visit?
> Wiesław: My wife prepares everything our son-in-law likes. They get everything; yes, my wife prepares the table here. The table is overflowing.
> Wioleta: We are waiting for him. Cos you wait, as if for guests. And you want to prepare; you want to cook. And it varies when we're at home, just the two of us usually, right? And when they come, [we serve] all the best, obviously! (A_PL_33G)

Some narratives included metaphors of a five-star hotel, spa, or all-inclusive holiday to emphasize the parental effort to host their children in a special way. These practices of care served the parents to express love for their offspring:

> Magdalena: And when they were about to visit, everything was prepared for them in their rooms, little boxes with gingerbread and juice in every room (…). Then they enjoyed it; they said, "even a 5-star hotel wouldn't prepare things like mom does". (A_PL_26G)

While the French material does not include images of abundance and food overflowing, it contains narratives about preparing for the children's visits and adapting to their needs. For these parents, the children visiting and taking care of them implies a change in the habits acquired since the children left, as the organization of shopping and meals established for two people is no longer sufficient:

Claude: For example, for meals, when there are just the two of us, we need a cheese board and bread, and then that's it. When we got Lothaire and Romane back during the lockdown, we had to put all the food logistics back in place because it's not the same thing now that we have our two teenagers at home! (...) When the kids leave home, there's almost nothing left to do. It becomes very light. The difference in food and laundry management is really important! (A_FR_19)

Similarly, in the Polish example below, when the daughter visited her parents, they changed their daily habits and routines to adapt to her needs:

Gracjan: Odd, but nice, too! Because when our daughter comes, there's always a great commotion! We're not in this mode anymore.
Zdzisława: And everything needs to be changed for the time of her visit.
Gracjan: Yes, yes, yes.
Interviewer: What do you need to change, for example?
Zdzisława: The fridge supply. And we have to cut down our smoking. And turn on the heating. She's always cold, and we're the opposite. And this is something we can't agree upon. She always feels cold, and we're hot. (A_PL_31G)

What's more, Zdzisława and Gracjan not only prepared their daughter's favourite food but also changed their eating habits during her visit, fearing her criticism:

Zdzisława: (...) She started to follow a diet, I mean, a way of eating. And now we go shopping with that in mind, but not yet according to what she precisely said. That's why, when she's visiting, we adapt to what it should be.
Gracjan: Yes. So the child terrorizes her parents (...).
Zdzisława: Yes, precisely. When she arrives and sees that this isn't right, that isn't right; she looks askance at as. (A_PL_31G)

Intense hosting may serve to please the child and court their favour. The quotation below demonstrates how Celina and Adam prepared for their son's visit, cleaning the house thoroughly (they used the phrase "like for the Pope's visit") and cooking the best meals, hoping the son would appreciate that:

Celina: But the fact is that our love is deep, so you feel like running around with a cloth [and cleaning].

> Interviewer: And you don't usually prepare for guests this way, do you? Is this some premium treatment, more than for an ordinary guest?
>
> Adam: I think so, yes—it's this desire that your child sees this [effort], a desire to court their favour. (A_PL_2G)

Agnieszka observed with surprise that when her adult sons visited her, she "switched guest mode on".

> Agnieszka: I switched this guest mode on. I made his bed, for example. When I used to change their bedsheets in the past, I did not put the pillow-case over the bedding; I only put the cases on the beds and said, "change the sheets", but now I changed it as if he was a guest. I'd do that for a guest, so I did it for him. And I checked if his room was tidy. (A_PL_1G)

Sometimes the intense model of hosted meetings involved a sense of duty and responsibility for the entire visit and resulted in the strain and tiredness of hosts (usually hostesses, to be more precise). Basia's narrative below demonstrates the shift from being a household member into a guest whose visit is a meticulously planned event:

> Basia: When [children] come to visit, I have an odd feeling that we have to sit and talk as we do with guests; we need to elaborate a plan; maybe we should go out, do something. In the past, we'd wander around the house, but now they are guests, and we have to anticipate what we will be occupied with. In the summer it's less trouble, cos we can go to the garden, barbecue, something's happening. But in the autumn, I think: damn, maybe we should suggest going somewhere... When our older son visits, we like to talk, and he always comes up with some scientific topic, and there are discussions till late at night, and his girlfriend is there, too. But when Piotrek comes, I feel obliged to organize this, and I feel a bit tired. (A_PL_4G)

Similarly, but to a lesser extent, Angèle organized her schedule according to the presence of her children:

> Angèle: I adapt my timetable slightly to the fact that they are there. Typically, when they're here, you don't go out. So if I have things planned, I try to clear my diary, more or less. It depends a bit on the duration of the activity and on how busy it is. Typically, if they're all here, we won't go to dinner with our friends, or go away for the weekend. (A_FR_19)

The guest status acquired by the children exempts them from participating in domestic tasks, thus creating an additional asymmetry in their exchanges. Similarly, the Polish interviews demonstrate that in some cases the long-standing custom of the children's involvement in household duties while spending leisure time without their parents has now changed into a new model of being together while visiting the family home. The mother cleans, cooks sophisticated dishes, and spends time with children-guests in intense interactions. At the same time, children have gained the status of "special guests" with additional privileges (such as demanding more cleanliness):

> Dorota: They were here as guests but in slightly different roles. And there was dinner, and I'd been thinking about what to cook since Thursday; I called them to ask what they felt like eating. After a month, Marcin said: "mom, this bathroom is really..."—and I say, child, when am I supposed to clean if I go to work all week, and then I host you? Cos in the past, when they lived here as household members, it was like, Marcin cleaned the little bathroom, someone cleaned this, someone else that, and it went on, they had their duties. And now, this role has changed; they are here to visit their mom. I feel I lack time for simple household chores, cos it was like this: mom, what are you doing? Come here; we'll watch a movie. And we watched Harry Potter, and everything was left behind. (A_PL_9G)

Traditional hospitality is based on the assumption that the relationship between the host and the guest is asymmetrical. The host is the one who cares, feeds, provides, and bestows while the guest receives these gifts. However, the degree of symmetry/asymmetry in contemporary domestic hospitality is varied and influenced by cultural and class patterns and the context of hosting (a spontaneous coffee/birthday/barbecue, etc.). Generally, to balance the host–guest relationship, revisits and little gifts from guests are standard practices. Guests are usually expected to express gratitude, discretion, and tactfulness and to respect boundaries of privacy (e.g. restrain from opening cupboards, entering rooms uninvited, or staying too late).

The discussed examples of adult children's visits demonstrate that while "hosting" defines parents' practices correctly, children do not adopt the guest's role. Parents also feel that the term "guest" does not truly represent their children's position. Compared with popular domestic hospitality rules, adult children's visits to their parents seem to reach the far ends of the asymmetry spectrum. The most extreme cases of asymmetry are when parents intensify the role of the ones who give (time, food, and care), while children remain the ones who receive (or even give up practices that used to balance the asymmetry in the past). Before departure, adult children were usually expected to engage in housework. Having moved out, children may abandon even symbolic practices of involvement while not taking on guest duties (bringing gifts, asking for a revisit). However, their involvement in the interaction and expressions of gratitude demonstrate a shift in the parent–child relationships. In contrast to the first type of visits, where children remain uninvolved and self-absorbed, this kind of encounter allows parents to have an intense, focused interaction with their children. While parents, particularly mothers, tend to feel burdened with housework that accompanies these encounters, their children's attention makes the effort worthwhile.

Informal Visits: When Adult Children and Parents Become Friends

In this section, we present some examples of visits when the children are treated and behave as "home guests" or "informal guests", moving towards symmetry and partnership within intergenerational relations. This specific character of familial intimacy can be observed in the level of informality of adult children's visits: meals may be eaten in front of the TV, as in the olden days (Cappellini & Parsons, 2012a, b), even though the children are now guests:

> Interviewer: Do you feel these meals differ from those you had when you lived together?
> Anna: Yes, because they enter [home] as guests rather than household members. It's absolutely informal because we don't bother with the big table, but we put everything on the coffee table, and for example, we turn on a football match, which they came to watch. But this isn't an ordinary meal, but I cook something everyone likes, it's more. (A_PL_12G)

Children are not received as guests and do not behave as guests: they visit their family homes "empty-handed", snoop through cupboards, and eat out of the fridge; they never ask for permission and stay as long as they like. The difference may also be observed in how children move around the house. Contrary to "real" guests, they feel free to do and take what they like. What is important, the parents not only accept this but also enjoy it. One of the mothers used the expression "home guest" to emphasize that children can treat their parents' home as their own:

> Dorota: They are guests-non guests. No—they are different guests, home guests (…)
> Interviewer: And this difference between guests and non-guests, what is it?
> Dorota: No strain, definitely.
> Interviewer: They can pour themselves a drink, take something from the fridge.
> Dorota: They have to. It's their home. (A_PL_9G)

Moreover, children do not need to be invited to their parents' house. They can even give late notice of their arrival. Many of them still have keys to their parents' house:

> Carole: Yes, yes, they have keys to the house, they have their own room, so there you go.
> Erwan: Yeah, it hasn't changed. (A_FR_40)

While in many aspects diverse, these visits were characterized by their declared ordinariness. Parents emphasized that their children's arrival never involved any revolution in domestic life; they used expressions such as "normal", "ordinary", and "usual". These visits, however, often involve new patterns rather than returning to the old ways. Both parties are usually more attentive and engaged in the interaction, and the relationship is more symmetrical and partner-like.

The transition of children from household members into "home guests" can be a chance to extinguish earlier tensions and conflicts and move towards a more harmonious parent–child relationship. Disputes over performing household chores are over since adult children are no longer required to do housework. Adult children, freed from the baggage of the role of a child from whom something is expected, were more willing to interact with parents. Some parents explicitly admitted that the relationship with their children after they moved out was more harmonious and that interactions, though less frequent, were more intense (de Singly & Ramos, 2010):

Agnieszka: Before, one would feel more obliged—me at least—to control and think about what they should do (…) and now I no longer worry about it. (A_PL_1G)

In some situations, greater involvement of adult children in interactions with parents and housework may be an attempt to repair former difficult relationships. In this family, the daughter, who used to rebel and refuse to do household chores, now does her best to be on good terms with her parents. When she visits, she takes over the work and prepares breakfasts and dinners for the family. She is a "full" household member now—while before the departure, she seemed to be a half-member. The daughter may even sometimes take on the role of host:

Honorata: It has dramatically changed because, as I've mentioned, one needed to put a lot of energy into getting her to work. She used to finally [work], but [she always said] "later, later" and made a face. And now, all by herself, she says: "okay, mom, I'll do everything here". She makes these meals, initiates [them], and wants to host us. She says she's making pancakes in the morning and asks what time we will get up; for example, when she stays over for the weekend, she says: pancakes at 10, and she goes downstairs. Or she can come to my bed and bring me a cup of tea (…). So now it's better than it used to be because, you know. No, she doesn't feel like a guest; she's entirely a household member now. (A_PL_24G)

Such visits involve new patterns rather than returning to the old ways. Both parties are more attentive to each other and more engaged in the interaction. While not earned with effort or sacrifice, visits are more festive than family meals were before the departure. Parents—particularly mothers—released from the burden of housework may fully engage in the encounter. Children have a chance to present their new abilities (e.g. cooking sophisticated food), and they sometimes bring up topics they never used to. The relationship seems less hierarchical and more partner-like:

Agnieszka: More relaxed, because one controlled [children] before—"Is your homework done, have you revised for school?"—and now we just talk about things, relaxed and without a sense of obligation.
Jan: They cook on their own; everyone boasts of their culinary achievements, shows, and talks. (A_PL_1G)

In some families, children's visits resembled hosting close friends, who engage in cooking and cleaning together with the hosts. In these cases, children were involved in housework; sometimes, they even took on the cooking and initiated social practices such as board games:

> Honorata: When Natasza texts me, it's always: "Dixit"? And we know she's coming (…). So, really, it's nice, and we make pizza, or Natasza cooks something, we go shopping with her, and she makes something (…) she creates something nice. (A_PL_24G)

In this section we highlighted cases where adult children transition from being perceived as mere "visitors" to a more integral part of their parents' households, resembling "home guests" or "informal guests". These visits, while ordinary, bring forth new patterns and increased engagement, fostering harmonious parent–child bonds and potential reconciliation of past conflicts.

Rare Visits and Rejected Invitations as Signs of Weakening Intergenerational Bonds

Finally, it may happen that an adult child does not want to take any role (a guest or a household member) despite the parents' efforts. Visits are sporadic—to parents' frustration and disappointment. In some cases, children seem to refuse to accept the burden of their parents' sacrifice.

Marzena and Maciej tried the strategy of devoted hosting by cooking vegetarian dishes (which neither of the spouses likes) for their daughter, but to no avail. The daughter prefers to cook with her friends:

> Marzena: I cooked dinners, and I cooked something for her separately. On Sunday, Saturday. But then there were a lot of refusals; she didn't want to come. And she sometimes visits her grandmother, but recently she went to her grandma but refused to eat because she said she would cook with her friend. (…) And she didn't want to [eat] at grandma's place. (A_PL_6G)

Gérald and Fabienne explains the infrequency of their daughter's visits by referring to her need for more independence:

> Fabienne: Jacinte well, she was 18, and I think that was her wish to…
> Gérald: Not to come and see us.

Fabienne: It was also her will to, to… Well, to take advantage of it too, to take advantage of it to live on her own and to take off, you know. (A_FR_2)

Sabrina also stresses the need for her child's autonomy:

Sabrina: But we thought he was going to come home more often because he has the opportunity but in fact no, I think he needed his autonomy. (A_FR_29)

Polish parents have never raised the question of autonomy. When visits were rare, Polish parents sought other excuses to persuade the researcher and themselves that the frequency of visits was not evidence of weak bonds. Pragmatic ("objective") reasons were usually given, such as the universal "lack of time" or being overworked:

Agnieszka: But actually, there's never anything like they say: let the parents drop in for a coffee in the afternoon. No, there's nothing like this; we don't go there; instead, they come by when they feel like it.
Jan: But I feel it results from something—and I begin to worry—from overworking. He and his wife both—work, work (…)
Agnieszka: They work a lot; it's kind of crazy. (A_PL_1G)

As we can see, efforts by parents to host their children with special gestures, such as preparing meals, may not always yield the desired outcome, as their children prioritize other activities. The reasons for infrequent visits vary, with some adult children seeking greater autonomy, while others cite practical reasons like lack of time or being overworked.

CONCLUSIONS

Domestic hospitality in the family context has rarely been a subject of academic interest. In addition, it has not been studied in relation to the problem of the empty nest transition as part of the family life cycle. Our chapter contributes to existing literature by juxtaposing the practice of entertaining and the notion of hospitality with the process of role transition in families with adult children who have recently moved out.

The analysis of Polish and French interviews demonstrates that families balance different levels of continuity or change in family relationships.

Although new arrangements and roles also emerge, our study rather shows continuity of interaction patterns. In particular, we observed the continuity of asymmetrical relations when the adult children returned to the role of a little child who bore no responsibility for the visit or even family relations and remained unengaged in interactions with their parents. In these cases, the parents–children relationship had not transitioned. In their parents' eyes, children remained uninterested and uninvolved. As a result, parents felt frustrated and irritated, even though they could potentially derive satisfaction from the temporal performance of the role of a caring parent.

Another type of visit was presented when adult children came to their parents as "real guests". The role of a guest transformed the parents–children encounter into a more formal one, demanded more work from the parents as hosts, and encouraged the children to demonstrate ritual forms of behaviour characteristic of a visit. The festive character of these visits involved less intimacy in family relations. Children could come with their partners and meet their siblings or other family members; the visits were less frequent, and the occasions were usually more special. The encounters were defined as "events" that needed particular framing.

The third type of encounter involved the most evident transition of the parents–children relationship. A new form of family intimacy emerged, which included the novel role of an independent adult child. While parents freed themselves from the burden of service and care practices, their interactions with children gained a more symmetrical character, which both parties could experience as satisfactory. Either the children took part of the responsibility and effort off their parents' backs or both parties decided to give up on feasts and careful cleaning, leaving space to spend quality time together. The latter solution helped both parties enjoy the visit without the burden of intense hosting or preoccupation with the daily grind. Reciprocation and more symmetrical involvement in the encounter also increased the chance of gender balance. Usually more burdened with housework, mothers could fully engage in the meeting rather than focus on physical and emotional work related to orchestrating an event.

The last model of parents–adult children encounters is characterized by a significant reduction in the frequency of their meetings. Increasingly independent children usually distance themselves from their parents, which responds to their needs and is socially accepted as a step towards adulthood. However, this process is not necessarily sharp, definite, or irreversible. The French GGS survey showed that the frequency of adult children's visits is dynamic (Régnier-Loilier, 2006). After a period of relatively frequent and regular visits of younger adult children, still financially and emotionally dependent on their parents, encounters become rarer. This situation might be painful for the parents, as it demonstrates that children prefer to distance themselves. Parents often seek justification for infrequent visits to protect the positive image of their relationship with their children. We observed some Polish-French differences in this regard. French parents tended to refer to their children's need for autonomy. In contrast, Polish parents interpreted rare visits instead by referring to external factors, such as their children's heavy workload or dietary preferences. The argument of professional career as a barrier to regular intergenerational contact was also confirmed by the GGS survey, which demonstrated that adult children who engaged in ambitious careers lived further away from their family homes (Régnier-Loilier, 2006). The frequency of contact may increase again when grandchildren are born.

In some cases, more than one pattern of visits may be found in a family. Depending on the context and occasion, families may adopt a more relaxed and informal visit style (type 3) and a more organized and festive one (type 2). However, the proposed typology generally suggests that these styles are dynamic and prone to change rather than coexist. Families tend to lean towards one hosting style, which may evolve over time. Type 1 is most characteristic of the first phase of departure (when children are still dependent on their parents, e.g. studying), but in some cases, it may carry on even when children live independently. The other types of visits referred to children with various life situations—studying, working, living with a partner, a spouse, or alone.

The results present how the process of children's departure is related to the evolution of family relationship patterns and is reflected in the situation of a visit. First, we may interpret adult children's visits as an encounter of two culturally varied interaction patterns. The first pattern relates to intimate family relations, characterized by close bonds and reciprocity, dependence, and imbalance. The other one refers to the situation of a visit, characterized by different rules of politeness and ritual exchange. The combination of these two logics helps examine parents and their children as continuing their family relations and taking on new roles. It may demonstrate and reinforce parents/hosts—children/guests unbalanced relations. However, the cultural frame of a visit situation may also help to repair and rebuild family relations (see also Chap. 7 in this book); the cultural requirements of politeness, respect, and attentiveness related to hospitality may be used as a tool to reconfigure family relationships with the help of a ritual. In a culturally sanctioned way, the encounter may also be released from the tensions of duties, daily grind, and expectations related to the roles of parents and children, and it may move towards festivity or even role transgression.

Different ways of organising and experiencing adult children visits presented in this chapter deliver only some of the complex and nuanced processes of the constantly emerging relationship between parents and their adult children after the children have moved out. While there are apparent differences between families, differentiation of interaction patterns and preferences within one family can also be observed, and their interdependence and dynamics are worth further investigation.

References

Allerton, C. (2012). Making guests, making 'liveliness': The transformative substances and sounds of Manggarai hospitality. *Journal of the Royal Anthropological Institute, 18*(1), 49–62. https://doi.org/10.1111/j.1467-9655.2012.01760.x

Aronsson, K., & Gottzén, L. (2011). Generational positions at a family dinner: Food morality and social order. *Language in Society, 40*, 405–426. https://doi.org/10.1017/S0047404511000455

Bachórz, A. (2013). *Rosja w tekście i w doświadczeniu. Analiza współczesnych polskich relacji z podróży*. Nomos.

Blichfeldt, B., & Gram, M. (2017). Domestic hospitality, gender, and impression management among Danish women. *Food and Foodways, 25*, 1–21. https://doi.org/10.1080/07409710.2017.1272294

Bloch, N. (2021). *Encounters across difference: Tourism and overcoming Subalternity in India*. Lexington Books.

Boas, F. (1888). *The Central Eskimo*. Louise Hope and the Online Distributed Proofreading Team.

Brannen, J., O'Connell, R., & Mooney, A. (2013). Families, meals and synchronicity: Eating together in British dual earner families. *Community, Work & Family, 16*(4), 417–434. https://doi.org/10.1080/13668803.2013.776514

Brunet, F., & Kertudo, P. (2013). Adapter la ville aux modes de vie des familles contemporaines. Enquête sur les moments familiaux partagés à Paris. *Recherche sociale, 205*(1), 6–101. https://doi.org/10.3917/recsoc.205.0006

Candea, M., & Da Col, G. (2012). The return to hospitality. *Journal of the Royal Anthropological Institute, 18*(1), 1–19. https://doi.org/10.1111/j.1467-9655.2012.01757.x

Cappellini, B., & Parsons, E. (2012a). Sharing the meal: Food consumption and family identity. *Research in Consumer Behavior, 14,* 109–128. https://doi.org/10.1108/S0885-2111(2012)0000014010

Cappellini, B., & Parsons, E. (2012b). Practising thrift at dinnertime: Mealtime leftovers, sacrifice and family membership. *The Sociological Review, 60*(2), 121–134. https://doi.org/10.1111/1467-954X.12041

Céroux, B., & Crépin, C. (2013). Rapports aux loisirs et pratiques des adolescents. *Revue des politiques sociales et familiales, 111*(1), 59–64. https://doi.org/10.3406/caf.2013.2750

Cohen, E. (1988). Authenticity and commoditization in tourism. *Annals of Tourism Research, 15*(3), 371–386. https://doi.org/10.1016/0160-7383(88)90028-X

de Singly, F., & Ramos, E. (2010). Moments communs en famille. *Ethnologie française, 40*(1), 11–18. https://doi.org/10.3917/ethn.101.0011

DeVault, M. L. (1994). *Feeding the family: The social organization of caring as gendered work.* University of Chicago Press.

Doja, A. (2011). Customary laws, folk culture, and social lifeworlds: Albanian studies in critical. *Perspective, 2,* 183–199.

Doja, A. (2014). From the German-speaking point of view: Unholy empire, Balkanism, and the culture circle particularism of Albanian studies. *Critique of Anthropology, 34*(3), 290–326. https://doi.org/10.1177/0308275X14531834

Duval, D. T. (2003). When hosts become guests: Return visits and diasporic identities in a commonwealth eastern Caribbean community. *Current Issues in Tourism, 6*(4), 267–308. https://doi.org/10.1080/13683500308667957

Fiese, B. H., Foley, K. P., & Spagnola, M. (2006). Routine and ritual elements in family mealtimes: Contexts for child well-being and family identity. *New Directions for Child and Adolescent Development, 2006*(111), 67–89. https://doi.org/10.1002/cd.156

Finch, J. (2007). Displaying families. *Sociology, 41*(1), 65–81. https://doi.org/10.1177/0038038507072284

Gotman, A. (2001). *Le sens de l'hospitalité, Essai sur les fondements sociaux de l'accueil de l'autre.* Presses Universitaires de France.

Gram, M., Hogg, M., Blichfeldt, B. S., & MacLaran, P. (2015). Intergenerational relationships and food consumption: The stories of young adults leaving home. *Young Consumers, 16*(1), 71–84. https://doi.org/10.1108/YC-01-2014-00422

Habermas, J. (1991). *The structural transformation of the public sphere.* MIT Press.

Herzfeld, M. (1988). *The poetics of manhood.* Princeton University Press.

Herzfeld, M. (2012). Afterword: Reciprocating the hospitality of these pages. *Journal of the Royal Anthropological Institute, 18*(1), 210–217. https://doi.org/10.1111/j.1467-9655.2012.01773.x

Hogg, M. K., Folkman Curasi, C., & Maclaran, P. (2004). The (re-)configuration of production and consumption in empty nest households/families. *Consumption Markets & Culture, 7*(3), 239–259. https://doi.org/10.1080/1025386042000271351

Horolets, A. (2014). *Konformizm, bunt, nostalgia: Turystyka niszowa z Polski do krajów byłego ZSRR*. Universitas.

James, A., & Curtis, P. (2010). Family displays and personal lives. *Sociology, 44*(6), 1163–1180. https://doi.org/10.1177/0038038510381612

Kotowska, I. E. (2019). Generations and gender survey Poland wave 1 & wave 2. *GGP*. Retrieved February 16, 2023, from https://ggp.colectica.org/item/int.ggp/3509fa64-9615-47c4-bcb0-296c230a9f75

Lashley, C., & Morrison, A. (2001). *In search of hospitality*. Routledge.

Lashley, C., Lynch, P., & Morrison, A. J. (Eds.). (2006). *Hospitality: A social lens* (1st ed.). Elsevier.

Matyska, A. (2013). *Transnational families in the making: The polish experience of living between Poland and Finland during and after the cold war*. Acta Universitatis Tamperensis.

Maunaye, E. (2001). Quitter ses parents: Trouver la bonne distance. *Terrain. Anthropologie & sciences humaines, 36*, 33–44. https://doi.org/10.4000/terrain.1168

Maunaye, E. (2002). Passer de chez ses parents à chez soi: Entre attachement et détachement. *Lien Social et Politiques, 43*, 59–66. https://doi.org/10.7202/005186ar

Maunaye, E. (2006). Entre recherche d'autonomie et besoin d'accompagnement. *Territoires, 472*, 14–16.

Mauss, M. (1992). The gift: The form and reason for exchange in archaic societies. *Man, 27*(2), 431. https://doi.org/10.2307/2804090

Ochs, E., & Shohet, M. (2006). The cultural structuring of mealtime socialization. *New Directions for Child and Adolescent Development, 2006*(111), 35–49. https://doi.org/10.1002/cd.154

Ochs, E., Pontecorvo, C., & Fasulo, A. (1996). Socializing taste. *Ethnos, 61*(1–2), 7–46. https://doi.org/10.1080/00141844.1996.9981526

Pitt-Rivers, J. (1972). *The people of the sierra* (2nd ed.). University of Chicago Press.

Portela, M., & Raynaud, É. (2019). Comment se composent les ressources des jeunes? Le dossier illustré par l'enquête nationale sur les ressources des jeunes (ENRJ). *Revue française des affaires sociales, 2*, 23–52. https://doi.org/10.3917/rfas.192.0023

Rancew-Sikora, D. (2015). Opowiadanie w społecznym układzie stołu. Analiza konwersacyjna spotkań rodzinnych. *Studia Humanistyczne AGH, 1*, 25–43.

Rancew-Sikora, D. (2021). *Gościnność—Rozstanie z ideałem Socjologiczna analiza znaczeń i praktyk przyjmowania gości*. Scholar.

Rancew-Sikora, D., & Skowrońska, M. (2022). Adult children move out: Family meals and reflections on parental self-sacrifice at the moment of transition. *Sociological Research Online, 28*(2). https://doi.org/10.1177/13607804211065050

Rancew-Sikora, D., & Żadkowska, M. (2017). Receiving guests at home by nationally mixed couples: The case of Polish females and Norwegian males. *Studia Migracyjne – Przegląd Polonijny, 166*(4), 61–86.

Régnier-Loilier, A. (2006). À quelle fréquence voit-on ses parents? *Population & Sociétés, 427*(9), 1–4. https://doi.org/10.3917/popsoc.427.0001

Régnier-Loilier, A. (2019). Generations and gender survey France wave 1 & wave 2. *GGP.* Retrieved February 13, 2023, from https://ggp.colectica.org/item/int.example/88be4983-72a2-4061-a80d 8af881265a7b

Scabini, E., & Cigoli, V. (1997). Young adult families: An evolutionary slowdown or a breakdown in the generational transition? *Journal of Family Issues, 18*(6), 608–626. https://doi.org/10.1177/019251397018006003

Selwyn, T. (1996). *The tourist image: Myths and myth making in tourism.* Wiley.

Shryock, A. (2008). Thinking about hospitality, with Derrida, Kant and the Balga Bedouin. *Anthropos, 103*(2), 405–421. https://doi.org/10.5771/0257-9774-2008-2-405

Shryock, A. (2009). Hospitality lessons: Learning the shared language of Derrida and the Balga Bedouin. *Paragraph, 32*(1), 32–50.

Silverstein, M., & Bengtson, V. L. (1997). Intergenerational solidarity and the structure of adult child–parent relationships in American families. *American Journal of Sociology, 103*(2), 429–460. https://doi.org/10.1086/231213

Simoni, V. (2017). Hosts and guests. In *The SAGE International Encyclopedia of travel and tourism.* Sage.

Skowrońska, M. (2014). Przyjmowanie gości w przestrzeni domowej jako problem granicy między publicznym a prywatnym. In M. Łukasiuk & M. Jewdokimow (Eds.), *Socjologia zamieszkiwania* (pp. 156–178). Sub Lupa.

Skowrońska, M. (2019). Czuj się jak u siebie, ale bez przesady. Kontrola przestrzeni i opieka nad gościem – dwa wymiary asymetrii władzy w sytuacji gościny. In B. Mateja-Jaworska & M. Skowrońska (Eds.), *Gość w dom. Współczesne praktyki przyjmowania gości* (pp. 97–130). Wydawnictwo Naukowe UAM.

Skowrońska, M. (2020). Klasowy wymiar gościnności: Zróżnicowanie dyspozycji organizujących praktyki gościny. *Kultura i Społeczeństwo, 64*(1), 25–59. https://doi.org/10.35757/KiS.2020.64.1.2

Sørensen, N. U., & Nielsen, M. L. (2021). 'In a way, you'd like to move with them': Young people, moving away from home, and the roles of parents. *Journal of Youth Studies, 24*(4), 547–561. https://doi.org/10.1080/13676261.2020.1747603

Stefánsson, V. (1913). *My life with the Eskimo.* Macmillan Company.

Trommsdorff, G. (2006). Parent-child relations over the lifespan: A cross-cultural perspective. In K. H. Rubin & O. B. Chung (Eds.), *Parenting beliefs, behaviors, and parent-child relations. A cross-cultural perspective* (pp. 143–183). Psychology Press.

Znaniecki, F. (1938). Socjologiczne podstawy ekologii ludzkiej. *Ruch Prawniczy, Ekonomiczny i Socjologiczny, 18*(1), 89–119.

CHAPTER 7

Return to the 'Full Nest'—Re-Cohabitation in Times of the Pandemic in France and Poland

Sandra Gaviria, Magdalena Herzberg-Kurasz, and Magdalena Żadkowska

INTRODUCTION

The phenomenon of adult children returning to their family homes, known as 'boomeranging' (Mitchell & Gee, 1996), has been increasing in several European countries and North America (Clemens & Axelson, 1985; White, 1994; Cherlin et al., 1997; Newmann, 2012; Bouchard, 2014; Gaviria, 2020). Often, modern parents seem to be sympathetic to the return of their residentially independent adult children. The return of

S. Gaviria (✉)
Université Le Havre Normandie, (UMR IDEES), Le Havre, France
e-mail: sandra.gaviria@univ-lehavre.fr

M. Herzberg-Kurasz
Social Sciences Department (Institute of Sociology), University of Gdańsk, Gdańsk, Poland
e-mail: magdalena.herzberg-kurasz@ug.edu.pl

M. Żadkowska et al. (eds.), *Reconfiguring Relations in the Empty Nest*, Palgrave Macmillan Studies in Family and Intimate Life, https://doi.org/10.1007/978-3-031-50403-7_7

141

adult children reflects the condition of the labour market, the availability and prices of housing, as well as the emotional difficulties that young people encounter in their life course and is no longer considered stigmatising for the young person or the parents as it was 20 years earlier. On the contrary, a young person returning home is considered a victim of a society which is lacking in the opportunities and resources it offers (Maunaye et al., 2019).

In Poland, pre-pandemic, we had a lack of studies concerning 'boomeranging' (Żadkowska & Herzberg-Kurasz, 2022). It might be related to the fact that the transition to an empty nest is a 'family matter'; young adults in Poland (Szafraniec, 2017) have to rely on the support of their parents and along with insufficient youth policies the data about their return is scarce (Krzaklewska, 2017). The process of leaving the home is called a mixture of 'old' (sequential—Arnett, 2000; Galland, 2003) and 'new' (prolonged/emerging) patterns to becoming an independent adult (Szafraniec, 2017; Sarnowska et al., 2018). Poland is seen as a 'northeastern' regime characterised by unfavourable market opportunity structures, an underdeveloped private rental sector, a lack of coherent youth or housing policies, and retrenched expenditure for social protection (Szafraniec, 2017).

The COVID-19 pandemic also had a strong impact on the situation of women (Hank & Steinbach, 2021). The extent of the impact on women's burden at home and the psychological, economic, and housing consequences for the young generation (Chevalier, 2021; Santos et al., 2022) will be seen in upcoming data in the next few years, although the tendencies of an increasing crisis are already there (Alon et al., 2020; Braveman, 2020; Collins et al., 2021).

The changes in dynamics of the transition to adulthood in Poland are getting more and more similar to situations observed elsewhere in Europe and the USA (Arnett, 2000; Galland, 2003; Benson & Furstenberg, 2006; Van de Velde, 2008; Gillespie, 2019). There are more studies on young adults not leaving home, who are reprimanded for being overly carefree or

M. Żadkowska
Social Sciences Department (Institute of Sociology), University of Gdańsk, Gdańsk, Poland

Centre de recherche sur les liens sociaux (CERLIS, UMR 8070), Université Paris Cité, Paris, France
e-mail: magdalena.zadkowska@ug.edu.pl

irresponsible or have admitted to being victims of structural factors (Krzaklewska, 2017).

As other European studies show, both in Poland and in France the emerging adulthood dynamic is also dispersed and desynchronised (Galland, 2003; Beaupré et al., 2006; Settersten et al., 2015; Boguszewski & Piszczatowska-Oleksiewicz, 2017; Kudlińska-Chróścicka, 2019; Winogrodzka & Sarnowska, 2019; Pustułka & Buler, 2022). The phenomenon, called 'boomeranging', changes the departure of adult children and reveals its dynamic character.

In France, prior to the COVID-19 pandemic, studies show (Gaviria, 2016) that the return of young people to the family home is an increasingly widespread phenomenon that is no longer an exception on the path of young people but a more likely possibility than was the case in the past. In Poland, 'boomeranging' processes have not been studied systematically (cf. Krzaklewska, 2017; Szafraniec, 2017; Żadkowska & Herzberg-Kurasz, 2022) as they have been in France, where the injunction to autonomy for young people is stronger and the departure of the child is considered a crucial step into adulthood (Gaviria, 2016, 2020; Maunaye et al., 2019). The parents who were surveyed are representatives of a generation that did not consider the option of returning to their family homes. At the same time, most of them declare that their home is open to the return of adult children. In the first phase of our study in 2019, before COVID-19, parents' gave theoretical assurances that their adult children could always return home (by saying 'This is always their home!' and 'They can always come back!').

BOOMERANG IN THE COVID PERIOD IN FRANCE AND POLAND

The goal of the chapter is to compare the worldwide phenomena of adult children returning home during the times of the COVID-19 pandemic in the context of France and Poland.

The COVID-19 pandemic has affected many families in the world. Along with pandemic restrictions, many young adults who had been living on their own—working, studying, engaging in intimate relationships—returned and started residing in their family homes again. The motives for return were varied and included their financial situation, health, safety, and family obligations (Gaviria, 2022; Żadkowska & Herzberg-Kurasz, 2022).

What seems to be an international phenomenon is that family life during the COVID-19 pandemic was intense, limited to immediate family members, and experienced 24 hours a day because of health restrictions and confinement.

Our research interest focused on several questions. To what extent did the return lead to the restoration of the previous form of relations between family members? How did the families organise themselves for the appropriation of the space of the house? How were family relations changed and conflicts managed? Did the return bring unexpected experiences or effects on family relationships?

To investigate the characteristics of returns home in the times of COVID-19, we analysed 78 in-depth interviews, 25 in Poland (18 joint with mothers and fathers, 6 individually with mothers, and 1 individually with fathers) and 53 in France (5 individually with fathers, 4 joint with mothers and fathers, and 44 individualy with mothers). The interviews were collected within corpus B, C, and D (the only one designed to study the influence of COVID-19). The majority of the population is made up of parents with children who were under 25 years old, were students, or were beginning their working lives. For many of them, especially in the French sample, independence was mainly residential and not financial. The interviews were conducted in Polish and French at different times after the first lockdown. First, the interviews were analysed separately in Poland and France. Then, the common themes were chosen to conduct coding and comparative analysis.

Results

The returns of adult children were sudden and unprepared. They also strongly influenced the routine of empty nests, including new practices of couples (parents together) and individuals (mothers and fathers/women and men separately), in many dimensions showing what had really changed before the return as a consequence of the empty nest experience. The main challenges were related to the fact that on the one hand the adult children had started the process of developing independence, while on the other the parents had begun the process of transitioning to the empty nest phase. Our comparative analysis shows that for families in both countries, the difficulties of living together with children who return home and the attitudes towards the return were very similar. In the example of France and Poland, we found that cultural and socio-demographic differences might not be crucial for changes in the parent–children relationships.

To answer our research questions, the main focus of the analysis was based on three themes which relate to space (1), practices of sharing household duties and changing routines (2), and reflection on the additional value of a sudden return (3). All three themes were analysed in relation to arranging and negotiating remote work and studying for all of the household members, as well as setting new rules within the family and taking care of the quality of life in the time of crisis.

Readapting the Space

Polish and French narratives about children's returns demonstrated many similarities regarding the use and change of the space of the home, during the time of the confinement. In both Poland and France, the idea of occupying specific spaces at home weakened in favour of more flexible arrangements since it was regarded as a temporary change before returning to normal. Young people, especially, seek a space to maximise their school or professional work. The families were thus forced to rethink and reorganise their living space to adapt not only to professional requirements (telecommuting and online meetings) but also to educational expectations (online training or children's school) and leisure activities (for example, practising their sport online).

For the parents, the priority remained the academic or professional success of the child and guaranteeing good working conditions for all. As a result, some families maximised the 'comfort' of those who had more difficult or intense studies such as medicine or preparatory classes.

The period of living independently had accelerated the children's transition to adulthood. Parents needed to learn to respect their children's growing need for autonomy, privacy, and independence as young adults. The parents had changed too. Many of them had developed new habits and new spaces in the home, either for themselves (cf. Chap. 12) or for the couple (cf. Chap. 9). The change of both parties made the returns a challenging task. These cases illustrate that emerging adulthood leads to a recomposition of the parent–child relationships. Parents need to acknowledge and accept their children's new status as adults, which is not always easy.

With their experience of independent living, the children began to use their room differently, treating it more like their own place behind a closed door. This was influenced by the need to combine the room function as a place to study, a place to work, and a training spot, all carried out remotely, as well as a space to meet online with friends and spend intimate time as a couple, a place to relax, and sometimes a place to eat alone, in those households where meals were no longer held together and were eaten in some cases in someone's own room/space. In the story of Kazimiera (53 years old) and Tomasz (59 years old), their second daughter Bogna (22 years old) was in her second year of university when the COVID-19 pandemic started. When Bogna returned, she introduced some changes compared to previous behaviour. Before her departure, she did not close the door to her room as family life happened in all spaces. After coming back she did not return to her previous role. Her growing independence was manifested in the use of space. Her departure was a significant moment of transition into adulthood. The daughter with her job and need to study had her own rhythm:

> Kazimiera: It has become a closed room. Because actually at this point Bogna just seems so much more grown up, right? She has her friends, her colleagues, her acquaintances and her likes. And the door to the room is closed, [while before] it was always open. Anyway, she also taught remotely and her mum taught in the other room remotely. So that door just had to be closed. But it stayed that way... Bogna would go into her room and just start locking the door, which is something wow, right? "Bogna has the door locked!" And we had to learn to knock on the door, because you used to just walk in. **Well, but respecting her adulthood, her familiarity, her privacy, well at this point you knock on the door, which was completely absent before, when she lived with us.** So that's what makes this time different. (A_PL_22P)

A new form of family life emerged: being together but detached from each other. Parents emphasised the separateness, independence, and autonomy of their adult children. They had to accept that their children's use of space was now different because of their development in the process of emerging adulthood. They declared that they respected their increased need for privacy as in Maria's (50 years old) testimony about Monika's return (20 years old):

> Maria: But in general, she's a bit different, she's at home, but she's a bit more independent, I would say more adult, right? It's a bit like... her autonomy is different. She emphasises here that she is with us, but we also have to

respect her rhythms, she closes herself off, she needs isolation, she needs to be alone up there, and when she wants to she comes down. So sometimes it is the case that on some days she is a guest at our place downstairs, right? So we are together, but a bit separate, I would say. (B_PL_2P)

The father, Tadeusz (53 years old), confirms they could afford the new arrangement because of the size of their house. Their second daughter Monika (20 years old) had just started university in the autumn of 2019 and was back home after half a year:

Tadeusz: The changes over the year that I would point out are, yes, firstly a certain rearrangement of functions in the house, which I mapped out here. I mean, my younger daughter Monika's room, after she moved to Poznań, was adopted by my wife as her office. And it was such a change, well a concrete one. Without any renovation work, but a complete change of furniture, some repainting and adaptation of functions. (...) And then our daughter, after she came back from Poznań, well her room was already occupied for another function, so she took the attic. But there was no problem because this attic, which had been the older daughter Katarzyna's, was still empty. So she moved into the attic, with some misgivings at first, some reluctance, she didn't have any good associations, but she soon found that it was a good place, such an isolated place, where she had her world, her peace and quiet. Also, it was such a major rearrangement for sure, a functional change in the house. (B_PL_2P)

It was easier to come up with a solution that reconciled both the pragmatic and the identity-related needs of both parties when the rooms to which the children returned had stayed unchanged or only been slightly transformed (see Chap. 5). In some families, the departure of the child did not mean a reappropriation of the room by the parents. It was preserved so that the child always had a home to come back to. This was the case of Marin, whose father said:

Claude: Ah no, no. We left it as it was because we think that he should be able to come back whenever he wants and even when we welcome him during the holiday periods and so on, we prefer him to have his room so that he feels good in his room so that he feels at home. We did well because, during the confinement period, he came back to live for two months so it was much better for him to have his room back and to feel comfortable. (D_FR_5)

However, both in France and in Poland, in many cases (see Chap. 5), the child's room had gone through a partial or complete change of function and a renovation. In the case of Mathilde, the older daughter, when she returned, the parents asked Juliette, the younger sister, to free up her room, which had been Mathilde's room. The mother, Valerie, explained how a large house helped to create a good atmosphere despite tensions between the two sisters:

> Valerie: In the end… even if at the beginning the relationship was strained between the girls because Mathilde had her habits, she preferred to spend time alone, well, we all got closer and… We did a lot of things together, although spending 24 hours a day together is difficult (…). Fortunately, we had enough space to separate. When I think about big families who live in small flats, oh dear, it must have been very hard for them. (D_FR_16)

In some cases, the parents had made new use of the room as is the case of Maël. His mother, Béatrice, explains that as parents their intention was not to keep the room for their child intact. But in the end, they tried to fit in with Maël's needs:

> Béatrice: So when Maël moved out, we… Charles and I decided to make a sports room because, well… we're all athletes in the family. We wanted to have our own sports room, without having to go to the gym. But then Maël came back and had to have his room back. (D_FR_28)

When Maël returned, at the beginning he shared the room with his brother but, finally, he decided to move back into the space of his former room without really appropriating it. The mother recognised that he no longer had a space at home but that he had the right to the living room like everyone else. The rooms were devoted to individual needs and activities, and the living room became a space of pleasure activities performed together:

> Angèle: It went very well. The children were in their rooms. And then when we were eating they came out to eat. Thierry and I don't have a room so we are always in the living room. At that time during confinement, we were worried, we were stressed about covid. We wondered what to do, so I watched TV all the time to find out. And then afterwards we would watch a series on tv, we were fans of that during the lockdown. At 4 pm we ate biscuits and watched a show together, an unusual habit for us. We liked it very

much. After some quality time together, the kids went back to their room. (D_FR_20)

Some changes in the child's room after the departure were directly related to the small space (square footage) of the house (apartment). The absence of the child made it possible to implement those changes leading to increased comfort for the parents remaining in the empty nest—a private bedroom for the couple (in some cases, for the first time, which they had always looked forward to), a sports activities room, an office, an 'own room', a relaxation room, a guest room, a storage room. That was the situation Magda experienced when she came back to a rearranged home:

> Barbara: the moment the child moved out of her room a bedroom was created which my husband and I had always wanted to have, this room was totally transformed including replacing the furniture, bed, wallpaper as well as carpets. It doesn't resemble her room at all. (…) When Magda came back she stayed in this room, the so-called guest room, which my husband and I had occupied before, because we decided that we now had our bedroom, we had already got used to being in it, so it stayed that way. (D_PL_202)

In such cases, when the houses were smaller, the family tried to find a solution. The returning young adult could occupy a guest room, a sibling's room or another quickly arranged place to live. Suddenly, the house became crowded, and the number of people waiting in line for the bathroom increased. In some cases, parents gave their returning children their former rooms that had already been refreshed and transformed for their own use. In large apartments (houses), wherever it was possible, adult children were given a privileged space, which was often a separate part of the house.

Although the (re)discovery of the child's private space was the main issue in relation to the re-adaptation of the space, families also needed to (re)create shared spaces to gather the family together again. It was challenging for them as they needed to readapt to the space they had already modified to their needs. On the other hand, some felt nostalgic and sentimental, living with their kids and knowing it was only for a restricted time:

> Sandra: I think the best moments were the meals outside on the terrace, it wasn't particularly hot but the weather was nice. It was a bit 'out of this world', we felt like we were on holiday but we weren't. Everything was a bit

different and it gave a lightness, you know. I found those moments particularly special. (...) It will probably never happen again. (D_FR_36)

The shared space was therefore important to cherish this exceptional moment of the sudden return.

Changing Domestic Practices

The second theme that emerged in the analysis of 'being a family again' in the times of 'boomeranging' was domestic chores and everyday life practices of parents that changed after their adult children's departure. The change that happened in the household was a trigger for various tensions and conflicts. As mentioned above, a large flat or house offered the possibility for people to separate, thus limiting the opportunities for conflicts to erupt over individual needs regarding leisure time as well as work or study.

The distribution of domestic duties turned out to be a problem in many households. Nevertheless, the children were grown up, and more independent and the problems seemed less important than in the past when the division of chores evoked many challenges. The empty nest brought a lot of relief in relation to domestic tasks. Women, especially, seem to have lost the space they regained in the empty nest (cf. Chap. 12). The couples had developed individual and/or joint practices (cf. Chaps. 9 and 10). After the children's return, women were the ones who mainly carried out housework. The sudden change in the number of habitants created an additional burden as in the case of Alexane with her son Athis:

> Alexane: Yeah, how can I put it, um? Well, it was... Sometimes I would tell him to come and, for example, start cooking dinner. Or do things in the kitchen. Well, he would always say: "wait, wait, wait". And that annoyed me, for example, you know. Because I'm telling you, he was there as if he was on holiday, as he couldn't go anywhere else. And I wanted to make his life easier too, you know? (D_FR_13)

Along with studies showing the overload of domestic duties that touched women all around the world during COVID-19 lockdowns, we have also noticed in both countries that the return of young adults caused an overload of domestic responsibilities for women. Mothers suddenly felt like they had returned to the starting point. What makes it so very gender sensitive is that fathers noticed their wives' overload (like Franciszek,

59-year-old father of Jerzy, 27 years old, and Ewa, 28 years old, who moved back to their family home from Berlin and Poznań, respectively, where they had been working, and were starting to work remotely) but did not intervene:

> Franciszek: A bit too much confusion. On the other hand, I will say that my wife is a bit exhausted after such a weekend because she's trying to please everyone—a dinner, a coffee, this and that and you know… Admittedly our daughter helps a lot, but, you know, my wife is always on the move all the time. And then when they leave, it's so. (B_PL_9G)

> Agnieszka: I had got used to not having to cook such big dinners, and suddenly it was "oh God, I have to bring sacks of food again" because they always ate a lot and I had to cook again. How I laughed afterwards, I said: "Go back to Warsaw, I'll have a rest". But no, in the first phase, when none of us knew if there would be corpses on the streets, well, I felt somehow safe that they were at home. (B_PL_1G)

The time apart significantly modifies the parent–children relationship. Emerging adults are very susceptible to change. Pursuing an education, exploring a new social environment, and making new friends—all of these factors inevitably distance them from their family of origin. If, as in the example below, the distancing also involves the child's aspirations to climb the social ladder higher than their parents, tensions arise:

> Emanuelle: Let's say that Astrid being a big, literary girl and… and having a much higher level of education, has difficulty sharing moments with me because she thinks I'm not educated enough for her, that's it. Let's say that Astrid has a rather high ego and is very pretentious. Few people are at her level. That's it, she has a rather high ego. So it's a bit difficult for me to have discussions with her because whatever subject we discuss, I'm never up to it, I never know enough. Anyway, given her rather high ego, she feels that she can't have discussions with me. So, no, I didn't go to university like her, but I'm not that stupid either [laughs]. I may not be as educated, but I think I'm a very intelligent person, and I'm someone you can talk to. But that's the way it is. I adapt and I try to smooth things over because personally I'm a person who hates conflicts, so I prefer to smooth things over and avoid any quarrels or arguments, I adapt, and I go with the flow. Otherwise, we would be in conflict all the time. So, I share few things with Astrid. (D_FR_48)

At the time of the adult children's return, food-related practices reflected the tensions and emotions happening at home. Adult children often returned with new eating habits (for example, a vegetarian or a vegan diet). Separation from their parents and living on their own led to new eating routines and habits, novel ideas, and inspirations showing an increase in children's independence. Karol (21-year-old son of Iwona and Konrad) exemplifies this situation:

> Iwona: Our son Karol, I mean I won't say he's fully vegetarian, but he's rather determined to not eat meat. So, in general, **he kind of forced us to do it that way** (…). So that's how it is. And we do it according to his rules. But I think it's going to stay that way, although my husband is complaining! The husband is complaining. (B_PL_7G)

New eating habits were sometimes quite authoritatively imposed by adult children. What is interesting is that there were some families where parents went along with these changes without objecting, even if they weren't particularly happy with them (for example, Kazimiera (53 years old) and Tomasz (59 years old) with their second daughter Bogna (22 years old):

> Kazimiera: She pops into the kitchen and she's, for example, trying to smuggle in her food and her menu, right? Because "Mum, I need to lose weight" or "You know what, Mum, let's do something", no?
> Tomasz: I wouldn't say it was a diet!
> Kazimiera: It was a diet too, among other things.
> Tomasz: I wouldn't say it was a diet, it didn't work on me!
> Kazimiera: You're resistant! So she just manifests her adulthood by saying, for example, "I'm eating breakfast later" or "I'm not eating that", which surprised us too, right? **Because until now we've done everything together and it was the same, and now it's just different.** (A_PL_22P)

The new practices can be interpreted as parents' acceptance of the transition into adulthood.

Additional Value of a Sudden Return

The third theme is related to an unexpected opportunity to spend time together again with all the children at home. For some families, it was a gift. They admit that after getting used to the empty nest phase, they never expected to get back to the good old days. They underlined the strengths of this unexpected period. They also seemed willing to return to parenting roles, despite the housework burden (especially for women) and the negotiation of space and daily practices.

The return allowed for moments of sharing time and a sense of a reunion with the old good times:

> Françoise: Well, since my son was gone, I have seen how much was missing at home. And since I was afraid that my son would go back after the first confinement, I took full advantage of him. He helped me with meals at home, we played board games as a family, and we had debates as a family. The atmosphere at home was perfect. What changed for Francis was the fact that he was with his family, whereas when he lived alone, he was missing us. (D_FR_18)

The pandemic significantly changed the quality of family time, as in the case of Elżbieta (53 years old) and Piotr (49 years old), who enjoyed the opportunity to have their adult children back at home. Their daughter Paula (31 years old) unexpectedly decided to spend the whole of the pandemic in Poland in their house (after having been independent for more than eight years and living in Italy), and their son Tomasz (22 years old, who had moved out of the parental house one year earlier, but just to the apartment next door) was at their place all the time:

> Elżbieta: These were such past moments [in the present], the kind of moments that **I would never have expected to still occur in my life** (...). That we were all in the same situation and had to sit at home—**that was special.** And there never used to be a willingness to spend four months in the family home on her part, nor would there really be that idea to sit. We wanted to sit and spend time together, and it was just a great experience. (B_PL_11P)

Despite having to survive conflicts and negotiations, the atmosphere of the 'full house' trend turned out to be rewarding. The end of the day was often a precious moment together:

> Delphine: So we were happy to meet up in the evening, because, well, in the evening I'd come home and we'd all eat. We were also able to play board games and things like that. They sometimes even did yoga with me, because I was doing it on video with our teacher, we weren't allowed to go... so several times the three of us did it. They also went running during the day.

(…) It was quite positive. I have remembered the positive in any case (laughs). (D_FR_26)

In some exceptional cases, when the departure had been related to family conflict, the return could be a moment of reconciliation:

> Claudia: Given that it was confinement, it was quite difficult to go and do some activities, but, on the contrary, it didn't prevent us from getting closer to Jennah. We were able to have some small meals together. I think it was just the two of us getting together and watching a couple of films together, really, just keeping ourselves busy as best we could. During the confinement, the main thing was to keep busy so as not to fall into something quite depressive. Well, we spent our time together keeping busy, and then with the whole family, we had a lot of dinners, family meals, and aperitifs. Really, it was quite fun. (D_FR_27)

For some mothers, it was a moment of reflection concerning their children's earlier departure from the family home. Their return during COVID-19 changed their perspective, highlighting the changes that had taken place. This unexpected and unplanned time spent together helped them cope with the guilt some parents felt about the empty nest (cf. Chap. 13). Some families (for example, Elżbieta's family) could only dream about such 'holidays':

> Elżbieta: And there never used to be any readiness on her part perhaps to spend four months in the family home, nor was there that compulsion to sit as we wanted to sit and spend time together, but **this was a great experience**. (B_PL_11P)

It was finally the other, better, side of the pandemic. Felicja and Gustaw (both 57 years old) have three children (Klaudia, 19 years old; Karol, 26 years old; and Leon, 25 years old), who came back home during the second lockdown. For all the restrictions and threats caused by lockdowns, the arrival of the children was a blessing:

> Gustaw: Three months of something, I think, right? May, June… three months. That's how it all worked out, they probably wanted that too, a bit of independence, because that first pandemic period was such that we were basically at home a lot too, right?
>
> Felicja: That's right! We were just mostly together, weren't we?

Gustaw: In a way a boon! That other side of the pandemic. (A_PL_29G)

For the women who were missing their past family life, this moment allowed them a form of inner serenity—for example, Irena (53 years old), mother of Marta (25 years old) and Kasia (27 years old), who returned home to stay for several months:

> Irena: I just... I don't know, somehow it all helped me so much, I don't know if it was just time or the fact that they were still here? So somehow all this, all of my tensions were released, to be honest. (B_PL_4P)

Some women, like Ela (49 years old), mother of Mariusz (22 years old), are aware of the next steps and the nest becoming empty again, but now, compared with the first departure, they feel prepared:

> Ela: But he's back and it's great—it's just great. And as we're starting to make some noises about him moving out, it's hard for me again, but now I think I'm calmer about it, and I know it has to be that way. I think it's because I know that I'm able to get used to it, whereas he won't be living so far away because he'll be living in Gniezno. (B_PL_1P)

The boomerang experience can be interpreted as a second chance to rebuild the family, confirming the family's unconditional solidarity with its now-adult and independent members.

CONCLUSIONS

The COVID-19 pandemic contributed to the emergencies and unplanned situations that were exploited by families in a variety of ways.

We have shown the family arrangements made to enable re-cohabitation in the times of COVID-19. They had to be rearranged because of two processes that were going on. First was the process, already started, of developing independence by emerging adults and the second was the parents' process of transitioning to the empty nest phase. The return demonstrated that the period of living apart had changed both parties, the children and the parents, and it was not possible to return to the same habits and relationship patterns. We observed these changes by analysing modifications in the home space and in domestic practices. The analysis shows that the greatest challenge for the parent is to respect the growing independence of their children (who need to be separate individuals, need to cook and eat differently, etc.). At the same time, families experienced moments of the 'good old times'—shared moments during meals, playing board games, watching movies, and so on. While parents also felt burdened with additional work and the necessity to reorganise space and habits, they also enjoyed the temporary return to the full nest. Interestingly, this period helped to make the process of departure smoother and easier. After a period of missing their child, they could derive satisfaction from an intense relationship with their children, which they felt prepared them to say goodbye again. What is more, parents realised that the empty nest released them from tensions and additional work. Of course, some will remember mainly sitting around the table together and being a family while others—the children's mess, worries, nerves, arguments, and tension.

For some mothers, it was a moment of reflection concerning their adult children's previous departure from the family home. The COVID-19 return changed their perspective, highlighting the changes that had taken place. This unexpected and unplanned time spent together helped them cope with their guilt or anxiety about the empty nest (cf. Chap. 13).

The phenomenon of boomeranging caused by COVID-19 shows that family solidarity on an everyday life basis can be easily awakened. It was the experience of both studied countries and happened beyond the quality of family relationships.

REFERENCES

Alon, T. M., Doepke, M., Olmstead-Rumsey, J., & Tertilt, M. (2020). The impact of COVID19 on gender equality. *National Bureau of Economic Research, 26947*, 1–37.

Arnett, J. J. (2000). Emerging adulthood: A theory of development from the late teens through the twenties. *American Psychologist, 55*, 469–480. https://doi.org/10.1037/0003-066X.55.5.469

Beaupré, P., Turcotte, P., & Milan, A. (2006). When is junior moving out? Transitions from the parental home to independence. *Canadian Social Trends, 82*, 9–15.

Benson, J. E., & Furstenberg, F. F. (2006). Entry into adulthood: Are adult role transitions meaningful markers of adult identity? *Advances in Life Course Research, 11*, 199–224. https://doi.org/10.1016/S1040-2608(06)11008-4

Boguszewski, R., & Piszczatowska-Oleksiewicz, M. (2017). *Pełnoletnie dzieci mieszkające z rodzicami*. CBOS. Retrieved February 5, 2023, from https://www.cbos.pl/

Bouchard, G. (2014). How do parents react when their children leave home? An integrative review. *Journal of Adult Development, 21*(2), 69–79. https://doi.org/10.1007/s10804-013-9180-8

Braveman, P. (2020, April 14). *COVID-19: Inequality is Our pre-existing condition.* UNESCO Inclusive Policy Lab. Retrieved March 5, 2023, from https://en.unesco.org/inclusivepolicylab/news/covid-19-inequality-our-pre-existing-condition

Cherlin, A. J., Scabini, E., & Rossi, G. (1997). Still in the nest: Delayed home leaving in Europe and the United States. *Journal of Family Issues, 18*, 572–575. https://doi.org/10.1177/019251397018006001

Chevalier, T. (2021). Varieties of youth transitions? A review of the comparative literature on the entry to adulthood. In A.-M. Castrén, V. Česnuitytė, I. Crespi, J.-A. Gauthier, R. Gouveia, C. Martin, A. M. Mínguez, & K. Suwada (Eds.), *The Palgrave handbook of family sociology in Europe* (pp. 575–589). Palgrave Macmillan.

Clemens, A. W., & Axelson, L. J. (1985). The not-so-empty-nest: The return of the fledgling adult. *Family Relations, 34*(2), 259–264. https://doi.org/10.2307/583900

Collins, C., Landivar, L. C., Ruppanner, L., & Scarborough, W. J. (2021). COVID-19 and the gender gap in work hours. *Gender, Work and Organization, 28*(1), 101–112. https://doi.org/10.1111/gwao.12506

Galland, O. (2003). Adolescence, post-adolescence, youth: Revised interpretations. *Revue Française de Sociologie, 44*(5), 163–188.

Gaviria, S. (2016). La génération boomerang, devenir adulte autrement. *SociologieS, 2016, 2–13.* https://doi.org/10.4000/sociologies.5212

Gaviria, S. (2020). *Revenir vivre en famille. Devenir adulte autrement.* Editions Le bord de L'eau.

Gaviria, S. (2022). La vuelta a casa en tiempos de pandemia: nuevas formas de convivencia. In A. Santos, E. Ballesté, C. Feixa, & A. Sanmartín (Eds.), *Hacia una segunda crisis en la juventud? Socialidades juveniles en tiempos de pandemia* (pp. 43–57). Centro Reina Sofía sobre Adolescencia y Juventud, Fundación FAD.

Gillespie, B. J. (2019). Adolescent intergenerational relationship dynamics and leaving and returning to the parental home. *Journal of Marriage and Family, 82*(3), 997–1014. https://doi.org/10.1111/jomf.12630

Hank, K., & Steinbach, A. (2021). The virus changed everything, didn't it? Couples' division of housework and childcare before and during the Corona crisis. *Journal of Family Research, 33*(1), 99–114. https://doi.org/10.20377/jfr-488

Krzaklewska, E. (2017). W stronę międzypokoleniowej współpracy? Wyprowadzenie się z domu rodzinnego z perspektywy dorosłych dzieci i ich rodziców. *Societas/Communitas, 2*(24), 159–176.

Kudlińska-Chróścicka, I. (2019). Stawanie się osobą dorosłą w czasach płynnej nowoczesności w doświadczeniu wielkomiejskich młodych dorosłych. *Przegląd Socjologii Jakościowej, 15*(4), 34–60.

Maunaye, E., Muniglia, V., Potin, A., & Rothé, C. (2019). Le domicile familial comme ressource? Expériences de recohabitation dans les transitions vers l'âge adulte. *Revue française des affaires sociales, 2*, 143–166. https://doi.org/10.3917/rfas.192.0143

Mitchell, B., & Gee, E. M. (1996). Boomerang kids and midlife parental marital satisfaction. *Family Relations, 45*, 442–448.

Newmann, N. K. (2012). *The accordion family: Boomerang kids, anxious parents, and the private toll of global competition*. Beacon Press.

Pustułka, P., & Buler, M. (2022). First-time motherhood and intergenerational solidarities during COVID-19. *Journal of Family Research, 34*(1), 16–40. https://doi.org/10.20377/jfr-705

Santos, A., Ballesté, E., Feixa, C., & Sanmartín, A. (Eds.). (2022). *Hacia una segunda crisis en la juventud? Sociedades juveniles en tiempos de pandemia*. Centro Reina Sofía sobre Adolescencia y Juventud, Fundación FAD. https://doi.org/10.5281/zenodo.6351483

Sarnowska, J., Winogrodzka, D., & Pustułka, P. (2018). The changing meanings of work among university-educated young adults from a temporal perspective. *Przegląd Socjologiczny, 67*(3), 111–134.

Settersten, R. A., Jr., Ottusch, T. M., & Schneider, B. (2015). Becoming adult: Meaning and makers for young Americans. In R. Scott & S. Kosslyn (Eds.), *Emerging trends in the social and behavioral sciences* (pp. 1–16). Wiley.

Szafraniec, K. (2017). The contemporary context of youth socialization: The specificity of post-communist countries. *Polish Sociological Review, 2*(198), 167–187.

Van de Velde, C. (2008). *Devenir adult. Sociologie comparée de la jeunesse en Europe*. Presses Universitaires de France.

White, L. (1994). Coresidence and leaving home: Young adults and their parents. *Annual Review of Sociology, 20*, 81–102.

Winogrodzka, D., & Sarnowska, J. (2019). Tranzycyjny efekt jojo w sekwencjach społecznych młodych migrantów. *Przegląd Socjologii Jakościowej, 15*(4), 130–153. https://doi.org/10.18778/1733-8069.15.4.07

Żadkowska, M., & Herzberg-Kurasz, M. (2022). "Boomeranging covidowy" – o powrotach dorosłych dzieci do domów. Perspektywa rodziców. *Przegląd Socjologii Jakościowej, 18*(1), 40–61. https://doi.org/10.18778/1733-8069.18.1.03

Animals in the Empty Nest: Recomposition of Family Roles

Magdalena Anita Gajewska, François de Singly,
Magdalena Żadkowska, Christophe Giraud,
Marianna Kostecka, and Sophie David–Goretta

INTRODUCTION

In light of emerging family studies, humans often treat pets "like family members" (Smith, 2003; Konecki, 2005; Doré & Michalon, 2017; Irvine & Cilia, 2017; Doré et al., 2019; de Singly & Morand, 2019). Not only do animal companions have first names, share the living space with

M. A. Gajewska (✉)
Social Sciences Department (Institute of Sociology), University of Gdańsk, Gdańsk, Poland
e-mail: magdalena.gajewska@ug.edu.pl

F. de Singly • C. Giraud • S. David–Goretta
Centre de recherche sur les liens sociaux (CERLIS, UMR 8070), Université Paris Cité, Paris, France
e-mail: francois@singly.org; christophe.giraud@parisdescartes.fr; sophie.david.goretta@gmail.com; sophie.david.goretta@gmail.com

159

M. Żadkowska et al. (eds.), *Reconfiguring Relations in the Empty Nest*, Palgrave Macmillan Studies in Family and Intimate Life, https://doi.org/10.1007/978-3-031-50403-7_8

humans, and co-create intimacy by witnessing daily life, but they also build strong emotional bonds with their caregivers (Serpell, 1996; Franklin, 1999, 2006; Bekoff, 2000; Bakke, 2007; Montag & Davis, 2020). The intensity of this human–non-human relationship and related practices varies widely (de Singly & Morand, 2019). One process responsible for an intense relationship may be parentification, which facilitates the accommodation of differences between the species within the family community (Konecki, 2005: 34). Animals are present in family photos (Carlisle-Frank & Frank, 2006); people talk "to" their pets and also talk "for" them (Sanders, 1999). People recognise the ability of pets to share intentions, feelings, and other aspects of family life (Irvine, 2004; Carter & Charles, 2013; Carter, 2015). The practices of caring for animals (i.e., feeding, walking, protecting, caring for, and other responsibilities) create intimate and familiar relationships.

Animals are often seen as emotional support for humans and at the same time as "fur babies" (Greenebaum, 2004; Blouin, 2008, 2012, 2013), so the terms "mom" and "dad" are commonly used to refer to the caregiver's role (Miller, 2011; Shir-Vertesh, 2012; Charles, 2016). Research on animal companions has recognised that animals not only participate in "making" the family (Charles & Davies, 2008; Power, 2008; Shir-Vertesh, 2012; Charles, 2014) and reshaping daily family practices but they are also seen as sources of emotional support (Irvine, 2004; Mamzer, 2015; Charles, 2016). And finally, like with other family members, animals often become irreplaceable, such that the death of the animal companion is met with grief and mourning (Charles & Davies, 2008). Being recognised as a family member allows the animal to be an active social actor and reshape the trajectory of family life (Żadkowska et al., 2022). Despite research showing that animals correct their behaviour by

M. Żadkowska
Social Sciences Department (Institute of Sociology), University of Gdańsk, Gdańsk, Poland

Centre de recherche sur les liens sociaux (CERLIS, UMR 8070), Université Paris Cité, Paris, France
e-mail: magdalena.zadkowska@ug.edu.pl

M. Kostecka
Faculty of Sociology, Adam Mickiewicz University, Poznań, Poland
e-mail: markos10@amu.edu.pl

adapting them to imposed norms (Irvine, 2004) and that they bond with humans, we are not able to know how being part of a human family affects them and what communication problems they face (Topál et al., 1998; Thielke & Udell, 2017).

The latest studies show that in Europe dogs live with humans in 24% of households, while in 26% there is at least one cat (FEDIAF, 2022). An animal companion lives in 46% of European households—there are almost 93 million dogs and over 113.5 million cats. Statistics on the number of dogs and cats in the countries where our project is being implemented confirm the European indicators: in Poland, there are 6.5 million dogs and 4.1 million cats living in households, while in France there are 7.5 million dogs, and 15.1 million cats as well as 106 million small mammals, birds, fish, and reptiles.

The appearance of animals in the family occurs at different times in a family's life. It may be when the children are mature, after a divorce or separation, or when the children leave home. First, the presence of an animal companion in the family may be permanent, at least for one of the spouses. Second, animals (sometimes starting with fish and a hamster and eventually opting for a dog) very often appear in the home at the request of the children. Examining the relationship between children and their caregivers has been likened to examining the relationship between "other sentient animals" and their "owners" (McLaughlin, 2019: 10). Nowadays, sociological studies concerning couples who plan not to have children and those whose children have already moved away emphasise the role of animals (Carter, 2015; Laurent-Simpson, 2017a, b; Leow, 2018; Gouveia & Castrén, 2021; Mikołejko, 2023; Owens & Grauerholz, 2019). The independence of children for a couple whose life together was based on caring for children can be a lifelong challenge. To simplify the work of reconverting marital relationships (see Chap. 9), they may choose a new care object, a new family member. Parental couples whose attachment style has been mediated by an object of mutual concern can, by imposing this role on an animal, protect their relationship from crisis and continue their existing intimate lifestyle, assuming responsibility for the animal together. In such a context, animals can be seen as a substitute for children (Doré et al., 2019).

METHOD

In this chapter, we analysed the accounts of French and Polish parents whose children have left home and who have a pet at home.[1] The Polish corpus is composed of 28 couples. These households had 25 dogs. In some of them, there was also a cat (three of them), a parrot (two of them), or an aquarium with fish (two of them). In three families, there was only one cat. Of these households, eight included only a mother (sometimes in a new relationship, corpus B and C—see Chap. 11). The French corpus is composed of interviews that were conducted during the 2022–2023 academic year in the Bachelor of Social Sciences programme at Université Paris Cité. For this chapter, 15 interviews with adults living in households whose children had left were analysed (corpus E). In the French corpus of 15 interviews, there are more families with dogs (nine) than with cats (six). None of them have a dog and a cat. Only one family has two dogs. Slightly less than half (7 families out of 15) already had a pet before the empty nest, so this is a possible conversion of an already-old relationship with the dog or cat. Six other families took a pet shortly after the empty nest. And in two others, the empty nest coincided with the death of a dog and the arrival of a new one.

In the presented study, we focused on thematic analysis (Boyatzis, 1998; Braun & Clarke, 2006). We included in the study corpus those interviews in which the theme of animals is linked to the theme of loneliness, change in the previous care routine and couple relationships. Thus, the corpus of our analyses included those interviews in which topics related to the recomposition of the parental role appeared and could provide a basis for an analysis of the "interspecies foster" child. These topics arose after we asked the question about what role animals play in an empty nest. Specifically, we asked how the departure of the children affected the place and function that the animal had for the adults. The children fulfilled several functions for the parents. Their departure partly disorganised parental roles and identities. We, therefore, examine how animals may, or may not, be in some way a functional equivalent of children for adults (Merton, 1997).

---

[1] Some authors refer to these as "interspecies families" (Kirksey, 2015; Owens & Grauerholz, 2019; Laing, 2021). But here these families no longer have children at home.

THE FUNCTIONS OF A PET AFTER THE CHILDREN HAVE LEFT

Parents can experience "gaps" after the children leave. The above-mentioned gaps arise when the responsibilities of parenthood disappear from everyday life (Chaps. 3 and 4). What we have learned from our research, which is described in other chapters of this book, is that the departure of children creates important forms of something lacking or emptiness for the parent(s):

1. For parents, children used to be a daily presence at home. They were present when they came home from work (fathers usually came home later than mothers). The departure of the children causes them to feel lonely (see also Chaps. 13 and 14). This need for solitude and recognition doesn't have to be strictly related to the children. Sometimes the children filled a need for adult presence and recognition (de Singly, 1996). The activities performed by the children or with the children are gone so there is a need for a new companion for the individual or couple.

2. The presence of children at home is a source of shared activities. This can consist of shared games or movies. It can also be outdoor activities: shopping or jogging with a child can be a moment together very much appreciated by a parent. Children bring shared moments, and things are done together. And their departure often leads to abandonning these activities that only made sense when done together: here, women, who are the ones who mainly organise and accompany the children's free time, are the first to be affected by this lack, but men too, to a lesser extent, can share sports activities or games (Champagne et al., 2015). In their book *Les chômeurs de Marienthal*, Paul Lazarsfeld and his team (1981) showed the importance of salaried employment for the structuring of the entire daily life of workers in the 1930s in Austria. The empty nest studies show how much the presence of children used to structure parents' everyday lives and women in particular (see Chap. 3).

3. Children are an opportunity for couples to collaborate, to work together. Attention given to the children is sometimes such that the couple spends little time together in private. The team is mainly a parenting team. When the children leave home, the couple may find it difficult to find common interests which they can collaborate on, to form a conjugal team (see Part 2).

All these functions are not equivalent, but the animal can unite them. It can simultaneously support personal recognition, bring a daily rhythm of activity and be a companion during activities or support to the couple. One can suppose that the attachment to the animal will be all the more important as it fulfils several functions at the same time.

An Animal Companion as a Vector of Affection

An animal can be particularly appreciated as a companion in the home that helps break the feeling of loneliness that invades parents when they come home. The animal can thus be a source of communication for the adult. In this function, the animals are functional equivalents of a (small) child or a husband/wife.

Adam, 49 years old, states that the animal will function as a substitute after their child moves out, making the house less empty; there is someone to care for and sadness and loneliness are less frequent:

> Adam: And it's kind of cool that we see her as a family member that we can continue to care for, we have our girl. It's very edifying, even in the context of just caring for animals—an empty house also allows for much deeper care for the animal. And besides, this relationship the animal has with these other parents makes these parents also feel less lonely, as they have an animal. And these emotions related to the child are poured into the animal—by all means, I recommend it. (B_PL_2G)

Myriam, 57 years old, a secretary, lives with her husband and has three children. She talks about their cat, Hermes, who arrived when the children were young (11 years ago). This woman got closer to the cat after the children left. She admits this:

> Myriam: It is perhaps to compensate for the emotional attachment that I no longer have with my children. The lack of communication, to take care of someone, to talk and discuss. Yes, that's it. To buy him little things, to please him, to keep me busy in fact". She adds: "And it's true that sometimes I'm all alone when my husband comes home late, with Hermes and... and the first thing I do when I get home, I wonder where he is. So, I look for him everywhere, I talk to him, and he meows. Sometimes I feel like he answers me when I call him. (E_FR_5)

When the children leave home, it creates an opportunity to get closer to others, that is, to those household members who remain. It not only minimises the distance but also intensifies the relationship. Emotions and attachment to animals become more strongly felt.

Sophie, a mother, and college teacher (her husband is a doctor) has a cat called Arya, who arrived when her two children moved out. Her arrival was not planned, but once her two sons had left, she appreciated having Arya: "It feels less empty". She talks to her "like to a baby". When asked about her role towards the cat, Sophie answers that she considers herself more "a parent" and "not an owner". Sophie talks to her cat, and she tells her about her day:

> Sophie: Oh yes I look completely crazy [she acts as she does in front of her cat]. Finally, yes it is a little as if I were speaking to a baby, even worse, since I do not think that I even spoke to my children like that. (E_FR_6)

The cat, Arya, helps fill the contact gap she feels when she comes home from school while her husband stays late at work. But as she notes, the cat doesn't fulfil all the functions of children:

> Interviewer: Do you think it helped you, with the kids being gone?
> Sophie: Oh yes, a little bit, well it feels a little less empty when I come home. Well, it doesn't replace the children, but yes, it does make it less empty. (E_FR_6)

This woman insists on the "limits" of this cat's status in the house: she is not allowed to eat leftovers or go into the bedroom. She also has doubts about her cat's interest in receiving affection. Another possible contribution the animal can make is to bring affection to the adult. It is a question of designating a certain form of attention to the adult, of valorisation of the cohabitation which can pass through physical demonstrations (request for cuddles, caresses). Animals can be seen as sources of cuddles.

For Valerie, 38 years old (upper class), married to a banker, petting and cuddling seem to be more important in the relationship with her cat than its mere presence or communication. She feels that the cat understands what she needs and that it is there for her. Her son left home, and Valerie took in a cat, Ficelle. She suffered a lot from the departure of her son:

Valerie: Ficelle allowed me to mitigate the pain that I felt when my son left. Thanks to him, I found affection, love and fun again. It filled a huge void after my son's departure. It's terrible to say, but today, without warmth, without this cat, without Ficelle, I would be very, very sad. (E_FR_1)

She specifies that for three or four months, right after her son's departure, it was hard. Not so much because of the void of activities but because of the absence of someone who counted and for whom she counted:

Valerie: Empty moments in the house [the cat didn't arrive right away]. So, I tried to fill it with activities like yoga, the gym, and that kind of thing. But it was too difficult. There was a cruel lack of affection in my home, even though of course my husband brings me affection, I'm not saying otherwise, but there was still a cruel lack of affection in my home. This cat brought me courage after the departure of my son, and warmth in the home. (E_FR_1)

Valerie's husband comes home later than her in the evening. In the meantime, she takes care of her cat:

Valerie: Well my little one, he comes directly. As soon as I am in bed, he comes to pamper herself near me... He feels when I need affection, he comes directly to me. (E_FR_1)

She insists: "I need the cuddle every day as soon as I get home from work". When she wants to cuddle, she talks to her cat with "a rather silly voice, as if she were talking to a baby... I tell him about my day, and how I feel. But I also ask him questions" (E_FR_1). Ficelle seems to bring this woman a form of personal recognition (de Singly, 1996). She feels understood by her animal. He replaces her son who has left, but also secondarily her husband, who is only present late at night. She does not have a determined "place" (a child's place or spouse's place) but fills the function that children and a spouse ensure, each in their own way, of someone to talk to and someone to touch and hug. Some women admitted that being with an animal provides a positive emotional experience. Agnieszka has three sons. All of them are adults, and the last one moved out recently. Agnieszka is 52 years old, and her husband, Jan, is 55. She works in governmental administration, and the husband runs his own company. The couple's dog plays a very important role at home after the children's departure (we will present it later on in the chapter), and it starts with emotionality and affection:

> Agnieszka: The dog, even if it is big, is a bit like a couch potato, it likes to be petted and cuddled. So, you can pour out all your positive emotions on the dog, pet it and talk to it as you would to a child. The dog is a kind of concentrator of positive emotions. (B_PL_1G)

Some men also expressed the importance of the bond with an animal in their emotional lives like Robert, who is married to Krystyna and has two children (Jan and Maja).

> Robert: Well, my children say that dad finally has a child. They say that dad never spoke so sweetly to them! (A_PL_13G)

Mieczysław (53 years old, a professor at a university) and his wife Irena (53 years old, a librarian) live with a cat. One of their daughters left her cat with them. Mieczysław admits that the cat is a kind of substitute for their children.

> Mieczysław: (...) There's no denying that it's a household member, in the sense that cats usually are, such a strange, different household member. A substitute for someone, kind of. And you have probably also met with such couples, who, for example, did not have pets, suddenly the children moved out and it turns out that they have pets, which are just such a substitute sometimes for children, grandchildren and so on. Meaning, if it is there, it is there, if it is not there.... ok such an animal is like a child, sometimes it is fun, sometimes it is annoying, etc. I don't feel so terribly attached that if they take it away, there will be despair, and if they don't take it away, there will be despair too, in the sense that I don't know what I will do—I'll just worry about it later. (B_PL_4P)

The choice of a "baby" animal can provide an opportunity for even more important work since it is then also necessary to "educate" it, to impose regular rhythms on it (whether it is for a dog or a cat). For this function, cats and dogs seem to be equivalent even if some cats (adults) can lead an independent life and go out of the house quite freely (if there is a cat flap). They still fill the gap.

An Animal as a Vector of a New Composition of Everyday Life Routine

The departure of a child signals the end of activities that were done precisely because they had meaning for both parent and child, in an intergenerational way. Some women mentioned several times that they lost their appetite for "doing" once the children were gone, and the meaning of certain practices disappeared (Chap. 3). Children and parents played the "companion" role that is missing in empty nests, but animals may have the function of providing a structured daily activity for a parent. Having an animal implies a set of regular tasks: preparing food for it, taking care of cleaning its kennel or basket, playing with it, and even taking it out. The animal is considered more like a child or even a small child, because, unlike teenagers, it will not open the fridge to feed itself. These conditions allow an adult to think of themselves as an animal "parent".

Animals in an empty nest become important companions during everyday activities. The duties associated with them determine the rhythm of the day. Spending free time with them can become a source of satisfaction and fulfilment. But before that happens, all actors, human and inhuman, must learn to integrate with each other, setting a new everyday life for each other. Their presence gives new meaning to ordinary activities, such as crossing the corridor or using the toilet, such as in the case of Kazimierz's dog, who had just arrived in their home. And the three of them are learning to live together. The dog and his actions bind them together in an interspecies community. He follows Kazimierz or Krystyna and spends time with them wherever they go. Kazimierz (59 years old, has a secondary education and works as a chemist) and his wife Krystyna (58 years old, a sensory integration therapist) took a dog from an animal shelter:

> Kazimierz: And the dog has become such that he just—whoever is in the house follows him. He's already starting to try to do it too, and he's already moving around, so to speak. It is not, so to speak, well it is funny. Well, we just treat it as funny and as the fact that even though the dog may have had a turbulent life, certainly not easy, well, and at the moment it's sort of gaining normality. (B_PL_12P)

Orelle is a nurse (like her mother, her father was a labourer) and has a husband (whose parents were restaurant owners). As a child, she dreamed of having a dog but her father always refused. She got one with her husband and children. This dog, Nido, died very soon after their daughter left home. Now a dog named Lucky lives with her and her husband:

> Orelle: The biggest blow was the death of Nido. When he died, I was lost. I had just started to get used to not seeing Lily anymore, and then this happened... I had no reference points anymore because I used to adapt the dog's outings to Lily's schedule, I had nothing... In the morning, you don't go out with the dog to smoke your cigarette. When I make food, it's for two and not three. In the evening, I don't have Nido in my bed before Frank [her husband] comes... I couldn't move on because the daily routine reminded me of it all the time. (E_FR_2)

Orelle feels lost:

> When you have a child, you do everything according to them, so when you find yourself without, you no longer have a base, a centre that motivates you. And this base I still had a little with Nido, but with his death, I had nothing. And now I have Lucky who has given me back my little daily routine. (E_FR_2)

Orelle wants to continue to build herself up in her home as a useful person for others. Without others, she finds herself without a role, without activity, in daily life without orientation (see Chap. 14). And this presence for certain women like Orelle gives them structure even though she has a demanding professional activity. This woman does not want to lock the new dog into the old pattern (Nido's successor), "Lucky must have his own life". She calls him Lucky. "Lucky is a good symbol for a new life". Orelle also gives him a nickname:

> Orelle: He is still my Lulu, my baby. I can't help it. And he is still small, I have the right to call him my baby [laughs]. (E_FR_2)

This new little pet gives a rhythm to her existence at home.

Edyta is 45, and her husband is a football coach and needs to coordinate his personal and family life around his professional life. Edyta was really devoted to raising her sons but now they are adults and have moved out. One of her ideas for managing the situation of the nest getting empty was adopting dogs. She decided not to have a third child and became "a dog mother" to regulate the new situation—with all the challenges it brings:

Edyta: I adopted a dog two years ago, and then another—I have four already. I'm active in foundations where we help animals—and it's such a time for me that when no one is around and everyone is off somewhere having fun, riding their bikes, these dogs give me such a break. My husband laughs because I drink very little alcohol, and he said that when they all moved out, we would start drinking—out of grief. Of course, we were joking. I don't know—until a few years ago, I regretted not having a third child. I still envy those mature moms who are 40, because now that I'm 45, I didn't decide to take that last step. Somewhere in the back of my mind, I had it, but I was afraid, and now I regret it terribly. When I see mothers who have grown-up children, like I had 5 years ago, the oldest son was 18, I think, really—you regret it. I'm looking for a solution, and maybe these dogs will give me one. (B_PL_51P)

An animal can be a companion for certain activities. This is especially true for owners of some large dogs. The physical needs of these animals are opportunities to go outside, to go for walks, and to get into trouble with other dogs in the streets. For Sabrina, a single mother with two children, her dog was definitely taken after the departure of her elder son, to fill the gap:

Sabrina: I preferred a dog to another animal because I find that with a dog the bonds are much stronger. I wanted to be able to spend time with him, to share strong moments, especially walks. And I can indeed take a dog almost everywhere, well it doesn't belong everywhere of course, but a dog is like a companion. (E_FR_3)

The term "companion" can refer to a spouse, a friend, or a grown child with whom one does an activity together. Some women, for example, said in the survey that they go shopping a lot with a grown-up child. But there are also those like Bogumiła for whom training a dog is just as much a pleasure as shopping with children:

Bogumiła: Skiing is another thing we have in common, and I train dogs with my daughters on the Kejtrówka. Our dog won first place in the tricks category. I enjoy such dog and walking games, and it's happening. Well [it's like] going shopping together. (A_PL_10G)

The dog that appeared in Agnieszka and Jan's house was meant to help the couple spend time actively, time that had been shared with the children until then:

Agnieszka: We were aware that things were going to get weird, and I thought to myself, "So what, we're going to just come home and look at each other sitting on the couch? So we're going to get a dog and we're going to have to take care of him" and that's clearly what it is because a dog isn't a Yorkshire Terrier, it's a dog that needs to be taken on long walks. And he's got to fill the gap left by the kids. (B_PL_1G)

Xavier is a teacher who lives with his wife, a midwife. They have two daughters. One of the daughters (Amber, the younger one) got a dog, Fazou, for her fifth birthday. Fazou died two months before this interview, and the gap he left confirms the dog's role in the family:

Interviewer: He was a full member?
[Xavier answers without hesitation]
Xavier: Oh yes, yes because many things were organised around him. It was a strong bond, so obviously that was missed when he passed away. (E_FR_4)

The importance of the role played by an animal in a family is especially evident when the decision to adopt (or buy) a new dog or cat is made due to the death of an old one.

An Animal as a New Vector of "Bonfire" in a Couple's Life

Once the children are gone, the animal can finally become a new object of collaboration for both parents. It obliges them to coordinate themselves to keep it, to take it out, to feed it. Some couples find they have little to talk about in the evening at dinner when they are alone (see Chap. 10). An animal can become an indispensable object of attention which the couple talks about, which the attention of both spouses is focused on. It plays the role that used to be played by a child.

Agnieszka and Jan (described above) conduct two separate lives under one roof. On an everyday life basis, they can, however, act as a parental couple in situations related to their dog:

Agnieszka: Well, if he wasn't here, it would be a little strange indeed. But now you have something to do, something to talk about. Before, you used to discuss what the children had done, and now you say what the dog has done. (B_PL_1G)

Agnieszka and Jan are sharing their experience of having a dog together, consciously considering the role of a dog or a cat in their home as a method to prepare for and survive when the house was going to become empty, with just the two of them left inside:

> Agnieszka: In my opinion, it is a method that can make the nest not empty, if someone has not had such a dog before. Because it keeps the subjects busy. We laugh at ourselves when we talk about him like he were a child. Well, we talk about him too much, well, but there are several topics. Besides, it's like this—we both work long hours, my husband comes home at 6–7 pm, that's when he comes home, I have always prepared a meal, well he eats that meal, but then he goes for a two-hour walk with the dog, so he has left, but it's not that he has gone just anywhere, I simply know that he has gone out with the dog, so I can do something else myself. (A_PL_1G)

Since Celina (a 49-year-old beautician) and Adam's (a 49-year-old manager of a reception desk) son moved out, the role of the kitten, Mira, has changed. She gets more attention and affection and has moved to the centre of the couple's relationship:

> Celina: I think we love her more because we say we have a cat baby. Also, Mira is more loved. My husband plays with her, which is unusual because we never did that when we had cats. Mira just talks to him and discusses. Come, you will show yourself to me. I'll show you! There she is, that's our lovely Mira. I am pretty, yes, our black Pearl. And this game is fun because she comes and sits down. And she doesn't talk to me there, she talks to the birds, but when he comes, she starts talking! Just meow, meow, meow! And they have this fish thing, a kind of toy on a piece of string and she hooks him up so that I should sit there, and they should play. And Adam says, "Well, now 5 minutes for you, we can play!". Well, and they play every day. Also, it's fun, well the cat has benefitted, I think. (B_PL_2G)

Now that the children are gone, there is more time and at the same time a need to perform care practices. Especially women share this need. They focus more on healthy and hygienic practices; they do more of the "care work" for the animals, but among the women, they also describe attachment between their husband and animal. The traditional gender order—triggered by the presence of an animal—might also be functional for the couple. She takes care of their nutrition and health, and he walks the animal and plays with it. Even though women care for the animal more, it remains an object of marital focus for the couple. For other couples, such a division does not exist. Activities related to animals are more equal, but they are also a continuation of their human parenting. As in the household of Zofia (a 44-year-old professor at a university) and Leszek a (45-year-old owner of a construction company):

> Zofia: I ended up shaving him, combing his hair, cutting off all his dread-locks and finding two wounds from confrontations with other animals. Because here, unfortunately, there's no way out through the fence, and the neighbour has dogs that are very aggressive, so our dog needs special treat-ment... But it's very interesting because it's back to being the focus of our attention. (B_PL_3P)

Ela (50 years old, lawyer) and Wiesiek (51 years old, navigator engineer) adopted a new cat immediately after their previous cat died. They needed a cat as they knew how important the role of a cat was for the two of them, especially after their son moved out:

> Ela: This cat spends most of his time—he has his basket in the living room, just like the previous one by the way, and it's a new joy for us because when we have a creature in the house, there's always a lot of laughter. Also, he entertains us mainly in the living room because he comes on the couch, cuddles, and stays, he is so sociable and very cool. (B_PL_1P)

An analysis of the practices connected with animals and adults in couples reveals a form of the gendered division of domestic work. Care practices were mentioned and performed more often by women. In contrast, men were more likely to play and walk with the animals. Thus, it appears that culturally assigned gender and parenting roles are reproduced in this arrangement. The division of pet care responsibilities in some parental couples follows the traditional division of caregiving roles. With or without the reproduction of gender roles, these activities aim not only at look-ing after the animal's well-being but also at reconstructing the forms of closeness that were formed within the parental couple. For example, a simple request to feed the cat, addressed to the husband, is a message in which the value of shared responsibility, of which an animal has become the axis, is put to the test. Accepting this request and feeding the cat shows the strength of the "conjugal We", even if it is transmitted through the practice of the "parental We" (de Singly, 2021). We can consider that tak-ing care of an animal is to introduce and take care of the common value of shared intimacy that is reproduced in everyday life by conjugal couples. It is not only the household chores and caregiving practices that affect partners in the process of (re)becoming a married couple. It is also the experience of the joy and pleasure of having a dog or cat. The cuddling, the petting, the love, one's recreation in the company of a pet. The animal helps to support the couple's relationship and create bonds and attachment styles, including with the animals.

CONCLUSION

This chapter aimed to show what roles can be played by an animal in an empty nest and how these roles can transform the couple's arrangements and the "nest" itself. We wanted to do this by referring to three main gaps that arise after children leave home and what the role of animals is in reconfiguring these aspects of parenting and living in a couple.

Examining the statements of the study participants, we noticed that the presence of an animal in the house can make it no longer feel so empty and that certain practices of family life and the life of the couple can be preserved. A cat or a dog can become a companion which minimises the feeling of loneliness by its presence. They can also structure a temporal rhythm within the household, of a time organised according to activities for others. The animal, like the children, can provide this rhythm, especially for parents who are very involved in caring for their children. Finally, the third gap is related to the functioning of the couple. Some parents function primarily as "collaborators" who are focused on one activity: raising children. The animal can become a new focus for the couple. New activities with animals, which did not exist before, can be developed.

The place occupied by an animal varies according to what was missing after the children's departure. Thus, the animal can require this work that the children needed. To put it differently, the animal might not take the "place" of the children but only fulfil some of "the same aspects of parental life" that the children had, which does not strictly concern the role of a child.

REFERENCES

Bakke, M. (2007). Między nami zwierzętami. O emocjonalnych związkach między ludźmi i innymi zwierzętami. *Teksty Drugie, 1/2*, 222–234.

Bekoff, M. (2000). Animal emotions: Exploring passionate natures: Current interdisciplinary research provides compelling evidence that many animals experience such emotions as joy, fear, love, despair, and grief—We are not alone.

Bioscience, 50(10), 861–870. https://doi.org/10.1641/0006-3568(2000)05
0[0861:AEEPN]2.0.CO;2

Blouin, D. D. (2008). *All in the family? Understanding the meaning of dogs and cats in the lives of American pet owners* [Doctoral dissertation, Indiana University]. Indiana University ProQuest Dissertations Publishing.

Blouin, D. D. (2012). Understanding the relationships between people and their pets. *Sociology Compass, 6*(11), 856–869.

Blouin, D. D. (2013). Are dogs children, companions, or just animals? Understanding variation in people's orientations toward animals. *Anthrozoös, 26*(2), 279–294.

Boyatzis, R. E. (1998). *Transforming qualitative information: Thematic analysis and code development.* Sage.

Braun, V., & Clarke, V. (2006). Using thematic analysis in psychology. *Qualitative Research in Psychology, 3*(2), 77–101. https://doi.org/10.1191/1478088706qp063oa

Carlisle-Frank, P., & Frank, J. M. (2006). Owners, guardians, and owner-guardians: Differing relationships with pets. *Anthrozoös, 19*(3), 225–242. https://doi.org/10.2752/089279306785415574

Carter, M. (2015, June 19). What's so wrong with 'pet parenting'? *HuffPost.* Retrieved from https://www.huffingtonpost.co.uk/marie-carter/pet-parenting-whats-so-wrong-with-it_b_7079174.html

Carter, B., & Charles, N. (2013). Animals, agency and resistance. *Journal for the Theory of Social Behaviour, 43,* 322–340.

Champagne, C., Pailhé, A., & Solaz, A. (2015). Le temps domestique et parental des hommes et des femmes: quels facteurs d'évolutions en 25 ans? *Economie et statistique, 478,* 209–238.

Charles, N. (2014). 'Animals just love you as you are': Experiencing kinship across the species barrier. *Sociology, 48*(4), 715–730.

Charles, N. (2016). Post-human families? Dog-human relationships in the domestic sphere. *Sociological Research Online, 21*(3), 1–12.

Charles, N., & Davies, C. A. (2008). My family and other animals: Pets as kin. *Sociological Research Online, 13,* 69–92.

de Singly, F. (1996). Le soi, le couple et la famille, Essais et recherches. *Sociologie du travail, 39*(1, 123–125.

de Singly, F. (2021). The family of individuals: An overview of the sociology of the family in Europe, 130 years after Durkheim's first university course. In A.-M. Castrén, V. Česnuitytė, I. Crespi, J.-A. Gauthier, R. Gouveia, C. Martin, A. M. Mínguez, & K. Suwada (Eds.), *The Palgrave handbook of family sociology in Europe* (pp. 15–43). Palgrave Macmillan.

de Singly, F., & Morand, E. (2019). Sociologie d'une forte proximité subjective au chat, au chien. *Enfances, Familles, Générations.* https://doi.org/10.7202/1064510ar

Doré, A., & Michalon, J. (2017). What makes human–animal relations 'organizational'? The de-scription of anthrozootechnical agencements. *Organization, 24*(6), 761–780. https://doi.org/10.1177/1350508416670249

Doré, À., Michalon, J., & Monteiro, T. (2019). The place and effect of animals in families. *Enfances Familles Générations, 32*.

FEDIAF. (2022). *European pet food. Annual report.* Retrieved March 2, 2023, from https://europeanpetfood.org/about/annual-report/

Franklin, A. (1999). *Animals and modern cultures: A sociology of human–animal relations in modernity.* Sage.

Franklin, A. (2006). Being dog conscious: A post-humanist approach to housing. *Housing, Theory and Society, 23*(3), 137–156.

Gouveia, R., & Castrén, A.-M. (2021). Redefining the boundaries of family and personal relationships. In A.-M. Castrén, V. Česnuitytė, I. Crespi, J.-A. Gauthier, R. Gouveia, C. Martin, A. M. Mínguez, & K. Suwada (Eds.), *The Palgrave handbook of family sociology in Europe* (pp. 259–277). Palgrave Macmillan.

Greenebaum, J. (2004). It's a dog's life: The elevation from pet to "fur baby" status in the age of applause. *Society & Animals, 12*, 117–135.

Irvine, L. (2004). *If you tame me: Understanding our connection with animals.* Temple University Press.

Irvine, L., & Cilia, L. (2017). More-than-human families: Pets, people, and practices in multispecies households. *Sociology Compass, 11*(2), e12455. https://doi.org/10.1111/SOC4.12455

Kirksey, E. (2015). Multispecies families, capitalism, and the law. In I. Braverman (Ed.), *Animals, biopolitics, law* (1st ed., pp. 175–194). Routledge.

Konecki, K. (2005). *Ludzie i ich zwierzęta. Interakcjonistyczno-symboliczna analiza społecznego świata właścicieli zwierząt domowych.* Scholar.

Laing, M. (2021). On being posthuman in human spaces: Critical posthumanist social work with interspecies families. *International Journal of Sociology and Social Policy, 41*(3/4), 361–375. https://doi.org/10.1108/IJSSP-09-2019-0185

Laurent-Simpson, A. (2017a). Considering alternative sources of role identity: Childless parents and their animal "children". *Sociological Forum, 32*(3), 610–634.

Laurent-Simpson, A. (2017b). 'They make me not want to have children': Effects of pets on childless people's fertility intentions. *Sociological Inquiry, 87*(4), 586–607. https://doi.org/10.1111/soin.12163

Lazarsfeld, P., Jahoda, M., & Zeisel, H. (1981). *Les chômeurs de Marienthal.* Les Éditions de Minuit.

Leow, C. (2018). *It's not just a dog: The role of companion animals in the family's emotional system.* University of Nebraska.

Mamzer, H. (2015). Posthumanizm we współczesnych modelach rodzin: zwierzęta jako członkowie rodziny? In S. Grotowska & I. Taranowicz (Eds.), *Rodzina wobec wyzwań współczesności. Wybrane problemy* (pp. 151–176). Oficyna Wydawnicza Arboretum.

McLaughlin, P. (2019). *If animals are like our children let us treat them alike: Creating tests of an animal's intelligence for determinations of legal personhood.* Library Faculty Publications. Retrieved April 15, 2023, from https://commons.law.famu.edu/library-facpub/13

Merton, R. K. (1997). *Eléments de théorie et de méthode sociologique.* Armand Colin.

Mikołejko, Z. (2023, January 7). Nowa rodzina. Dlaczego zwierzęta zastępują nam dzieci. *Gazeta Wyborcza, 2003,* 26–29.

Miller, A. (2011). Just don't call me mom: Pros and cons of a family law model for companion animals in the U.S. *Humanimalia, 2*(2), 90–114.

Montag, C., & Davis, K. L. (2020). *Animal emotions: How they drive human behavior.* Punctum Books.

Owens, N., & Grauerholz, L. (2019). Interspecies parenting: How pet parents construct their roles. *Humanity and Society, 43*(2), 96–119. https://doi.org/10.1177/0160597617748166

Power, E. (2008). Furry families: Making a human-dog family through the home. *Social & Cultural Geography, 9*(5), 535–555.

Sanders, C. R. (1999). *Understanding dogs: Living and working with canine companions.* Temple University Press.

Serpell, J. A. (1996). Evidence for an association between pet behavior and owner attachment levels. *Applied Animal Behaviour Science, 47*(1–2), 49–60. https://doi.org/10.1016/0168-1591(95)01010-6

Shir-Vertesh, D. (2012). Flexible personhood: Loving animals as family members in Israel. *American Anthropologist, 114,* 420–432.

Smith, C. (2003). *Moral, believing animals: Human personhood and culture.* Oxford University Press.

Thielke, L. E., & Udell, M. A. R. (2017). The role of oxytocin in dog-human relationships and potential applications for the treatment of separation anxiety in dogs: Oxytocin and separation anxiety. *Biological Reviews, 92,* 378–388.

Topál, J., Miklósi, Á., Csányi, V., & Dóka, A. (1998). Attachment behavior in dogs (Canis familiaris): A new application of Ainsworth's (1969) strange situation test. *Journal of Comparative Psychology, 112*(3), 219–229.

Żadkowska, M., Bieńko, M., Gajewska, M., Mizielińska, J., & Stasińska, A. (2022). *Exploring interspecies family life practices with animal companions.* In Paper presented [not published] at the conference in Warsaw.

PART II

The Couple in 'The Empty Nest'

Redefining a Couple's Relationship in the Empty Nest: The New Honeymoon

Filip Schmidt, Marta Skowrońska, Magdalena Żadkowska, and Christophe Giraud

INTRODUCTION

Most studies on the empty nest phase try to answer whether some aspects of life (particularly spousal relations, parental relations, and general life satisfaction) have changed after adult children's departure. They also often analyse whether these aspects have improved or deteriorated. In the

F. Schmidt (✉) • M. Skowrońska
Faculty of Sociology, Adam Mickiewicz University, Poznań, Poland
e-mail: fschmidt@amu.edu.pl; marta.skowronska@amu.edu.pl

M. Żadkowska
Social Sciences Department (Institute of Sociology), University of Gdańsk, Gdańsk, Poland

Centre de recherche sur les liens sociaux (CERLIS, UMR 8070), Université Paris Cité, Paris, France
e-mail: magdalena.zadkowska@ug.edu.pl

© The Author(s), under exclusive license to Springer Nature Switzerland AG 2024
M. Żadkowska et al. (eds.), *Reconfiguring Relations in the Empty Nest*, Palgrave Macmillan Studies in Family and Intimate Life, https://doi.org/10.1007/978-3-031-50403-7_9

chapters that make up this part of the book, we propose instead to view the transition to the empty nest phase as a transformation of two interdependent types of relationship: between parents and children and between partners. Drawing on the concept of the family as a dynamic network of interdependencies, we show that the transformations of changes in these relationships are mutually contingent and that the transition to the empty nest can be accompanied by different, sometimes conflicting, meanings and emotions.

In this chapter, we first present four model scenarios resulting from the combination of different levels of interdependence between partners and between parents and children after departure. We then focus in detail on the scenario in which interdependence with children has weakened, while partner interdependence has been maintained or developed, described as the "new honeymoon". The opposite scenario of couples who are together but apart is presented in a separate chapter of this book.

Relief and Loss as Two Non-exclusive Forms of Experiencing Change

As Bouchard (2014: 71) notes, the psychological impact of children's departure from the parents' perspective is often described using one of the two dominant approaches. The first one is the "role strain–role relief" perspective, which suggests an improvement in parental well-being because the presence of children at home increased exposure to stressors. The second one is the "role loss" perspective, which demonstrates the decrease in well-being due to the absence of alternative roles of parents after the departure. While early studies rather demonstrated parents' decrease in life satisfaction, recent research suggests that the "empty nest syndrome" is rare, mostly due to parents' engagement in multiple roles and their alternative sources of self-definition (Mitchell & Lovegreen, 2009). However, the perspectives of loss and strain do not have to be treated as mutually exclusive but rather as relational concepts which can co-exist and influence each other. The term "empty nest syndrome" poorly

C. Giraud
Centre de recherche sur les liens sociaux (CERLIS, UMR 8070), Université Paris Cité, Paris, France
e-mail: christophe.giraud@parisdescartes.fr

reflects the complex mix of experiences and emotions accompanying this stage of life (Dare, 2011), and so does concentrating on one type of experience (strain vs loss) or measuring them on a unimodal scale.

Parent–Adult Children Relationships

While studies on loss and relief focus on the parents and their life quality, there is also a strong stream of research analysing the transformation of parents–children relations in the empty nest phase. Nowadays, parents are involved in their children's adult lives in many more ways than before (Lück et al., 2021: 99). Several models have been developed to explain various aspects of the transition of the parents–children relationship.

For instance, Bozhenko (2011) analysed separation level, communication strategies, and personal attitudes, while Aquilino (1997) studied emotional closeness, shared activities, support from children, and the level of control and conflict. Among the most influential studies into the dynamics of parents–adult children relations were the analyses of intergenerational solidarity, particularly by Silverstein, Bengtson, and Roberts (Bengtson & Roberts, 1991; Silverstein & Bengtson, 1997). Their contribution was identifying several aspects of solidarity: affectual, associational, consensual, normative, functional, and structural. Instead of only measuring a generalised level of solidarity, they focused on its different variants and models.

Distinguishing between different types of parent–child bonds and the patterns of their transformation in adulthood is very important. Still, to understand the transition to empty nesting and the different possible outcomes of this process, we need to understand how spousal and child–parent relationships are interrelated.

Manifestations of Interdependence

The term "interdependence" is most associated with the Actor-Partner Interdependence Model, in which individuals are interdependent in a family configuration because each one fulfils some of the others' needs for emotional support, financial and practical resources, and social recognition (Bouchard & McNair, 2016). In our view, this approach places too much emphasis on family as a cohesive group, and too little on how various individuals create configurations of interdependencies through their daily practices and interactions. The data we have collected suggests that families experiencing the transition to the empty nest are in the constant process of configuration of interdependencies. Rather than only measuring the level of interdependence by arbitrarily constructed scales, we have searched for manifestations of interdependence in practices by analysing qualitative empirical material. Referring partly to the intergenerational solidarity model (Bengtson & Roberts, 1991; Silverstein & Bengtson, 1997), we have distinguished the following aspects of interdependence: (1) material/economic, (2) practices-based, and (3) emotional. Each of these aspects divides into subtypes. Material/economic independence may mean that one person depends on another person's financial support or that material space (family home) binds people together. Interdependence manifested in practices means that people do things together or do different things close to one another, and/or they share their thoughts and confide in each other. It may also mean that people do things for one another or they take each other into account in their actions. Finally, emotional interdependence means that partners depend on each other's presence, they want to control each other, and/or they express their feelings (e.g. saying that they love each other or care about each other).

Family as a Dynamic Process and Empty Nest in the Context of the Life Course

While the early studies of the family life cycle often provided a set of universal and static phases through which a family has to go, the seminal works of Elder (1985, 1994, 1999) introduced the idea of the family life course as a dynamic process. This concept is based on two assumptions: (1) the shape of later phases is influenced by cumulative events of the earlier stages and (2) the lives and life courses of family members and other people are interlocked and intertwined (linked lives) and mutually influence each other (Trommsdorff, 2006). In recent years, there has been an increasing interest in the family as a dynamic process, which is shaped by institutional context and which undergoes transitions, following different trajectories rooted in the sociopolitical context (Konietzka & Kreyenfeld, 2021). The family is also seen as a dynamic network of interdependencies "in which individuals cooperate, but also hinder each other because of the social stress generated by the necessity of sharing existing resources" (Widmer, 2021: 61). These patterns of interdependencies, rather than household composition, determine the everyday functioning of the family and maintain the sense of we-ness (Widmer, 2021).

In the dynamic process of being a family, one of the most important transitions is "emptying the nest"—when the adult children leave the family home. The children's departure introduces significant changes to the family's network of interdependencies. This chapter aims to contribute to the existing literature and the notion of family as a dynamic network of interdependencies by analysing how interdependence between parents and children, and between parents as partners, affects each other.

We investigate how configurations of different strength and form of these interdependencies impact the reconfiguration of a couple's relationship after children's departure, combining the perspectives of children–parent and parent–parent (couple) relationships. Our thesis is that the reconfiguration of couplehood differs depending on the level of children-centredness of the parents and their level of partner interdependence. When children leave home, child-centred care practices significantly decrease, and decisions usually no longer need to be child-dependent. The transition to the empty nest phase may vary depending on how much the couple remains nevertheless child-centred and how much resources the partners have to maintain or develop the practices, emotions, and materiality that bind them together as a couple. Finally, we also include the theory of "displaying couple" (Finch, 2007). Regardless of the level of interdependence and child-centredness and the type of bond between the spouses, a couple is involved in "displaying" some aspects of couplehood/being a family to others (e.g. friends and family). We aim to investigate what different types of couples display and how this display is modified in the transition to the empty nest.

This chapter is based on 75 interviews with couples (dyadic in-depth interviews, corpus A) and 45 individual interviews with some of the spouses (corpus B). We analyse the reconfiguration of the couple's roles and practices (and meanings attached to them) in the transition to the empty nest. We also observe the level of child-centredness as an essential modifying factor and investigate what the couples decide to display. The analysis comprised individual coding using MAXQDA software and teamwork of all coders who compared and discussed their results. The first step in the coding process was to identify the manifestations of interdependence or the lack of thereof. In the next step, each couple was analysed concerning the qualitatively assessed level of parents–children and spousal interdependence and categorised according to the model we have developed before. The analysis included elements of inductive and deductive approaches. While we have, based on the previously developed model, discovered new, important themes that were added in the process, such as detailed elements of constructing and practising each scenario. The work by a team of four coders helped us increase interrater reliability.

THEORETICAL PROPOSAL

Table 9.1 presents four model scenarios for post-parental couples depending on the level of interdependence between them and between them and their children after the children's departure. We have not included interdependence before the departure in the typology for two reasons. First, all families in our sample had strong bonds with their children when they still lived at home, even if manifestations of these bonds differed. Second, the couples were almost always strongly interrelated before the departure because of their shared parental work even if they differed in other manifestations of spousal interdependence. Thus, the departure begins a significant transition of the network of interdependencies.

Type (I) features weak interdependence between parental couple and children and between the spouses. It refers to cases when the departure of children significantly weakens the parent–children interdependence and reveals that without the "children project" the couple has very little in common. In the case of type (II), the time and space freed by now-independent children are a resource rather than a threat to the marital couple. Partners either continue their strong bond or relearn how to live together after years of focusing on children. Type (III) describes couples with low levels of interdependence who remain strongly interconnected with their children even after their moving out. In this case, children usually live nearby and visit often. Thus, the couple may live as if (almost)

Table 9.1 Empty nest as the transformation of interdependencies: Four model scenarios

		Interdependence between spouses after the departure	
		Weak	Strong
Interdependence between parents and children after the departure	Weak	Together/apart (I)	New honeymoon (II)
	Strong	Dissolved in the family (III)	Parents and partners (IV)

nothing has changed and still work as a parental team. Their low levels of other forms of interdependence may not be revealed due to continued focus on children. Finally, type (IV) describes couples who continue intense levels of interdependence with each other and their children. Children's departure is not perceived as a shock, similarly to type (III). The difference between these two types is the presence of non-parental forms of partner interdependence in type (IV).

It is worth noting that the analysis of parents–children relations takes a dyadic perspective. In other words, we analyse the relationship between children and the parental team rather than individual parents. While acknowledging the entire matrix of the parents–children relationships would provide more nuance and complexity, this part aimed to focus on marital relations. For this reason, we have decided to give a more geneneralised picture of the interdependence between parents and their children.

The Specificity of the "New Honeymoon" Scenario

In this chapter, we investigate the couples who converted the released resources into strengthening the marital bond when their interdependence with children has weakened. We have named this scenario of the couple's trajectory in the empty nest phase a "new honeymoon" to emphasise the reinforcement of the conjugal bond.

Before the children's departure, couples work on their shared project—bringing up their children. Such projects demand time, effort, financial resources, and energy. However, couples differ regarding the intensity of their work and the amount of space they leave for their relationship. Sometimes the "children project" is an extension of the marital team, which retains the primary role. In other cases, the team is primarily parental, while the marital (conjugal) relationship is secondary (it has been "put on hold" for the time of the children's upbringing or has never developed). While the "new honeymoon" scenario refers to couples with strong levels of spousal interdependencies after the children's departure, this scenario may emerge during a longer process. Family relationships are processual and dynamic. Some couples begin the "new honeymoon" right after their children's departure. In other cases, a couple has to learn or relearn how to be together. After the departure, a couple may display low levels of interdependencies, but develop them in time, by undertaking new practices. On the other hand, the "new honeymoon" may only be a period, after which the partners start gradually to fall apart.

Several factors can facilitate or hinder the emergence of the new honeymoon scenario: the couple's history (experience of living together before the children were born), housing conditions and financial situation, workload, and the general amount of time for each other in the full nest phase. Respondents differ in whether and how long they had been a couple before the children were born. In some cases, spouses moved into the family home of one of the partners, significantly hindering the possibility of building a partnership and parental bond. For couples with fewer financial resources, the space of opportunity after the children's departure is usually more significant than in couples with ample resources. Excessive workload, commuting long distances, working abroad, or caring for other family members could also have made it very difficult for a couple to strengthen their relationship in the full nest phase. Some of the interviewees explicitly said that these factors had had a very negative impact on the marital bond. If time resources were limited, the relationship with children might be the only one parents were able to cherish.

First, we describe how reduced interdependence with children releases resources that tend to be used for the couple, even if this process is slowed by feelings of loss and guilt. We then describe how some "new honeymoon" couples rely on patterns of interdependence developed over the years, while others find a way to relearn how to be a couple, in many cases by recalling the couple's history. Finally, we describe two dominant ways of practicing the "new honeymoon" through shared daily activities and joint projects (Fig. 9.1).

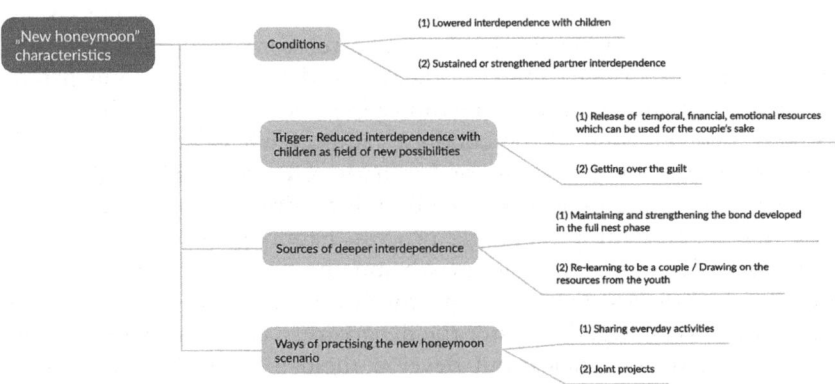

Fig. 9.1 Characteristics of the "new honeymoon" scenario

More Resources, Fewer Obligations: Common Experiences in Different Proportions

As we have discussed earlier, the emptying of the nest is usually accompanied by both sadness and relief, which are experienced universally, but to different degrees. Relief results from the release of resources that until now were focused on the child (cf. Giraud de & Singly, 2012). At the same time, along with the departure of the children, rhythms and activities that structured daily life and made partners work together disappear or weaken. When the interdependence with the child(ren) is not sustained, the partners need to redefine their time, attention, and daily activities—otherwise they may move towards the "together apart" scenario (see Chap. 10) or break up. In this chapter, we examine couples who succeeded and felt that the departure of their children strengthened them.

The departure of children releases various types of resources, such as finances, time, and emotional (no need to worry, care, or quarrel so much) and physical (cooking, cleaning, shopping, driving, etc.) supplies. Several couples have observed increased **time and financial resources**. While parents like to highlight that they "don't want to complain" about the children-related expenses or effort (this would threaten their role as carers), their narratives contain direct expressions of relief. One of the parents, Marcin, quickly calculates: 200PLN a month saved thanks to lower energy bills after the departure of his son and his girlfriend, giving almost 2500 PLN a year "for an extra trip" (A_PL_12G). His wife, Anna, adds that they also gained more time:

> Interviewer: And has your son's departure changed anything in your relationship, in the way you spend your free time? Do you have more time?
> Anna: Yes, we have more time because all the extra logistics have changed, so we have more time plus we're more focused on each other, there are no distracting factors. (A_PL_12G)

Kazimiera's narrative also demonstrates that she and her husband now take advantage of extra temporal, financial, and emotional resources. They can afford a weekend getaway without having to worry about money or time, and they spend their time "quietly"—without tension:

> Kazimiera: Above all, it's been more time for us. (…) I guess, this is **the best time for our marriage** (…) we are on our own. Adults, with **our own**

money (...). I know the girls will do fine, so we **don't need to provide for them** either. So it's just a normal, **quiet life with time for each other**— going to the **cinema, to the theatre, a weekend getaway** together. (A_PL_22P)

While the departure of the children usually instantly gives the parents more autonomy in time management, the release of the financial burden may take more time. Many parents still support their children after they move out, at least until they have got a permanent job. In France, in contrast to Poland, students have to pay university fees, which significantly prolongs the period of the parents' financial sacrifices. Valérie and her husband wait until their two daughters, who are still students, have a job so that they can start their projects:

Valérie: Then, afterwards, we would like to have projects for the house, you know, to do some work, some improvements, but we still don't have the budget because university fees are high, so it's a bit on hold. But yes, we have ideas on what we would like to redo, improve, change, but well... (A_FR_6)

In addition to time and money, an important resource couples take advantage of is the **release from obligation or burden,** expressed in recurring terms, such as the expression "we don't have to" [cook, worry, plan, etc.] and the words **"calmness", "peaceful", and "relaxed"**. Couples experience a general sense of freedom in managing their personal and marital schedules, which combines emotional and physical relief: "fewer obligations", says Mounir, and his wife agrees: "you are much freer to do what you like]" (A_FR_32). Other interviewees also mention their emotional relief:

Magdalena: When he moved out, we felt a sense of calm. Calm and that we didn't have to do anything (...) no obligation (...) we live peacefully, we do what we want. (A_PL_26G)

Maria: Mentally, it's certainly such a rest, that we can take care of ourselves a little selfishly. (A_PL_2P)

Sofiane: You take your time, you do a little bit of what you want, well "what you want" in quotation marks.
  Nour: You find another rhythm of life.

Sofiane: You find another rhythm of life. It's much more relaxed and it's our rhythm (…). (A_FR_39)

Calmness and relaxation also result from the release of tension. Stanisław admits that he has finally stopped worrying about his son. The constant fear that he felt ("he always messed around", A_PL_26G) made it difficult to focus on other aspects of life. Some parents also admit that their children's departure has eliminated a **considerable amount of tension** from the marital relationship. For many couples, children are the primary source of everyday conflicts. "Fewer nerves, I guess (…) We quarrel less often"— Stanisław says, and his wife Magdalena confirms: "tensions between us, like, you shouldn't have told him that (…) eternal misunderstandings. And now there's less of that…" (A_PL_26G).

Less stress and tension foster **various ideas for spending time together as a couple**, such as trips and outings. Erwan and Carole (A_FR_ 40), both executives, enjoy improvised weekends. When the kids were at home, the couple's involvement in the practices of care kept them from going away for a weekend. "They would have a party and wouldn't revise for school", "They wouldn't cook for themselves", they say. Everyday family logistics imprisoned them within a rigid timetable. Now they are happy to improvise. "[Their departure] left more room for improvisation, that's true. Because before, everything was logistics, we had to plan", Carole says.

Another aspect of the freedom offered by the absence of children relates to **intimacy.** While the presence of children made some partners careful about their nudity, the empty nest allows them to take a shower with open doors and walk around the apartment in just underwear. Clarisse and Sébastien compare the times when they are alone and are often less modest and the times when the children come back. Intimacy is expressed not only in body-related behaviour but also in conversation, which can no longer be overheard.

Clarisse: (…). If, in the evening, I feel like walking around in my nightie at home, I can do that. (…) But if your children are here, you're more likely to…

Sébastien: It's going to be more difficult, you have to be a little more careful (…) and then you also try to pay attention to how you speak and the dialogue you have. (A_FR_4)

So far we have presented clear cases of released resources that have provided space for couples. However, in some cases, the "new honeymoon" is a result of a longer process of gradual weakening of interdependence with children, a long-term accomplishment which needs to be renewed and sustained.

For instance, Magdalena and Stanisław (A_PL_26G) did not support their daughter's decision to move out. The mother objected to adapting her room for other purposes ("She may return!"). It took a long time before the parents stopped wondering each night if Dominica had got home safely from work. Finally, when they gained confidence that she was doing well and had a suitable partner, that fear was replaced by pride and calmness, allowing for more attention to be directed towards the couple. This story is one of many examples of the processual character of transitioning to the empty nest and shifting the attention from a parental to a marital relationship. Some narratives (Jadwiga and Cezary, Delphine and Didier) include reflexive work on this transition. Jadwiga employed the psychological narrative of healthy and unhealthy relationships to assure herself that she should move on:

> Jadwiga: So I decided I had to cut the umbilical cord because it was simply getting unhealthy. For me and for them, right? (A_PL_27G)

A sense of relief may also be accompanied by a sense of guilt, when parents feel that enjoyment may indicate an insufficient fulfilment of their parental role. Jadwiga, declaring that the empty nest is "the best time ever", quickly adds:

> Jadwiga: Although I'm not sure if it speaks well of us that we [feel good]. Because I have a feeling it may speak badly, but well... (A_PL_27G)

Similarly, a French couple who plans their conjugal activities, are wondering if their projects are not too far advanced. As they explicitly express, they are "in transition" rather than in the next biographical stage.

> Didier: But it might be a little early, the kids haven't gone far and been away long yet.
> Delphine: Yeah.
> Didier: (…) We're starting to realise that we're going to have a little more freedom, but to plan I think it's still a little early.

Delphine: We are in transition for the moment. (A_FR_26)

It is important to note that the transition process is fragile and reversible, as shown by the situation of Fabienne and her husband Fabrice, confronted with the return of one of their children for economic reasons, one year after their departure. The couple, who have been emancipated from the children for a year, returns to being a parental couple:

> Fabienne: when Jacinte left and before Athis came back (…) During that time (…) we were just a couple. We were still parents, but less so because there were no children at home. We started to establish little habits of going out to eat on Sunday in the afternoon or Saturday night from time to time. And it's true that when Athis came back, all that was a little bit out of place because we were back to being a couple of parents. (A_FR_2)

The departure of adult children from the family home not only brings about universal feelings of sadness and relief but also leads to the release of various resources, enabling couples to strengthen their relationships, experience greater autonomy, and rekindle intimacy. However, the transition to the empty nest is a dynamic process that may involve guilt, reflection, and adjustments, with some couples facing the challenge of reverting to their parental roles when adult children return home for various reasons.

BUILDING THE "NEW HONEYMOON" SCENARIO

We have discussed the increased temporal, financial, emotional, and physical resources as foundations for the "new honeymoon" scenario. We will now demonstrate two general ways of constructing it. The first is to maintain and strengthen relationship patterns that have been developed over the years. In this case, the departure is not experienced as a shock but rather as a chance to reinforce the relationship. The other way is to relearn how to be a couple—work out a new path for the relationship, which may take some time and demand effort. In some cases, this process involves using the couple's past (the period before children) as a relationship model to follow. Recalling romantic events from the couple's past and taking up activities that were put to one side for a while may help to strengthen the bond between the partners.

Maintaining and Strengthening the Bond Developed in the Full Nest Phase

While all the interviewed parents experienced the full nest phase as a time concentrated on the children, some couples managed to attend to their conjugal relationship. When partners found time for each other when the children were still at home, the empty nest phase does not come as a shock, but a continuing process of shifting the focus from family life to a dyadic relationship.

Fabienne and Francis are a French middle-class couple. They are respectively 50 and 51 years old. They have a 23-year-old daughter who is finishing her studies (she is in a master's programme). They report little change after their daughter's departure and explain that they have always been able to cherish couple time. "We have never put our life as a couple on hold", they say. This attitude clearly distinguishes them from the other two paths of building the new honeymoon scenario, both of which sideline the romantic relationship for the time of the children's upbringing.

> Fabienne: (…) Charlotte arrived (…) we asked one of our friends every Wednesday evening (…) she took care of the little one for us. (…) Although we had Charlotte, we didn't stop going to restaurants, movies, theatres, on trips, etc. (…) We never put our life as a couple on hold. (A_FR_20)

Similarly, a Polish couple, Zbyszek and Teresa, say they "like spending time together" and "don't mind the silence at home", noting that they have always found time for each other, even with the children at home:

> Teresa: We usually expected them [the children] to organise their time, and we organised our time in our way. (A_PL_5G)

Zosia and Leszek have always enjoyed each other's company, with the children and without. They declare they are never bored because they have always had shared interests. They also cherish memories of many years together:

> Leszek: Zosia and I have never been bored in each other's company (…). We simply have a shared life, common interests, common memories, because we have known each other practically since the beginning of high school. (B_PL_3P)

Marcin and Anna have always defined their relationship as central, despite their strong bonds with the kids:

> Anna: The empty nest [syndrome] appears when a family [couple] had nothing but the kids. (...) Since the beginning of our marriage, we have always assumed we're more important because it's us who're going to stay together till the end—that's the setup. (A_PL_12G)

Magdalena and Stanisław are convinced that their successful relationship after the children moved out results from maintaining their bond despite the very absorbing parenting process:

> Stanisław: And this is the most important, to spend time together.
> Magdalena: Even when the children are still here (...) because later when (...) the child moves out after 20 years, and we (...) lived apart all that time (...) it's difficult to say: now the child is gone, we'll be together. I think it doesn't work this way, you have to be together all your life to celebrate the couple time afterwards (...) when your paths have parted it's difficult to glue them together again. (A_PL_26G)

As we have demonstrated, some couples manage to prioritise and nurture their romantic relationship throughout their parenting years, making the transition to the empty nest phase less of a shock and more of a continuation in focusing on the couplehood.

Relearning How to Be a Couple

While paying continuous attention to the conjugal relationship in the full nest phase makes the empty nest transition a smooth and natural process, relegating marital bonds to the background results in the necessity to build the relationship anew. Couples who had a chance to live together for a more extended period before children arrived may use the empty nest as an opportunity to return to the practices and emotions from their youth. If the children took up all their time and attention in the full nest phase, they might now feel they want to pick up where they left off. Their narratives contain terms such as "recalling", "recollecting", "remembering", and "finding again".

Celina and Adam name the full nest phase a period of forgetting—a time when parents focus on their offspring while paying little attention to their own needs and interests. The empty nest, on the other hand, is a period of recalling and returning:

> Adam: We have time for ourselves. This element of concentration, which was there for 20 years, on which our whole life was focused, has gone. One forgets about one's own needs, passions and interests, and now is the moment when life is giving us such an opportunity to recollect them and start pursuing them again. (A_PL_2G)

Felicja recalls when she and her husband "spent a lot of time together" and "just took a backpack and went to the mountains" to get away from the drudgery of everyday life (A_PL_29G). Now, when the children are gone, they have returned to their passion. Clarisse and Sébastien started to ride motorcycles again as they used to do in their youth:

> Clarisse: what we stopped when we had the children, that is, the motorcycle, going away at weekends, we have taken all that up again (…) We have resumed our life as before. (A_FR_4)

Delphine repeats the word "find", which suggests retrieving something that was lost:

> Delphine: (…) we have started to feel… finally it's very pleasant to be together, uh, we are finding ourselves… we are finding ourselves together (…) it's not unpleasant in the end… also to find each other when you come home (…) we take time to prepare dinner together you know, we find each other a bit like… like when we were both newlyweds. It's kind of fun. (A_FR_13)

Some couples use the expression of returning to the early stages of their relationship. Jadwiga and Cezary name the experience of "leaving the house, locking the door and going somewhere alone" as their "second youth". Carole and Erwan mention "starting their youth again":

> Carole: Find ourselves as we were before, finally. At last, we can start our youth again. (A_FR_40)

In the process of learning how to be a couple again, reaching into the past may be insufficient, particularly if the couple had little opportunity to work on their relationship before their children were born. In some cases (particularly in the Polish sample—in Poland the average age of having children is lower), children arrived very soon, or the couple had to share an apartment with their parents or in-laws. In these cases, the interviewees admitted they hardly remembered being a couple without children—their entire relationship has always been integrated into family life. Moreover, even if a couple's past is a valuable resource, they may want to introduce new elements, because they are in a different stage of life, and their needs and attitudes have evolved.

Jadwiga (A_PL_27G) describes the birth of her daughter as one of the most challenging periods of her life, and "terrible exhaustion". Financial and health troubles forced her to live with her elderly father and her husband to spend most of the year working abroad. This, combined with further problems, led to a temporary break-up. It was only when the children moved out that the value of the relationship was rediscovered. It took some time, but now, the interviewee says, is their "best time ever".

Clarisse and Sébastien, whose narrative contained elements of returning to their youth, found that the sense of "being newlyweds again" resulted from a process of relearning how to be a couple. Years of focusing on having children meant that the spouses had little chance to work out how to live together:

> Interviewer: But now that the three children are gone, (…) what has changed most in your life (…)?
> Clarisse: Learning again. Learning to live together again.
> Sébastien: Learning to live as a couple again (…) finding a certain bond, a certain dialogue (…) You didn't have that kind of relationship anymore because the priority was the children, and logically, like many people, you put your life on hold. When you no longer have the children, you have to resume this relationship and bring it back to life so that you can actually live again, live as a couple. (A_FR_4)

Thus, couples who have put their marriage on hold may find their children's departure to be a significant turning point in their married lives. The empty nest phase can be a chance to make up for lost time. For a long time, Sofiane and Nour were geographically and maritally separated. Their moments together as a family were often marked by tension, particularly between the father and one of his sons. Now is the time for marital renewal:

Nour: We are trying to discover activities that we have not tried together because when the children were small, we went to Disneyland, we did more activities related to the children. It's true that we left our relationship a bit behind, so the fact that we're both together now allows us to do activities together. I think when we go on trips, we'll be able to discover many activities. (A_FR_39)

The process of relearning can be challenging. At first, it may feel like a shock, as Yves and Angèle observe:

Angèle: Oh, that was a shock. You know, sometimes we forgot to see each other and spend time together when we had to look after the kids. And here we are, the two of us, face to face. So, it's weird, really weird.
Yves: Yeah, it is. But at the same time it's cool to be together again now that we don't have the kids. It's like being a young couple again. You know.
Angèle: Right, but it's also different; it's still a new phase in our lives. Let's say we've rediscovered each other. (A_FR_19)

There may be feelings of insecurity or anxiety before the couple is comfortable with the new way of being together. For many years, children were one of the parents' main topics of conversation. Now the partners may be uncertain whether they will find anything to talk about. Before going on their first holiday without the children, Edyta's husband (B_PL_51) made a list of topics to discuss to avoid uncomfortable silences:

Edyta: We always went on holiday with our children. And there came a time when our sons went away for seasonal jobs. And we said, OK, we're going to go on our own, because it's time to relax. (…) my husband made a list of things to talk about, because these holidays were always with and about the children. (…) We didn't even take out the bit of paper with the topics. (…) It was a moment we were terribly afraid of and it turned out to be one of the best trips, such total relaxation. (B _PL_51)

In the sometimes-challenging process of rebuilding a couple, the partners may find that a "return to their youth" is not only difficult, but that it would also not be in line with the new biographical stage. Sexual fascination can be transformed into a friendship, as in the example of the couple Celina and Adam:

Adam: This is a completely different dimension of our relationship. Until now we have been parents, now we are starting to be partners again (…).

Celina: (…) We are more connected by such a deep friendship, a very big one, than by some sexual impulses, I would say. (…) It's beautiful that we have gone from the raptures of falling in love, that is, these emotional things, to great, deep feelings and to friendship… I think that's how it is, that it's beautiful. (B_PL_2G)

Concerned that their relationship might be going in a different direction than they would have liked, the couple decided to do some conscious work on the evolution of their bond. They even took part in a workshop on partner relationships:

Celina: We're both in our fifties. And at that age, there's something that many relationships get to [where] the wife becomes such a housewife, she strokes her husband's head, and he becomes some kind of a child. And I didn't want that, (…) before we both digested it, understood it, we had such a month where…. we each analysed for ourselves how it was (…), and after that month it turned out that we needed it very much, it worked for us, and we grew much, much stronger together. (…) We even went on a course about partnerships and relationships in general. And that was a great help to us (…). (B_PL_2G)

As a result, they felt the need to renew their marriage vows. They did so informally, by the sea, just the two of them. It was a symbolic way of starting a new chapter in their relationship:

Celina: (…) we wrote such beautiful vows to each other, from the heart. And we read them to each other on this beach, and it was windy, and we were standing like this, imagine (…) It was such a meaningful moment… I've had two weddings before, but they can't compare to this moment (…) And it was beautiful, and we had our own wedding again, just the two of us. (B_PL_2G)

For some couples, the transition to the empty nest phase involves a process of relearning how to prioritise and nurture their romantic relationship, often marked by returning to past interests and emotions, while others may find it challenging to adjust to this new phase of their lives.

PRACTISING THE HONEYMOON SCENARIO

We have discussed released resources as the foundation of the "new honeymoon" scenario and three ways of constructing it. We will now focus on practising this relationship model, demonstrating in detail how couples reinforce or rediscover their bond. We will analyse two types of practices: sharing everyday activities and developing future projects.

Sharing Everyday Activities

The resources freed up by the children allow the parents to invest their time, money, and attention in activities they can do together. These might be walking (Teresa and Leszek, Felicja and Gustaw, Zofia and Leszek), cycling (Kazimierz and Krystyna), mushrooming (Magdalena and Stanisław), eating out (Cezary and Jadwiga), motorcycling (Clarisse and Sébastien), or other practices:

> Teresa: We have bought Nordic walking sticks and we go for walks, we bought bicycles some time ago, so we are trying to fill this free time and to spend it in as active a way as possible (…). (A_PL_5G)

> Krystyna: I'll say this—we can be more physically active now because when I come back from work I don't have to look after the kids, I just have to find time for a bike ride or something. That is a big change. (A_PL_12P)

> Zofia: Leszek calls and says, 'Listen, Zosia, let's go for a walk at 13:30 today. We have three hours (…) so we agree to spend this free time, which is scarce, together and we are very happy about it. (B_PL_3P)

> Cezary: My wife used to cook a lot. (…) And (…) now sometimes it's even like we're sitting together and she's like 'you know what, get dressed, we're going out for dinner' and we go out for dinner. (A_PL_27G)

Some couples found it necessary to give up or reduce activities they enjoyed. They replaced them with others in order to be able to share them with loved ones. Couples Magdalena and Stanisław and Jadwiga and Cezary show that when interests differ, one mechanism for increasing interdependence is to consider and compromise with the partner and their preferences:

Stanisław: I don't go fishing, do I? Because my wife doesn't like it.
Magdalena: But we go mushroom picking!
Stanisław: We love to go and pick mushrooms. But fishing, I don't leave her, I don't go fishing all Sunday (...) When we go to see my parents or her mother, we go together.
Magdalena: (...) If we go for a walk, we go together.
Stanisław: Or even sitting at home having a drink, we sit together. (A_PL_26G)

Jadwiga: (...) we don't do sports, I can't ride a bike anymore (...)
Cezary: And by myself it's somehow not [fun]... Because if my wife could still ride a bike, then maybe the two of us could do it...
Jadwiga: Yeah, we'd definitely go cycling.
Cezary: Not alone though (A_PL_27G)

While time and money are important resources in encouraging new or intensified shared practices, what's crucial is the relief from the stress, tension, and dilemmas that come with doing family activities. Sometimes, when done without the presence of children, the same activity suddenly feels very different. Eating, watching television, walking, and other everyday practices have become "peaceful" for Cezary and Jadwiga because the children are no longer the subject or catalyst for conflict. In addition, without giving attention and care to the children, and without feeling remorse for not involving them, the couple can immerse themselves in these activities. Jadwiga and Cezary can finally go for a walk without feeling that they should ask their daughters to join them. They can also watch movies without constant interruptions:

Cezary: (...). Here, you know, we are sitting in front of the television, and my wife is doing something. Well, if our daughters were here, there would always be some questions. We would have to give some answers.
Jadwiga: Yeah, maybe our remorse that we didn't take them with us, right?
Cezary: Well, because that often happened, didn't it? '(...)
Jadwiga: (...) And somehow it felt so stupid [to go alone]. (A_PL_27G)

Valérie and Eric enjoy their walks along the coast and cycling. Their attempts to engage in these activities before usually failed—their children preferred city walks:

Valérie: Well, it's true that I was more focused on going to the city with Léa. The nature stuff was a bit too much for them.

Eric: Yes, they wouldn't do it. (…) We have started to go cycling together again or go for walks on the coastal path. (A_FR_6)

Sharing does not necessarily have to mean a specific activity such as the ones mentioned above. Anna and Marcin demonstrate that observing the world together, an exchange of thoughts, are very important for couples who have a strong bond:

Anna: We like to look—at people, at the world. We like to think. (…)

Marcin: (…) the most painful thing is when we can't comment on something with each other face to face. (A_PL_12G)

It is also worth noting that sharing activities does not exclude leaving some space for individual interests and personal space. Proportions of couple time and individual time differ, but the crucial element is to find a balance that satisfies both parties. Irmina and Ksawery go shopping and cook together, watch movies, and enjoy their little trips. They also respect each other's need to spend time separately—when the husband works in his study, the wife reads or goes for a walk. "We feel very good with each other", they say.

Irmina: We watch [name of TV show] together. Or some good films.

Ksawery: We make dumplings together because that's what I often do and it's quicker when my wife helps me.

Irmina: Well, [we watch] some nice TV series, we always watch together. That's in the evenings. What else do we do together? We like to go out together. But during the day? My husband goes to the studio, and I sit, read or go to a concert, or go for a walk. (…) We go shopping together. (A_PL_30G)

Adam and Celina, who went on a relationship-related course, also found that time for oneself is important for them and that discovery helped them develop their bond:

Celina: And we noticed that it's very good to give ourselves a lot of space. (B_PL_2G)

For couples experiencing the empty nest phase, the freedom from parental responsibilities often leads to increased time, resources, and opportunities to engage in shared activities and strengthen their relationship, whether through physical activities, leisurely pursuits, or simply enjoying each other's company and personal space.

New Honeymoon as Joint Projects

Couples who enjoy doing everyday activities together may be able to strengthen or explore their relationship without having to introduce new projects into their lives. For some couples, however, new and unusual ventures are what attract them to this new phase of their lives. They give it new meaning and bring them together. Our interviewees engaged in various new projects: house renovations, long trips, summer houses, or moving house.

Eric and Delphine are planning a tour of France on electric bicycles, which they are in the process of buying:

> Eric: Then, as another project, we want to buy... both of us an electric bike (...). So we were thinking of rediscovering France on an electric bike (...).
> Delphine: This is our electric bike project. (A_FR_13)

They also dream of travelling to faraway places like the United States:

> Natalie: No, but another big project; it's our 30th anniversary. We said we would go...
> Eric: Maybe to the United States,
> Natalie: We talked about the American West, the big parks. That's a big project in the long run. But it has to happen before we're out of shape. (A_FR_13)

For some, the empty nest phase is the first time in their lives or the first opportunity in a long time to take a holiday together. For those who have travelled together in the past, it may be a time to go to places they did not visit when the children were at home. Holiday plans may include places that are further away, requiring financial and time resources that may have increased after the children moved out.

Magdalena: More castles to visit. I love castles. Well, it's that kind of further planning, that going away for weekends, exploring, being together. (...) It's such a break to visit something different. (...)

Stanisław: Well, I say, well, it's such a dream to go somewhere further away, to travel somewhere like that, isn't it? (A_PL_26G)

Marcin: To give you an example—at the moment we probably have the trip of a lifetime ahead of us, at least in terms of the financial burden and so on. We are going to the States. (A_PL_12G)

Many of the projects involve redesigning the family home. The family space can be renovated and even reorganised when the children leave. For Fabienne, who is inactive due to illness and whose children have left home, breakfast is the time when she meets her husband, who is still working, to discuss future projects.

Fabienne: We like to have breakfast together to talk about the next vacation... The next vacation, the news that we have children. Well, we're going to have a new kitchen installed, we've talked about it a lot before, and this time it's at breakfast, for example. (...) then in December, we will have for the first time in our life a kitchen arranged and equipped, here it is. And then in June, July, August and then the autumn which follows, we have the roof to redo, the bathroom (...). (A_FR_2)

A unique type of project is the purchase of a second house or plot of land, or even moving house.

Krystyna: But we have another passion—we bought a piece of land in [a rural area] and we go there at weekends. We have plans for what we want to do there, because it's a piece of land, some water and so on. Because we like to be outdoors, we like to ride our bikes somewhere, but we also like to go to the lake to swim and just sit there. (A_PL_12P)

Leszek: We had a goal, last year in May we bought this land, this year in November we are already going to be living there. So I guess this is kind of a life goal, this is kind of the next chapter of our life. I'm very happy about it and I think that's what the next decade of our life will be all about. (B_PL_3P)

These practices symbolically mark the transition to the next biographical phase. Just as young parents build the nest in preparation for a growing family, parents of adult children rearrange the nest to make room for the couple. Camille and Fabrice provide an illustration of this process. They are thinking about leaving the house in the country where their four children spent their childhood to settle closer to a big city. Their project includes children's visits, but does not put them at the centre. The couple is still two parents, but the emphasis is shifted towards the marital relationship.

> Fabrice: So we said to ourselves, maybe our next project will be to imagine our house (...) a house where we can live even when we are older, you know. Something (...) smaller, maybe, but modular at the same time, so we can still accommodate the children who visit, that's it. (A_FR_13)

The joint projects of couples are not without tensions, conflicts, or dilemmas. Sometimes they result from longer processes of negotiations. The development of joint projects also requires a reduction of interdependence with children and a focus on the couple, as the example of Magdalena and Stanisław shows. The decision about the sale of the family home is too difficult for them in this respect. Some time ago, the couple had a plan to move to a flat in a bigger city, to be closer to restaurants and cafes, but in the end they decided against it. Their house is like a refuge for their children, who like to visit and stay for longer periods, while the small size of the flat they were planning to buy might have discouraged the children from visiting.

> Magdalena: We even used to think about it, remember? When the kids had just moved out, that we'd sell the house and move into [...] a flat in a block, that it would be nice to go out somewhere, to a restaurant, to a pub in the evening, to go for a walk. Because that's what we used to do, that's how we felt free, when we were alone, to go for a walk, to go to a restaurant, to go to a pub, to go somewhere for a glass of wine! But then we found out that this house was a kind of refuge, a piece of land, a terrace. And the children, they're happy to come back here, they can barbecue and [how would they do that] there? (A_PL_26G)

Eric and his wife have similar dilemmas. On the one hand, they feel they should now be guided by their own needs and not those of their children. On the other hand, they would like their housing decision not to prevent their children from visiting them.

Eric: We don't want to live completely (...) far away from the children ()
[but] we don't want to build something according to the children. Because
they will live their lives (...) and at the same time we don't want to say "if
the children want to visit us, they have to travel 6 hours". (A_FR_ 13)

In the empty nest phase, couples often embark on new and meaningful
projects, such as house renovations, long trips, purchasing second homes,
or even moving to mark this transitional period and strengthen their relationship, with these endeavours requiring negotiation and adaptation to
the evolving dynamics of their family structure. In particular, new honeymoon couples consolidate around new "marital construction sites"
(Kaufmann, 2020) and find multiple ways to give meaning to the new
stage of life.

Conclusion

In this chapter, we have discussed the "new honeymoon" scenario, which
characterises couples who have used released temporal, financial, and
emotional resources to develop their relationship successfully. As we have
demonstrated, the transition to the empty nest phase is a complex process,
and couples may sometimes struggle before settling their new dyadic
arrangement. The transition process is certainly easier for couples who did
not "put their relationship on hold" after their children were born, but
found time for a conjugal relationship. In these cases, the children's departure feels less of a shock, and more like an evolution towards a new biographical stage or further development of the conjugal bond. Couples
whose lives revolved around the children need to relearn how to live
together when their major life project (raising the children) has ended. A
couple's past—recollections of romantic gestures and events—may help to
rebuild the bond, but it is usually necessary to add new elements to the
relationship. After many years, partners' needs and expectations of the
relationship have evolved, and a couple may need to adapt to a different
life stage. In addition, using resources from the past is possible if the couple had the opportunity to build a life without the children for some time
in their youth. In this respect, French and Polish couples differ. In France,
couples have more time to strengthen their dyadic relationship before having children. In Poland, in the generation we studied, it was common for
couples to decide to have a child more quickly. As a result, the couple was
quickly integrated into the broader family context.

In our analysis, we were also interested in how the couples use the resources freed up by the children and how they invest their time, money, and attention to strengthen their relationship. Some couples use the empty nest phase to develop bigger projects, such as long-distance trips, home renovations, and moving into a new house. Interestingly, however, in many cases, the activities have remained the same, but without the children's presence, they feel completely different. Without the tension created by children's needs and expectations, ordinary practices like walks or watching TV provide more comfort and relaxation.

It is worth noting that the process of relearning how to be a couple after many years of focusing on children may be a challenging task. One interviewed couple decided to attend a workshop that helped them understand their needs and how to communicate them. This example demonstrates that professional counselling may be very helpful for couples to strengthen their bond again in the empty nest phase.

Our study also demonstrates that the transition to the empty nest is a combination of mixed feelings, such as loss and relief, and enjoyment and guilt. The joy resulting from newly gained freedom merges with a sense of remorse when parents feel that proper fulfilment of the parental role should involve more of a sense of loss. In addition, reducing the interdependence between parents and children may last longer than expected. Moreover, the process of transition is not irreversible, and children sometimes return, which can disrupt the rebuilding of the couplehood.

References

Aquilino, W. S. (1997). From adolescent to young adult: A prospective study of parent-child relations during the transition to adulthood. *Journal of Marriage and Family, 59*(3), 670–686. https://doi.org/10.2307/353953

Bengtson, V. L., & Roberts, R. E. L. (1991). Intergenerational solidarity in aging families: An example of formal theory construction. *Journal of Marriage and Family, 53*(4), 856–870. https://doi.org/10.2307/352993

Bouchard, G. (2014). How do parents react when their children leave home? An integrative review. *Journal of Adult Development, 21*(2), 69–79. https://doi.org/10.1007/s10804-013-9180-8

Bouchard, G., & McNair, J. L. (2016). Dyadic examination of the influence of family relationships on life satisfaction at the empty-Nest stage. *Journal of Adult Development, 23*(3), 174–182. https://doi.org/10.1007/s10804-016-9233-x

Bozhenko, E. (2011). Adult child-parent relationships: On the problem of classification. *Procedia - Social and Behavioral Sciences, 30*, 1625–1629. https://doi.org/10.1016/j.sbspro.2011.10.315

Dare, J. S. (2011). Transitions in midlife women's lives: Contemporary experiences. *Health Care for Women International, 32*(2), 111–133. https://doi.org/10.1080/07399332.2010.500753

Elder, G. H. (1985). Perspectives on the life course. In *Life course dynamics: Trajectories and transitions* (1st ed., pp. 23–49). Cornell University Press.

Elder, G. H. (1994). Time, human agency, and social change: Perspectives on the life course. *Social Psychology Quarterly, 57*(1), 4–15. https://doi.org/10.2307/2786971

Elder, G. H. (Ed.). (1999). *Children of the great depression. Social change in life experience* (25th ed.). Routledge.

Finch, J. (2007). Displaying families. *Sociology, 41*(1), 65–81. https://doi.org/10.1177/0038038507072284

Giraud, C., & de Singly, F. (2012). *En famille à Paris*. Armand Colin.

Kaufmann, J.-C. (2020). Solidarność i zaufanie w parze. *Fabrica Societatis, 3*(2020), 35–40. https://doi.org/10.34616/129166

Konietzka, D., & Kreyenfeld, M. (2021). Life course sociology: Key concepts and applications in family sociology. In I. N. Schneider & M. Kreyenfeld (Eds.), *Research handbook on the sociology of the family* (pp. 73–87). Edward Elgar Publishing.

Lück, D., Ruckdeschel, K., Dechant, A., & Schneider, N. F. (2021). Family demography and values in Europe: Continuity and change. In A.-M. Castrén, V. Cesnuityte, I. Crespi, J.-A. Gauthier, R. Gouveia, C. Martin, A. Moreno Mínguez, & K. Suwada (Eds.), *The Palgrave handbook of family sociology in Europe* (pp. 85–106). Palgrave Macmillan.

Mitchell, B. A., & Lovegreen, L. D. (2009). The empty Nest syndrome in midlife families: A multimethod exploration of parental gender differences and cultural dynamics. *Journal of Family Issues, 30*(12), 1651–1670. https://doi.org/10.1177/0192513X09339020

Silverstein, M., & Bengtson, V. (1997). Intergenerational solidarity and the structure of adult child–parent relationships in American families. *American Journal of Sociology, 103*(2), 429–460. https://doi.org/10.1086/231213

Trommsdorff, G. (2006). Parent-child relations over the life-span. A cross-cultural perspective. In K. H. Rubin & O. B. Chung (Eds.), *Parenting beliefs, behaviors, and parent-child relations. A cross-cultural perspective* (pp. 143–183). Psychology Press.

Widmer, E. D. (2021). Family diversity in a configurational perspective. In N. Schneider & M. Kreyenfeld (Eds.), *Research handbook on the sociology of the family* (pp. 60–72). Edward Elgar.

CHAPTER 10

Redefining a Couple's Relationship in the Empty Nest: Together Apart

Marta Skowrońska, Filip Schmidt, Christophe Giraud, and Magdalena Żadkowska

INTRODUCTION[1]

In this chapter, we closely examine one of the trajectories that a couple may follow in the empty nest phase. In this scenario, the children's departure deprives parents of the major project they had been running together and reveals their otherwise weak bond.

---

[1] More theretical background to this chapter is found in Chap. 9.

M. Skowrońska (✉) • F. Schmidt
Faculty of Sociology, Adam Mickiewicz University, Poznań, Poland
e-mail: marta.skowronska@amu.edu.pl; fschmidt@amu.edu.pl

C. Giraud
Centre de recherche sur les liens sociaux (CERLIS, UMR 8070), Université Paris Cité, Paris, France
e-mail: christophe.giraud@parisdescartes.fr

© The Author(s), under exclusive license to Springer Nature Switzerland AG 2024
M. Żadkowska et al. (eds.), *Reconfiguring Relations in the Empty Nest*, Palgrave Macmillan Studies in Family and Intimate Life, https://doi.org/10.1007/978-3-031-50403-7_10

In family studies, the empty nest phase has been a subject of considerable exploration, with researchers traditionally focusing on how it affects spousal relationships, as well as overall life satisfaction (Mitchell & Lovegreen, 2009; Bouchard, 2014). They have sought to determine whether these changes lead to improvements or deterioration in these aspects of life. Another stream of research focuses on the transformation of the parent–children relationship (Aquilino, 1997; Bozhenko, 2011). In this chapter, we offer an alternative perspective. Rather than isolating these aspects, we view it as a complex transformation involving two interdependent relationship types: parents and children, and romantic partners. This approach highlights that changes in these relationships mutually influence one another, often resulting in diverse and sometimes conflicting emotions.

In contrast to the Actor-Partner Interdependence Model (Bouchard & McNair, 2016), which is rooted in game theory and social exchange theory and defines relationships in terms of satisfaction, our perspective defines interdependence as a process established through daily habitual practices. In this regard, we draw inspiration from the intergenerational solidarity model (Bengtson & Roberts, 1991; Silverstein & Bengtson, 1997) and the work of Widmer (2021), who describe family as a network of mutually oriented and functionally dependent individuals. Interdependence reflects how one member's actions significantly affect others within this network. This perspective emphasises that conjugal relationships should be understood within a broader relational context, acknowledging the influence of relatives, friends, and social networks. The patterns of these interdependencies, rather than household composition, shape family dynamics and foster a collective identity (Widmer, 2021).

The interdependence we discuss involves the substantial influence of one family member's decisions and actions on others within the family unit. Our objective is to analyse the transformation of relationships

M. Żadkowska
Social Sciences Department (Institute of Sociology), University of Gdańsk, Gdańsk, Poland

Centre de recherche sur les liens sociaux (CERLIS, UMR 8070), Université Paris Cité, Paris, France
e-mail: magdalena.zadkowska@ug.edu.pl

between spouses and between parents and their adult children while recognising the intricate web of interdependencies that characterises family life. Instead of relying solely on arbitrary measurement scales, we employ a qualitative approach to uncover manifestations of interdependence. These manifestations encompass various facets, including emotional bonds, material support, and shared practices. Through this multifaceted examination, we hope to shed light on the nuanced dynamics of family relationships during critical life transitions.

Our theoretical proposal introduces four model scenarios for postparental couples during the empty nest phase. These scenarios consider the levels of interdependence between spouses and between parents and children following their children's departure:

- Type I (together/apart): Weak interdependence between the parental couple and children and between the spouses.
- Type II (honeymoon): Strong interdependence between the parental couple and weak with their children.
- Type III (dissolved in the family): Weak interdependence between the parental couple but strong interdependence with their children.
- Type IV (parents and partners): Couples that maintain intense levels of interdependence with each other and their children.

In this chapter, we examine in detail Type I, "together/apart", which refers to couples whose interdependence has weakened after their children's departure. This model bears a resemblance to "living together apart" (LTA), a situation of estranged couples who carry on living under the same roof despite their desire to separate (Martin et al., 2011). However, the significant difference between the analysed model and LTA lies in whether the partners see themselves as a couple. While the LTA do not consider themselves in a relationship (some are divorced), together apart couples do. LTA primarily refers to situations where two adults continue to live together for financial reasons, housing difficulties, and sometimes "for the children's benefit" while defining each other as "roommates" or "tenants" (Ibidem). In this chapter, however, we will analyse married couples who continue to consider themselves spouses but whose level of interdependence is low and restricted only to some aspects.

In our analysis we draw upon 75 couples' interviews (dyadic in-depth interviews, corpus A) and 45 individual interviews with select spouses (corpus B). Our analysis involved individual coding with MAXQDA.

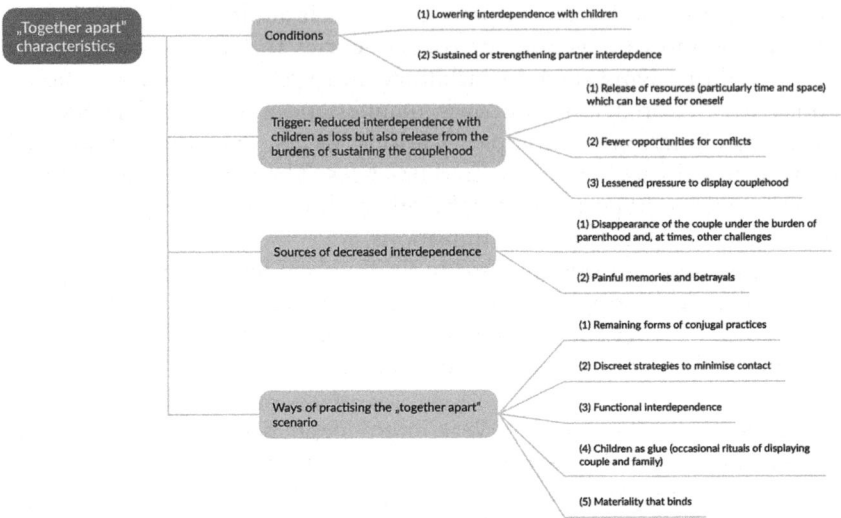

Fig. 10.1 Characteristics of the "together apart" scenario

First, we describe how reduced interdependence with children is experienced as a loss, but also frees the couple from some of the burdens of maintaining couplehood, reduces the opportunities for conflicts, and lessens the pressure to display couple. We then move to indicate the sources of low partner interdependence, which often are to be found in a quick disappearance of the couple under the burden of either parenthood or painful memories. Finally, we describe five dominant ways of practising the "together apart" scenario, which hold the couple together which are based on basic forms of conjugal practices, functional and material interdependence, but also discreet strategies of minimising contact and rare famiy reunions (Fig. 10.1).

THE SPECIFICITY OF THE TOGETHER APART SCENARIO

In another chapter of this book, we analysed couples who reconverted parental time into conjugal time after the children's departure. This chapter examines couples who have not used released resources to develop their relationship, while the interdependence with children has significantly weakend after their departure. Parenthood united the couple and gave them a sense of purpose and a joint project. The empty nest phase revealed how little they had in common beyond that. For years, the life of together apart couples revolved around the children—parents were busy taking care of them, talking about them, arguing with or about them. Children were the project that the spouses shared. Couplehood moved to the background, declining with time. The quotation below is an extreme example of this process. Emanuelle realises that her marriage existed only as a part of the family structure and never as an independent dyad:

> Emanuelle: We don't have time [as a couple] any more. In fact, we never had time for ourselves; we never took the time to have [uh] moments to ourselves; we never did.[2]

In some cases, the relationship was affected by difficult events and situations, which still hurt. In others, it is impossible to distinguish one particular factor. What unites all together apart couples is that the children's departure reveals the poor condition of the relationship, but the spouses stay together, nevertheless. This chapter will explore how the relationship is maintained despite difficulties and how the spouses lead almost parallel lives while displaying couplehood (Finch, 2007) to others.

The model scenario discussed in this chapter may only be a period of a longer process, which can move in different directions. Sometimes the couple has lived parallel lives for years, even with the children under their roof, but they managed to conceal it. Sometimes taking care of the children was a firmly uniting task, and only the empty nest displayed the otherwise weak levels of interdependence. In such cases, the departure of the children may come as a shock that even questions the point of the couple's existence. The future of these couples may also vary. When all aspects of interdependence (even financial/material) vanish, this scenario may finally lead to a separation or a divorce (see Chap. 11). However (at least theoretically), partners may overcome the crisis and find, for example, an activity they enjoy. Shared practices may strengthen the emotional aspects of interdependence. In some cases, the couple may thus move into the "new honeymoon" scenario (II). We should also emphasise that we are analysing model scenarios, whereas, in reality, couples may dynamically oscillate between different models, bearing the characteristics of more than one type.

---

[2] In this chapter, we do not use references that identify the corpus to which the interview belongs, that is, the codes used in the previous chapters. This decision stems from the particularly sensitive nature of the subject of analysis.

MORE RESOURCES, FEWER OBLIGATIONS

As the children's departure is a revelation of the state of the relationship, it might seem that the couple's experience will be one of loss rather than relief. But as we have noted before, feelings of loss and relief are not mutually exclusive; all parents experience some combination of both. Sadness and longing mix with a rest from responsibilities and tensions, as in Weronika's narrative below:

> Weronika: Not having to worry about cooking, whether the shopping is done, whether the fridge's full or not. If it's not (full), it's not a tragedy. I have peace of mind. But there is sadness because Maja is not here.

We will now analyse three aspects of relief: more individual time and space for the spouses, less conflict between the spouses, and no longer needing to display couplehood.

Departure as a Relief: More Time and Space for Oneself

We have already stated that the departure of children releases various types of resources: financial, temporal, emotional, and physical, which brings a sense of relief. As one of the interviewees, Anna, observes:

> Anna: It is certainly the case that you're more relaxed; you don't have to worry. You don't have to think about what to make for dinner, because even if there is no dinner, well, my husband will have whatever, a fried egg.

The main difference between new honeymoon and together apart couples is that the latter use the freed-up resources for individual benefit rather than strengthening their marital relationship:

> Katarzyna: It's as if the duties are over, the task is done, and everyone somehow runs off in their own direction into their other needs and interests.

Although there is more time and opportunity to be together as a couple, this opportunity is not exploited, Helena observes:

> Helena: Well... you seem to have more time, right? And just more opportunities, but we don't seem to use them, to be honest.

Relief comes from not feeling obliged to do anything. Parents no longer have to adjust their schedules to meet their children's needs and expectations. Even adult children demanded attention and support. Parents dropped them off, picked them up, did the shopping, planned and prepared meals, and spent time listening to and advising them:

Interviewer: Now that Zuza has moved out, do you have more time for yourself?

Felicja: Definitely, yes, yes. She was a very absorbing child, very absorbing in general. (...)

Researcher: Even when she was an adult before she moved out, those last years, was her presence here absorbing? (...)

Kazik: It was because you had to go and pick her up after a concert... Because of this, because of that.

In the past, parents often rushed home from work to eat a family meal:

Sebastian: Your family is waiting at home, so you are in a hurry. You go back and do what you can to get away faster, to get home from Cracow or wherever.

Children's presence was a glue that bound the family together. Their presence forced parents to sit down to shared meals. Today, a lack of this pressure brings relief, which may also mix with sadness and a sense of loss:

Weronika: There was dinner; dinner was waiting for dad, we were waiting for dad, well... Well, it's not like that now; it's changed. She kept us together, didn't she? Well, now she doesn't.

Cassandra: He can work even later hours. So he doesn't have to make excuses. I don't put pressure on him anymore (...) because the children are no longer here, so it isn't really a big deal for me. (...) When the children were here, it was a point of honour for me that we at least had dinner together.

The end of parental work reduces conjugal obligation in couples who exist mainly through their parental role and do not wish for or cannot reconvert this commitment into a marital one. The released resources are used to develop personal interests, as in the example below. Partners drift apart, but they mainly accept this fact:

> Felicja: We also live apart sometimes. I go away a lot. Actually, I go away every month, I go away for a week, two weeks (…) But he's fine at home alone, so to speak—no one bothers him, no one disturbs him.

Problems appear when partners have not developed any interests or passions—either shared or personal. If life focused entirely on the children, their departure brought mostly loss, as in the example below. Marta and Kazik felt a sense of emptiness after their children left home, as they had never had the chance to focus on themselves:

> Marta: In retrospect, I look at it as if our lives revolve around the children, and once the children are gone, it somehow ends.

Another challenge relates to differences between the partners regarding individual and shared time (independence vs interdependence). Maria and Wojciech's individual interviews provide two entirely different pictures of their relationship. The wife seems content with the current state of their relationship. She does not mind separate bedrooms and meals and focuses on developing her artistic passions, using the released space to realise her needs:

> Maria: I am in full bloom now—I am still young enough to be active professionally for many more years, so I can do many projects. (…) Sometimes we sit together and watch something, or each of us does something, but most of the time we're in our own rooms (…) each of us plans our own activities or hobbies (…) When my daughter moved out, we got our own living space, which we'd been missing all our lives. And at the moment I can say, for my part, that I am very happy with it. (…) Sometimes there are days when we hardly talk at all because we just pass each other by. (…) But it is also good to be alone.

On the other hand, her husband Wojciech is disappointed and frustrated by this relationship model. Although he also focuses on his interests, he does so with the feeling that he has no other choice:

> Wojciech: And there are days when my wife and I just say the proverbial "hello", right? And that's it. (…) Well, that's how we live: as flatmates, so to speak. It's sad for me. I don't know, the impression I get from my wife is that it suits her.

As we have demonstrated, together apart couples also experience relief, which results from increased time and financial resources along with a reduction in caregiving responsibilities. However, these newfound resources tend to be directed towards individual pursuits rather than strengthening the marital bond. Moreover, the extent of this relief varies depending on whether the partners have cultivated personal interests and their expectations regarding the relationship.

Departure as a Relief: Fewer Conflicts

Another source of relief comes from the lack of tension. Children's presence intensified interactions between the partners, who sometimes differed in their parental attitudes and values, and who often felt tired of negotiating various parental decisions. The quotation below demonstrates a typical quarrel between parents—when one accuses the child of something, and the other defends them. This pattern of fighting disappears when the child moves out of the house:

> Felicja: It's calmer now. There's no trigger...
> Kazik: Between you and me—that one is an attacker, one is a defender of the child and "what do you want from her" etc. (...)
> Felicja: And when she left, I said, honestly, Kazik, you could have...— and then we started. It continued. Now, because there are no more such issues, it's quieter.

Even when the parents were on the same side, some disputes—between brothers and sisters or between the children and the parents—affected the whole family structure. Releasing such tensions brings relaxation while reducing the intensity of interaction between the parents:

> Sebastian: When I look at it, there used to be such arguments, we used to shout, (...) there were such arguments. And now days are much quieter.
> Patrycja: The brats would sometimes put us on the spot, and you had to react; it would get in the way, and we'd have these discussions in a raised tone.
> Sebastian: Well, yes, such family quarrels.
> Patrycja: I don't want to argue anymore.

Similarly to other aspects of relief, this one may be mixed with loss—particularly when discussing various children-related issues was the primary interaction between a couple. Weronika admits with bitterness in the quotation below that she and her husband stopped quarrelling. Without their daughter, the couple hardly ever has a conversation, friendly or otherwise; they are "neither together nor apart":

> Weronika: And no, we don't have any arguments about it right now. No, no. We don't have any fights now (…). Each of us does their own thing. Or we do things together when we feel like it. My husband has gone into social activities, and as I said, I've gone into being alone (…) Well, but that's the way it is; we're neither together nor apart.

Hence, although the reduction in conflicts brings relief, it also signifies a broader decline in partner interactions, which can lead to feelings of emptiness.

Departure as a Relief: No Need to Display Couplehood

The absence of children significantly reduces the obligation to be a couple, previously manifested in various moments of everyday life. Without the need to display couplehood on a daily basis, the partners may also feel relieved. They don't have to eat together; they don't have to plan things together when no one is watching:

> Weronika: she has moved out, and now she is not at home, we don't have to pretend anything. (…) For example, we don't have to pretend that it's cool or warm when it's not, do we? Because it's not.

However, interdependence with the children does not disappear completely, which is an important reason why some together apart couples do not break up completely. We will discuss this further in the section "Practising parallel lives".

TRAJECTORIES OF COUPLES WITH WEAK INTERDEPENDENCE

While "honeymoon couples" may try to return to their past to search for the foundation of their bond, together apart couples do not like to recollect their past. In many cases, memories are painful. Recalling the past was a difficult part of the interviews, and details were rarely revealed to the researchers. Weronika's husband's affair of years ago still casts a shadow on the relationship. Jakub and Anna grew apart because of the time and effort the husband devoted to his ill grandmother, neglecting his wife and kids. Anna recalls:

Anna: When he leaves each weekend for a whole day, it's not... When he leaves once a week during such a difficult period, it's certainly... it's sort of forced me to begin to distance myself and organise this free day on my own, hasn't it?

Yet another couple experienced a crisis related to the husband's excessive workload. In other cases, partners cannot point to one event or specific reason for their relationship deteriorating:

Katarzyna: It's not because of anything that's happened. No, it's just that there are so many threads, and one by one, they start to break.

While the exact reasons may differ, couples often repeat several themes when discussing how their relationship developed. We will now present two cases from Poland, where relationship trajectories are very similar. Both couples (Felicja and Kazik and Weronika and Błażej) experienced a long period of partying, travelling, and romantic experiences before their children were born:

Felicja: Back then, we had the same lifestyle, you know, when it was just the two of us—we'd go away, have a weekend, go abroad, go to Prague, Italy, relax, you know—come home from work, have dinner or go to the cinema or go out on the town.

Weronika: My husband was a terribly social soul. We met on a trip; he was playing on his guitar (...)
   Błażej: I don't play it anymore. It gets dusted off at Christmas.
   Weronika: It was a very happy... apart from my struggle to have a baby (...), it was a very happy time.

Both couples experienced a considerable change in their lives after the birth of their children. Marked by illnesses and stress, the early years of parenthood were an enormous challenge. The various problems that couples encountered required them to sacrifice and give up their needs—particularly time for themselves as a couple. All their attention was focused on their children's upbringing. Weronika and Błażej struggled to have a child—long infertility treatment seriously affected the woman's health. She then suffered from postpartum depression. The couple's daughter became a sensitive child with sleeping problems:

> Weronika: I was also on drugs that weakened me, that destroyed me (...). I was so scared after the birth. In fact, I remember it now as a kind of postpartum depression. (...) I sat by the cot and looked to see if she was breathing.

> Weronika: She did not always want to sleep in her own room. She was so sensitive that it was difficult to put her to bed at night.

Felicja and Kazik's daughter's illnesses were frequent and severe, often requiring hospital treatment. Her health meant that the mother had to give up work, which contributed to her frustration and worsened the family's financial situation:

> Felicja: She got sick frequently and needed a lot of care—hospitalisation, because she got [illness description], (...) I have to be honest, I experienced [a lot] in that first period...
> Kazik: My life was turned upside down, and on top of that my wife was (...) out of work for six years.
> Felicja: I had to quit work (...).
> Kazik: She was on unpaid leave, so the finances worsened; let's not fool ourselves. (...)

In this period, conflicts began to arise. In the case of Felicja and Kazik, three issues came to the fore: differences in the approach to bringing up the children, working away from home, and the lack of support felt by one of the spouses. These problems are also repeated in other couples' narratives:

> Kazik: My relationship with my daughter, for instance, between the ages of 8 and 15, was somewhat diminished because I was working away from home, only coming home for weekends. (...)
> Felicja: Let's say it started to loosen up when Zuza started to get sick, and you thought I was making it up. And in general, I didn't feel any support from him, and I became distant because of that. And in general, with these problems, with the whole Zuza thing, I was alone (...) because he didn't see the problem, etc., etc., so he also isolated himself a bit.

In the case of Błażej and Weronika, the lack of support was compounded by a lack of trust. The husband betrayed his wife and moved out with his lover, resulting in the wife and daughter's mental health problems. After several months, the husband and father returned to his family, but his relationship with his wife remained tense:

> Weronika: (…) Well, he moved out with another woman.
> Interviewer: And this shocked your daughter, you said…?
> Weronika: Yes, she then got obsessive-compulsive disorder. Very serious.

When the children moved out, the two analysed relationships were already in a bad state. Unpleasant memories and unhealed wounds had distanced the spouses from each other. They have been drifting further and further apart for years, and the differences between their temperaments, tastes, and interests had widened:

> Weronika: We have a bit of an unfortunate situation in our marriage. It has only become apparent over time that we have different needs.

> Kazik: Yes, we are together, but a bit apart. (…)
> Felicja: I mean, we generally have different ways of spending our free time. I'm a very active person, and my husband is more of a couch potato.

While the two presented cases are not universal, they repeatedly demonstrate occurring elements of the together apart couples' trajectories. After their children are born, couples largely or entirely focus on them, sacrificing their needs and neglecting their own relationship. Other challenges—working away from home, financial difficulties, children's illnesses, and the necessity to look after elderly parents—add to the problems experienced by young parents. Differences in parenting attitudes and a perceived lack of support by one of the partners also make the spouses drift apart.

While in all cases, the children's departure reveals the poor condition of the relationship, couples differ regarding the intensity of this experience. If the spouses had already developed their own interests and learnt to live "together but a bit apart", the departure is not felt like a shock. If the partners (or one of them) concentrated on children right up to their moving out, the empty nest phase might be a challenge, at least at first. In most together apart couples in our sample, including the two cases examined above, the transition to the empty nest involved a sense of sadness and resignation rather than shock.

Anna openly admits that her relationship was in a bad state before, and she had already managed to develop a new form of being together—living parallel lives:

Anna: My life wouldn't change much [if i divorced]. Because I had/I've already arranged my life in such a way that I'm kind of living [my life] under the same roof, yes?

Similarly, for Lothaire and his wife Angèle, their two daughters' departure brought little change in their daily activities, which were already very separate:

Lothaire: We are not people who go out much... Museums, things like that, we never did... (...) most of our free time, [Angèle] spends in the garden, and I spend on the computer, to repair them, to... (...) it hasn't changed much.

Sandra uses the metaphor "fellow travellers" to describe the process of the couple drifting apart and finding their own paths. Long before the children were gone, the couple had learned to focus on their personal interests rather than couple activities and projects:

Sandra: We learned to be very independent of each other, and as I was telling you, since he's never here on weekends [his games are on weekends], if I didn't want to stay at home, I would do this, I would do that, I'm used to doing things alone, I'm not dependent on him at all to be happy.
Lothaire: Yes, yes.
Sandra: It's horrible what I'm saying, but that's what it is, we are fellow travellers.

However, the children's departure occasionally led to a sudden realisation of the state of the relationship. In the cases of Katarzyna and Olek, as well as Cassandra and Théo, women were very involved in family life, contrary to their husbands. As a result, they have not developed individual activity patterns and felt much more loss than relief in the transition process. In the full nest phase, women fought to increase their husbands' presence and involvement in family life and sometimes succeeded. Now that the children are gone, the house feels completely empty. The women's intense work is no longer needed. Both husbands distance themselves even more and provide no support to their wives:

Katarzyna: My husband was so much more involved (at work) because he was running his own business, so I was very much living the lives of the children. Some extra activities, windsurfing, judo, English, birthdays (...).

There was so much of that, practically every day, that I didn't have any space of my own (…). We did more shared activities [with the children]. And now it's like: If we don't have that, we don't even want to cook for each other.

Cassandra: For the last twenty years (…) I've been thinking about the others and only after that myself behind. So that means that when suddenly I find myself without my children, it's a shock because I have to think about myself because it's something I don't know how to do any more (…) and the person most likely to understand me, to listen to me and to feel and share my sadness and my loneliness, didn't [support me].

In summary, together apart couples tend to have complex trajectories marked by early challenges in their relationships exacerbated by the demands of parenting. Their children's departure often reveals the underlying issues and differing interests that have kept them somewhat apart, leading to feelings of sadness and resignation rather than shock. The cases of shock were exceptional and involved individuals deeply absorbed in family life, preventing them from recognising earlier signs of a relationship crisis.

Practising Parallel Lives

Why do together apart couples remain couples? While their general level of interdependence is low, some of its aspects protect the spouses from a break-up. Our study demonstrates that there are several such aspects. Couples still share some elements of their everyday lives. After years of living together, they have developed habitual practices that provide them with security and comfort. Moreover, their household is a well-functioning mechanism that they both sustain—each spouse has their duties and is experienced in performing them. Another aspect of interdependence is contact with their children, which can cement an otherwise weak relationship and provide an opportunity to "display family" to others. Financial/material interdependence is also the glue that binds the couple together.

Everyday Activities

The fundamental characteristic of everyday life is its routinised, automated, and intuitive character. By reproducing their daily practices, couples developed routine and regularity, which are sources of comfort and security. Choosing a well-trodden path feels more accessible and convenient than forging a new one. One interviewee, Sebastian, admits that comfort and habit are essential factors that keep his relationship, even if "deep retrospection" could lead to undermining the sense of the relationship:

> Sebastian: Well, you know, it's not the same feeling as 20 years ago (...) after the years together, well, there are other factors, well, comfort, habit. If you looked inside yourself and did a deep introspection and asked yourself that honest question, you would come up with a couple of things, yeah?

Spouses may also fear that separation would make everyday life more difficult, as Weronika does:

> Interviewer: Do you think it would be more difficult for you on your own?
> Weronika: I believe so. I think it would be.

We will examine the reasons for these difficulties, analysing two aspects of interdependence: remaining forms of conjugal practices and functional interdependence.

Remaining Forms of Conjugal Practices

In all the narratives of together apart couples, three activities were most commonly practised together, even if sporadically or in a restricted form: having meals, going on trips or holidays, and watching TV. Couples do not eat together daily, but they usually have a specific meal-related habit that has persisted despite their generally limited amount of shared activities. Felicja and Kazik, for example, mostly eat apart and have different dietary preferences, but they both enjoy and prepare several fish and vegetarian dishes together, which seemingly are comfort food to them:

> Felicja: But we do fish things together, some salmon—we have our flagship dish, and we actually make that together. We also prepare other things together—risotto, stuff like that.
> Kazik: But we both like herings, for example. If there are herrings, we eat it together.

Weronika and Błażej, who hardly ever sit together during the week, continue to have the weekend meals they used to have with their children.

While new honeymoon couples enjoy the new, dyadic form of the meal, together apart couples see it as just a continuation of family tradition, a remnant of an earlier ritual:

> Weronika: Saturday, Sunday, dinner is always like in the old days, we used to eat with Maja, now we eat together, that's how it is.

Together apart couples usually underline that their shared meals are radically less frequent but have not entirely disappeared. Maria and Wojciech, who hardly ever see each other during the week, regularly have lunch together at weekends:

> Wojciech: It varies. At the weekend, mostly. At weekends mostly just lunch. I'm talking about one meal daily, so at weekends it's lunch.

Eating out is also one of the things that people prefer not to do alone, just like going on vacation. It seems more convenient for couples to organise a trip together, just as they used to do. However, spending several days side by side can also be challenging when the relationship is in a bad state. In some cases, couples book two separate rooms. Felicja and Kazik justify this decision by referring to the problem of snoring:

> Felicja: We went to [a seaside village] two years ago. We were alone for a week.
> Interviewer: And what was it like?
> Kazik: Well, two separate rooms... unfortunately, I snore terribly.

Edyta and Kamil continue to go on holidays, although before their daughter's departure, they always travelled with her and never wanted to go alone. Throughout the entire period of parenthood, the couple only went somewhere without their child once—to a wedding reception. They now encourage their daughter to join them wherever they go, sometimes successfully:

> Edyta: Well, we were hoping she would come too.
> Kamil: It didn't work out.
> Edyta: Well, because two years ago (...) she did.

In cases of more profound relationship crisis, a holiday together—without other people, forcing a close examination of the state of the relationship—may be too challenging, as in the case of Anna and Jakub. Anna openly admits:

> Anna: I do not enjoy going on holiday with just my husband.

At the same time, going away alone is also challenging and involves various dilemmas that we will analyse in the following sections. Watching television and discussing political problems (provided the couple's political views are similar) is safer:

> Weronika: We like to talk about politics, for example. We watch political programmes because we share the same views. So this is also our platform for conversation.

> Jakub: If it's a ritual, it's more like we sit at 8 pm and watch news.
> Anna: Yeah, yeah.
> Jakub: (…) if somebody's late, you pause, you wait, and you have to sit together (…) and talk about it (…) well, it might not be a meal, but it's something.
> Anna: Yeah, it's a ritual.

In the narratives of together apart couples, despite their limited shared activities, three practices remained somewhat consistent: having meals, going on trips or holidays, and watching TV, signifying a continuation of family traditions rather than newfound intimacy.

Discreet Strategies to Minimise Contact

Couples who are together despite an apparent crisis oscillate between the need to be together in specific contexts and the desire to be apart and escape from their dyadic interaction. While they occasionally share a meal, a conversation or a moment of television, they also use discreet strategies to avoid excessive co-presence. The most popular method is working late:

> Katarzyna: My husband is rarely at home. Primarily he's working, (…) I think that's where he has his space, where he escapes, a kind of solitude (…) I am basically non-stop at work; I just can't imagine what I would do [without it].

Weronika: We've drifted apart a bit in how we spend our time. My husband has got into workaholism and social activities.

The most explicit about their dissatisfaction, Jakub and Anna, use various strategies to sustain the status quo without confronting their relationship's status (which would be "a big threat", Anna admits). They bought a dog, which the woman interprets as a "safety valve" as it gave the couple a legitimate reason not to go on holiday:

Jakub: We are not leaving because we have a dog, and there is no one to leave him with! (...).

Anna: Well, I don't know if it was on purpose, so that there would be an argument that we cannot go anywhere because now we have to take care of the dog, that it was a kind of safety valve so that the marriage would continue to function in the way it did. Because what if suddenly we were here alone and had to take care of ourselves? I think that could be a big threat to the relationship.

The pet adds to the long working hours, leaving the couple hardly any time together at home. When the husband is back from work, he is served dinner by Anna (eats alone), and right afterwards he leaves for a two- to three-hour walk with the dog. Anna feels safe—she's released from the necessity to spend time with her partner, while at the same time the reason for his absence is known and legitimate ("it's not like he's gone just anywhere"):

Anna: we all work long hours, so when my husband comes home at 6–7 pm, that's when he gets home (...) he eats his meal, but then he goes for a two-hour walk with the dog, so he's gone again, but it's not like he's gone anywhere, I just know he's gone with the dog so that I can do something else.

In addition to their workload and the dog, the couple has yet another "safety valve" (this time even defined as "luxury")—the husband spends one day of the weekend looking after his elderly mom:

Anna: At the same time, I still have the luxury, so to speak, that my husband has to look after his mother, so he is either out all day on Sunday or out all day on Saturday, so we basically have one day a week to spend together.

In this way, the couple is left with one hour together each day (spent on watching the news) and one day of the weekend, when they mostly find individual activities and do housework, which is analysed in the next section.

Functional Interdependence

Another binding element of everyday life is household duties, which couples share. The distribution of tasks and the fact that the partners have been doing the same jobs for years form a smoothly functioning household:

> Interviewer: And did you have anything that was a connecting element between you? Did you meet somewhere along the way?
> Kazik: Well, shopping.
> Felicja: Living together in the same house. The only thing we actually agreed on was shopping for the flat, some stuff here, appliances...

Sometimes, the role distribution persists even if other practice elements have vanished. Anna always cooked dinners for the family; her husband never learned how to cook. After the children's departure, the institution of shared meals has almost entirely disappeared. Although the couple does not eat together, the wife still cooks and serves dinner to her husband, who mostly eats it alone. She sits down for a little while as if suggesting that the ritual is complete and then leaves:

> Anna: We continue to have these rituals, that I make dinner, serve dinner, but to this day I have something like this, that if he comes back and I happen to be doing something of my own, I don't know, on the computer, reading or something, then I serve him dinner, but I don't sit with him while he eats, do I? I mean I do for a while, but then he finishes it by himself because he eats it for a long time and I get bored here.

Two individuals who perform their duties separately may maintain a smoothly running household according to a well-known pattern. These activities' repetitive and embodied nature may be a source of comfort. However, the division of tasks sometimes involves tensions. In the case of Edyta and Kamil, the inequality of this division has persisted for years and is unlikely to change. Although the wife is irritated that more work falls to her, the couple replicates the established pattern:

Kamil: I mean, my cooking skills are such that I can boil water.

Edyta: (...) My husband mainly takes care of the central heating so that the hot water is there. And the rest I do.

Kamil: I drive; I do the shopping.

Interestingly, however, in several cases, the departure of children helped partners realise the amount of inequality in sharing domestic tasks (in all cases, women were more burdened). With the children gone, women felt they could cook or clean less than before. In some cases (i.e. Jakub and Anna or Kazik and Felicja), it only meant that they worked less, while their husbands did the same amount, and the cooking or cleaning standards dropped. Yet, there were also situations when husbands got more involved in domestic tasks:

Patrycja: I used to do everything, both cooking and cleaning, and he rarely did. And now, for example, it is normal for me to leave the kitchen when we have finished eating and go into the living room, because we eat in the kitchen when there are just two of us, and he cleans up. (B_PL_11P).

Weronika: Housework, has anything changed? No, no, we share, my husband has taken over more.

New arrangements and modifications in domestic tasks can easily involve tensions, as in the case of Claude and Ambre. Despite her husband's slightly greater involvement in domestic duties, the division of labour appears unjust to Ambre. She feels burdened with the role of the household manager who continuously distributes tasks and has to give instructions:

Claude: I do everything that Ambre doesn't do.

Ambre: That's it. Well, he's getting off his ass a little more than before.

Interviewer: Oh yeah?

Claude: Well, I do the dishes.

Ambre: Yeah, that, on the other hand, he clears the table in the evening, and he cleans up because I make dinner. But no, I think I still do a lot of, um... You see, I can start cooking, he's not going to ask me "well, do you want a hand?". No, he'll be on his computer, you know. (...) it pisses me off because it's always me who has to ask.

Couples continue to share household duties, primarily for the sake of maintaining a well-functioning household, as it is more convenient to preserve existing routines than to undertake significant changes.

Children as Glue/Displaying Family

Another reason the spouses stay together is the idea of home and family, which becomes present when their children visit. "The children cemented our relationship. And the fact that it survived is because we had children", Anna says (A_PL_1G). While children cannot cement their parents' relationship on a daily basis, their visits and phone calls provide a reason for the couple to stay together. Talking about their children's visits, the interviewees start talking with energy and enthusiasm:

> Felicja: And then it's fun (...) sometimes we buy a cake, everything we like, so to speak, and we have a little party—well, with some pizza...
>
> Anna: It is very cheerful when they arrive. Nobody argues here and there are always some funny conversations, stories.

In some families, children continue to go on holidays with their parents, at least sometimes or for a part of the trip. Anna and Jakub almost gave up their holiday plans when their son decided not to go, but as he finally changed his mind, the three of them went to the seaside and had fun. Similarly, Edyta and Kamil plan their holidays, hoping their daughter will join them and modify their plans according to her needs:

> Interviewer: And how are you going to spend your next holidays? Do you already know? Will there be a trip at some point?
>
> Edyta: We have plans for [the mountains]. There is a chance that Julia will be more attracted to that than to [the lowlands].

Children also provide major conversation topics. While some couples feared that after their children's departure, they would have nothing to talk about, the children continue to deliver issues to debate:

> Helena: (...) I was a bit worried that we wouldn't really have much to talk about. Because when my daughters were here, to be honest, they almost completely filled the space. (...) but to be honest, there's always something

to talk about. There's always politics, there's always work... Plus our daughters, the same, there are a lot of topics.

The children's presence is important for together apart couples because they provide them with a sense of meaning—even after their departure, they are still a family, a unit bigger than the couple itself. Thanks to the children, they may display family to themselves and to others:

> Olek: We're not on a desert island—if the two of us were in some kind of isolated arrangement, then we could separate and do what we please. But we still have the children, so I can't imagine the kind of emotions that would cause us to separate. But undoubtedly, the children are the glue, they are the most important—I think so.

The value of family unity is powerful. Weronika, whose daughter Maja has even suggested that the couple should divorce, believes that despite this suggestion, Maja needs her parents together. In her view, her daughter would despair if family holidays and celebrations were to end:

> Weronika: I think she needs it. I think she needs it.
> Interviewer: Even though she suggested divorce?
> Weronika: Even though she suggested the divorce. But I think if we didn't have Christmas, dinner and all that, she would suffer a lot.

The enduring presence and significance of their children in the lives of together apart couples serve as a powerful glue, providing a sense of purpose and unity that keeps them together, despite the challenges they face in their relationships.

Materiality that Binds

In the case of one couple, the issue of finances and a home loan was one of the key elements sustaining the relationship. While the wife seemed to be happy with the model of living side by side, Wojciech, the husband, was deeply frustrated and was thinking of separating, but material issues were very much holding him back:

> Wojciech: Everything depends on me, including the mortgage. And it is not easy to solve. (...) First, I have to repay the loan, and second, I have to pay

alimony to my non-working wife for a while. So there is nothing left for me at the moment.

In addition, the house's materiality may be an essential element in a relationship. First, home is part of a broader idea of family analysed in the previous section. Jakub says that their home is a place to which he feels attached and to which their sons can always return and relate to memories and experiences of their childhoods:

> Jakub: Apart from my own attachment, this is the place where the boys will want to come with their wives and children and feel comfortable, that rooting and that kind of place where they grew up.

> Jakub: (…) coming home is such a warm feeling that I wouldn't want to deprive my children (of this place) under any circumstances.

Homes also give spouses a shared project—they may be constantly improved, renovated, or refurnished. Patrycja and Sebastian are unsure if they will have a shared bedroom or two separate ones, but they are both involved in the renovation project:

> Patrycja: Then we argued about who wants the bedroom where, and I think Sebastian is more inclined to go my way with the bedroom, I think we'll have it where I want it.
>   Sebastian: (…) We're doing two bedrooms for now, so we can end up having separate bedrooms.

Jakub and Anna are also busy renovating. While the result is their further distancing (two bedrooms instead of one), they are planning the work together:

> Anna: Well, we're doing the whole swap now. We're going to make my current bedroom into the guest room, and I'm going to go down to one of my son's rooms.

For some couples, housing and financial difficulties may be the reason to stay together. Still, sometimes it is the other way round: the house size allows the couple to comfortably lead two almost parallel lives. Anna likes her new separate bedroom very much. She finally feels relaxed and released of the tension related to sharing the room with her husband:

Anna: So these negative emotions were still there [in the shared bedroom]. And now, because, well, I'm alone here, it's actually quite an enclave, I must say, I never get angry here, it's always peaceful (...). There are no bad emotions in my room.

In some cases, financial considerations, such as home loans and the shared ownership of a house, can play a pivotal role in keeping a couple together. Additionally, the physicality and shared projects (Kaufmann, 2020) associated with their home can further strengthen their bond, offering a sense of stability and attachment beyond the relationship itself.

Future Plans and Dreams

Patrycja: In general, when I think about the future of our marriage, it's a bit boring. I mean boring to the point of saying, "and now what?"

Patrycja expressed a fear that many others must share—what next? While the "new honeymoon" couples love to dream of exotic holidays and summer houses, for together apart couples, thoughts of the future are rarely optimistic, so they rather avoid them. A popular strategy is to focus on individual plans. Olek is planning to set up his own media room to watch movies and listen to music as loud as he wants. Weronika is thinking about education and sports:

Olek: There's a place where we now have a projector and sound equipment. And I'm planning to make a place where you can watch a film, listen to music, or have a concert. That's what I'm going to do—those are my plans.

Weronika: Possibly find some more hobbies, broaden my interests, the university of the third age, more sports, swimming and things like that.

However, in developing individual plans, interviewees may encounter challenges. They are officially in a relationship, and excluding their partner from their projects may seem weird to others and even to themselves. It was difficult for Anna to plan a holiday by herself at first. She thought it might feel lonely and sad. It turned out differently and she learnt how to enjoy trips by herself. However, their friends may not understand why Anna and Jakub do not spend holidays together. Workload, again, is used as an excuse:

> Anna: And I had such a moment, such sadness, that I was alone... But then I was fine alone by the sea. I mean, I also know how to organise time for myself, and it no longer bothers me. Well, all our friends, however, go together, don't they? Of course, I can find an argument for friends (...) that my husband has to work now and cannot [go].

Felicja encountered another similar dilemma. She dreams of moving to the seaside and describes it as an individual project until asked whether her husband should live there with her. She is puzzled and unsure of what to decide. Finally, she comes up with a solution:

> Felicja: It would be nice to see each other occasionally, but [not] be together all the time... I'd prefer two separate houses close to each other.

Edyta also likes to plan her future house individually, motivated by moving closer to the city. She is tired of living in the countryside and the related transport poverty. She neither entirely excludes her husband from this plan nor makes her dreams dependent on his preferences:

> Edyta: Yes, I want to move. If he wants to, he can come with me. If not, he can stay in the countryside.

Are there thoughts of divorce? While never raised in dyadic interviews, divorce was sometimes discussed in individual interviews. Anna thinks about divorce about once a week, but not intensely, and she always convinces herself that it would make no sense:

> Anna: Thoughts about living apart, I would say I have them on average once a week, but they don't clutter up my life, yes? I just ask myself and say "well, no, I'll stay, it wouldn't be that different, and it would make problems".

Weronika admits she is unhappy in her marriage, and while her daughter encourages her to divorce, she does not feel ready to do it:

> Weronika: So I live my life, but I don't think I can take any big steps.

Wojciech has similar feelings, but he predicts that maybe one day, when his frustration is unbearable, he will decide to leave:

Wojciech: I get a bit tired of it. I'm getting a bit tired of it, I don't know if it's just that when I'm tired enough, I will decide to take some steps.

Finally, Katarzyna expresses dilemmas that accompany many other together apart couples. She is afraid to think of the future because she is unsure whether her relationship will survive. Both staying together and separating are uneasy thoughts. She still hopes things might improve but generally feels pessimistic. And she is afraid of staying alone:

> Katarzyna: I don't know if I can live with my husband. I don't know if I can live without him either—I don't know. But at the moment, it's like we're moving apart more than we're moving together. That may change, although I can't see any sign of it. And I don't want to be alone.

We have listed many reasons why together apart couples stay together, demonstrating how everyday practices, duties, children, and the house's materiality bind them. However, there is also one emotional aspect of interdependence we have not discussed, which relates to the fear of loneliness. The interviewed couples were, on average, 50–60 years old, and the ageing problem might not yet be dominant in their narratives, but it is starting to show. Katarzyna, quoted above, said: "I don't want to be alone". Jakub mentioned:

> Jakub: It's worth having someone there when you get older.

And although no one else raised this issue, as the years go by, the fear of getting old alone can be a powerful argument for why a relationship will last.

CONCLUSION

In this chapter, we have discussed the "together apart" couples whose interdependence weakened after their children's departure.[3] While parenthood mostly united the couple and provided them with shared practices and conversation topics, the empty nest phase revealed the poor state of their relationship.

---

[3] See Chap. 9 for theoretical foundation of this concept.

The trajectories of together apart couples are not identical, but key elements can be identified, similar for French and Polish cases. The children brought about a vast change in couples' lives, which began to revolve around caregiving practices. Partners stopped valuing their relationship and focused on the needs of their children. Other difficulties also contributed to their drifting apart, such as working away from home, financial problems, children's illnesses, or the need to care for elderly parents. Parents often had different parenting styles and attitudes, leading to conflict and tension. Emotional distance increased when one spouse felt deprived of the other's support.

While the departure of the children was challenging for all the parents, elements of relief and satisfaction were also observed, demonstrating that the empty nest transition is never simply a matter of loss or relief, but a combination of both. Even together apart couples, who rarely derive satisfaction from marital practices, may experience enjoyment in the empty nest phase due to their increased time to develop personal interests and reduced conflict and tension. In addition, conflicted or strained couples may feel relieved not to have to display couplehood in front of their children.

The couples interviewed differed in their experiences of transition, mostly related to whether they had had the opportunity to develop a model of "living together but a bit apart" and to be "fellow travellers" before their children left. If they had, the departure was not experienced as a shock. If the partners (or one of them) had never had a chance to focus on themselves, the sense of loss was more significant. In this second type of relationship, separation might be the next step of their life course.

We were interested in how couples maintain their fragile relationships. In other words, we wanted to find out what makes partners stay together despite an apparent crisis. We identified several crucial aspects of mutual interdependence. Partners stick to established ways and patterns of doing things, which is a source of comfort to them. For many, continuing habitual practices is easier and more comfortable than making radical changes in their daily lives. Partners maintain parts of their old routines such as Sunday dinner, weekend trips, holidays, or watching the news together. Deprived of the presence of their children, who used to be essential interaction partners, they limit these shared practices for fear of being left alone with their spouse for too long. They are aware that the silence that might prevail between them would expose the problems in their relationship and force them to have difficult conversations. They, therefore, use avoidance strategies, escaping to work, caring for other family members, or developing their passions. The issue of routines is also related to household management. Some couples are used to sharing responsibilities, which makes the household run smoothly. Children are also a vital bonding element for couples; their visits display the family anew. Children can also be a topic of conversation, making interactions more natural. Finally, an important bonding factor is materiality. There are times when financial and housing difficulties are an essential argument for not separating. In addition, the family home is a place of memories and children's visits and a symbol of the family. Thus, it would be too painful for some people to move away. The house can also allow some couples to undertake projects, such as renovations. In addition, the size of the house makes it possible to find separate enclaves for the couple to avoid each other's presence.

We also want to address a few methodological issues related to studying fragile couples. It is not easy to admit to oneself and to a researcher that one is in an unsatisfactory relationship. In this respect, the combination of DDI and IDI interviews was very helpful. The dyadic interviews helped the researchers to identify issues to be addressed in the subsequent IDI interviews. Respondents tended to open up much more in the individual interviews, which allowed us to identify most of the couples with weak ties. This is probably the reason why there was a predominance of Polish together apart couples over French ones, as the French study only included dyadic interviews. Another issue relates to the recruitment process. It is easier to recruit couples who are satisfied with their relationship than those who are not. Therefore, out of 75 couples, we only identified 7 Polish and 4 French couples with weak ties.

In this chapter, we have analysed together apart couples who stay together despite their unsatisfactory relationship. As we have mentioned before, however (see Chap. 9), couplehood is a dynamic process, which can move in different directions, including separation or divorce.

REFERENCES

Aquilino, W. S. (1997). From adolescent to young adult: A prospective study of parent-child relations during the transition to adulthood. *Journal of Marriage and Family, 59*(3), 670–686. https://doi.org/10.2307/353953

Bengtson, V. L., & Roberts, R. E. L. (1991). Intergenerational solidarity in aging families: An example of formal theory construction. *Journal of Marriage and Family, 53*(4), 856–870. https://doi.org/10.2307/352993

Bouchard, G. (2014). How do parents react when their children leave home? An integrative review. *Journal of Adult Development, 21*(2), 69–79. https://doi.org/10.1007/s10804-013-9180-8

Bouchard, G., & McNair, J. L. (2016). Dyadic examination of the influence of family relationships on life satisfaction at the empty-Nest stage. *Journal of Adult Development, 23*(3), 174–182. https://doi.org/10.1007/s10804-016-9233-x

Bozhenko, E. (2011). Adult child-parent relationships: On the problem of classification. *Procedia - Social and Behavioral Sciences, 30*, 1625–1629. https://doi.org/10.1016/j.sbspro.2011.10.315

Finch, J. (2007). Displaying families. *Sociology, 41*(1), 65–81. https://doi.org/10.1177/0038038507072284

Kaufmann, J.-C. (2020). Solidarność i zaufanie w parze. *Fabrica Societatis, 3*(2020), 35–40. https://doi.org/10.34616/129166

Martin, C., Cherlin, A., & Cross-Barnet, C. (2011). Living together apart in France and the United States. *Population, 66*(3–4), 561–581. https://doi.org/10.1353/pop.2011.0025

Mitchell, B. A., & Lovegreen, L. D. (2009). The empty Nest syndrome in midlife families: A multimethod exploration of parental gender differences and cultural dynamics. *Journal of Family Issues, 30*(12), 1651–1670. https://doi.org/10.1177/0192513X09339020

Silverstein, M., & Bengtson, V. (1997). Intergenerational Solidarity and the structure of adult child–parent relationships in American families. *American Journal of Sociology, 103*(2), 429–460. https://doi.org/10.1086/231213

Widmer, E. D. (2021). Family diversity in a configurational perspective. In N. Schneider & M. Kreyenfeld (Eds.), *Research handbook on the sociology of the family* (pp. 60–72). Edward Elgar.

CHAPTER 11

Recoupling Transitions in the Empty Nest: Women's Perspective

Magdalena Żadkowska and Christophe Giraud

INTRODUCTION

The processes of individualization give people different relationship scenarios to be taken into consideration. Couples choose between the "conjugal We," "family We," or both (de Singly, 2021). Freedom of choice influences decisions about divorce; the divorce rate per 1000 people in the second decade of the twenty-first century remains stable and indicates 1.6 in Poland (2019 data) and 1.9 in France (2016 data). 29.1% of

M. Żadkowska (✉)
Social Sciences Department (Institute of Sociology), University of Gdańsk, Gdańsk, Poland

Centre de recherche sur les liens sociaux (CERLIS, UMR 8070), Université Paris Cité, Paris, France
e-mail: magdalena.zadkowska@ug.edu.pl

C. Giraud
Centre de recherche sur les liens sociaux (CERLIS, UMR 8070), Université Paris Cité, Paris, France
e-mail: christophe.giraud@parisdescartes.fr

© The Author(s), under exclusive license to Springer Nature Switzerland AG 2024
M. Żadkowska et al. (eds.), *Reconfiguring Relations in the Empty Nest*, Palgrave Macmillan Studies in Family and Intimate Life, https://doi.org/10.1007/978-3-031-50403-7_11

marriages in France last more than 20 years, compared with 29.5% in Poland (Demographic Yearbook, 2020). Attitudes towards the permanence of marriage are also changing—strong supporters of divorce are three times as numerous as their staunch opponents (although 52% "don't support divorce, they allow it in certain situations"), and the percentage of the former is on an upward trend (Boguszewski, 2019). High divorce rates, interpreted from this perspective, reflect the increasing importance placed on the quality of marriage today and are seen as one of the factors transforming attitudes towards marriage (Paprzycka & Mianowska, 2019). In France, 30% of marriages celebrated in 1980 have ended in divorce (Bellamy, 2016: 3).

Applying the frame of life course studies (Elder, 1995; Dewilde, 2003; Aeby & Gauthier, 2021; Cooney, 2022), this chapter examines families with the experience of separation, divorce, or death of one of the partners before the transition to the empty nest. In most cases, children's presence was a glue that bound the family together until the children had grown up, but once children were teenagers or young adults, the marriage ended. We analyze the event of emptying the nest as a possible trigger for women to choose a new partner or to decide on the form of an actual relationship. The chapter aims to show the impact of the children's departure on the possible reconfigurations of women's intimate lives after the relationship with the child's father has ended. Do they start a new relationship? Does the recoupling story end up with cohabitation? And how does the children's departure influence this process?

Studies show that divorce brings different family readjustments to its members (Amato, 2010). Parental separation influences the parent–children relationships and the strength of their interdependence. After divorce, adult children's relationships with their mothers are affected less negatively than relationships with their fathers (Amato, 2010). French young adults who move out see their mothers twice as often as their fathers (Régnier-Loilier et al., 2009) and their attachment to their mothers is more secure (Carranza et al., 2009; Fraley & Heffernan, 2013).

The postdivorce repartnering, as a continuous process of family formation, is still an unstudied phenomena, although there are models to study this transition (Anderson & Greene, 2005). Anderson and Greene differentiate 9 potential transitions (that can occur in a different sequence and may occur together), in the postdivorce repartnering: (1) Dating initiation, (2) Child introduction, (3) Serious involvement, (4) Sleepover, (5) Cohabitation, (6) Break up of a serious relationship, (7) Pregnancy in the new relationship, (8) Engagement, (9) Remarriage (Anderson & Greene, 2005: 49). The model goes along with other studies, showing evidence that postdivorce repartnering trajectories are not straightforward (Hughes, 2000). Women have more difficulty than men in finding a partner after separation or divorce (Villeneuve-Gokalp, 1994). The woman's age at the time of the relationship's dissolution is a strong predictor of the likelihood of repartnering (De Jong Gierveld, 2004). Moreover, women with non-residential children have a higher probability of recoupling than women with children who are still at home (De Graaf & Kalmijn, 2003; van Eeden-Moorefield et al., 2007). The other gendered phenomenon is that women (widows) are more likely to choose to remain without a partner for intrinsic factors: a reluctance to resign from their new-found freedom (Davidson, 2001). Although shared parenting after separation and divorce is increasing, especially for the millennial generation (Flaquer, 2021), most children continue to live with their mothers after a divorce or separation (Langmeyer et al., 2022). The children influence their mothers' lives: being scared of changes caused by a new person in their everyday life, they "protect the family territory from intruders" (De Jong Gierveld & Merz, 2013: 1100). That is why people with children might opt for a non-cohabitating arrangement (e.g. LAT—see below), aware that they need to negotiate the family boundaries with their children (De Jong Gierveld & Merz, 2013).

After a breakup, the possible need to start a new relationship may clash with the need to maintain autonomy and a sense of obligation and connection to one's children. To reconcile these forces, the new relationship may take different forms, other than marriage. Nowadays, the couple's living arrangements can be organized differently (than getting married, cohabiting, or staying single) as: "free together" (Burkart & Kohli, 1992; de Singly, 2000), "alone together" (Amato et al., 2007; Turkle, 2011), and "living apart together" (Levin, 2004; Stoilova et al., 2017). Particularly Living Apart Together (LAT—cf. Levin, 2004; Roseneil, 2006) has gained popularity in recent decades (Lyssens-Danneboom & Mortelmans, 2014). Several studies are devoted to analyzing this type of relationship as very popular among young people (Haskey, 2005; Reimondos et al., 2011), showing that "dating LATs" often mean that it is "too early" or that people are "not ready" to cohabit (Duncan & Phillips, 2010). For people over 50 years old, specific variants of LAT are particularly common—"partner LATs" (Duncan & Phillips, 2010) or "committed LATs" (Ermisch & Siedler, 2008). While most couples see LAT as a temporary arrangement, other dyads consider it a permanent form, which provides autonomy and intimacy (Beaujouan, 2009). Studies show that LAT relationships let women develop a "female self" that combines "feminine" intimacy and emotional expression with "masculine" independence and competence (Lyssens-Danneboom & Mortelmans, 2014). Studies demonstrate that the preferences for LAT might be predicted by gender, age, education, and place of life—better-educated, older women, with older children, and residents of urbanized areas are more likely to prefer LAT to cohabitation (De Jong Gierveld & Merz, 2013).

In this chapter, we have analyzed the stories of 31 women who were widowed or divorced. The separations, in most cases, occurred when living with the children. The French sample consisted of 17 divorced women, all in recoupling status. In the Polish sample, there were 14 women in new relationships at the moment of their interview. Two women were widows, and the rest were divorced. The Polish and French women were between 49 and 62 years old and the majority had two children. Only two women did not have a higher education degree. The respondents lived in cities, towns, and in the countryside. In Poland, the interviews were conducted online in Polish, while in France they were face-to-face in French. For all the studied women, an unsatisfactory marriage or widowhood influenced their relationships with their children, and the dissolution between parents happened while the children were still in their care. The everyday presence of the children at home strongly influenced their intimate lives or the lack thereof. Our thematic analysis focused on how the children's departure (or lack of it) affected the women's ability to return to a new emotional and sexual life and how they changed (or did not) the recoupling arrangements. In our analysis, we use Anderson and Greene's (2005) "Nine potential transitions model in the postdivorce repartnering" (Ibidem: 49).

RESULTS: THE INFLUENCE OF CHILDREN'S DEPARTURE ON THE INTIMATE LIVES OF THEIR MOTHERS

"Emptying the nest" creates space for a new relationship or new personal life arrangements. All participants were in a recoupling situation at the moment of the interview (empty nest). As our respondents revealed, in the full nest (while children were still at home), the new relationship arrangements differed in terms of their presence and level of commitment (1) and women's attitudes towards cohabitation (2). With regard to the first of these differences, some women do not enter a new relationship in the full nest phase because of their children at home. They do not want their intimate life to influence their family life. Other women only have affairs (they are dating), very often in secret from the children, trying not to involve the children in new configurations. Finally, there are also women who consider their new relationship as "the one till death tears us apart" and whose children consider the new partner as an important person in their mother's and in their family's life. Secondly, female participants also have varied attitudes towards cohabitation. Many of them lead the Living Apart Together relationship for different reasons, including for the sake of the children or for their own preferences. Only in a few households did the new partner cohabit with the woman and her children, creating a reconstructed family.

It is important to underline that all participants were different in terms of the phase of their relationship. We encountered women at the very first stage of their new relationships ("dating") and also in relationships lasting several years and with "serious involvement." The adult children's departure influences **all** of the above mentioned family arrangements, giving women the possibility to start or change their intimate relationships. Considering the Anderson and Greene's model as the point of reference for the full nest, we will present five types of transition trajectories we have identified in our study (Anderson & Greene, 2005: 49):

(1) Dating initiation **➔ Empty Nest ➔** Dating & Sleepover

The first trajectory exemplifies recoupling that is relatively new and the influence of the children's departure lets women feel free to use the freedom they have gained.

(2) Dating initiation **➔ Empty Nest** → Sleepover → Child introduction → (Serious Involvement)

The second scenario presents the stories of new couples which were triggered by the children's departure. From the "dating couple" situation now, in an empty nest, couples get more and more committed.

(3) Dating initiation → Child introduction → Serious involvement (LAT) → **Empty Nest** → Cohabitation → (Engagement/Remarriage)

The third trajectory was met in long-lasting couples who started to recouple while their children were living with their mothers. To illustrate its complexity, we show more detailed stories.

(4) Dating initiation → Child introduction → Serious involvement (LAT) → **Empty Nest** → No Cohabitation/Committed LAT

The fourth pathway is also related to long-lasting couples. What makes these stories specific is that there are no plans to change the form of cohabitation after the children's departure. Participating women declare "Committed LAT" to be their final choice of relationship.

(5) No intimate relationship → **Empty Nest** → Divorce → Dating initiation (with possible further phases)

The last trajectory presents examples of women who have divorced and started new relationships only when their children were adults and had moved out. The space for recoupling opened up because of the children's departure as it is linked to formal dissolution with the father of the children.

None of our respondents shared a story about the "Break up of a serious relationship," which is presented in Anderson and Greene's model. And in all situations, "pregnancy" was no longer possible or planned— which is an important factor in decisions about living arrangements, for example in the repartnering stories of couples that are much younger than the women participating in this study.

Dating → Empty Nest → Dating & Sleepover

After a divorce, which happened in the full nest, some women go on dates or have a relationship with no commitment. They only enter ephemeral relationships hidden from the children. The presence of the children makes women feel not ready to start a committed relationship. When the children leave home, some of these women continue to conduct relationships that they do not call "being a couple." They declare they are single or dating "without a plan." Some of them sleep over at another person's place. Tamara represents such an example. She is having an affair and she calls it "situationship," a type of "in-and-out" relationship (Gouveia &

Castrén, 2021). The everyday life practices arranged in the space and time without her adult children around give her input to decide that she prefers to live alone, and as Tamara calls it to have "a relationship without a plan":

> Tamara: Now … I'm so involved in my children's lives and in the lives of my friends and, in fact, it's as if the relationship we have, the one where we meet once or twice a month … So to speak, it is connected with this empty nest … This is going to sound so strange, but I'm just getting started professionally, and I just wouldn't even want this freedom of mine, let's say, to be exchanged for such rituals of everyday life as cleaning and so on. And then there's also I guess that one thing, I don't really feel like getting to know or struggling with … Like I feel like getting to know my partner from the best side, maybe I do. I don't want to know if he can peel potatoes, surely he can, no? I don't want to know if, if I told him to vacuum today, would he do it or not do it, right? I'm also trying to build the kind of relationship where there's not so much room for checking in with myself. (C_PL_111, 57 y.o., divorced for 8 years, in "situationship")

The empty nest gives Tamara a sense of freedom she doesn't want to lose. A new relationship would mean another form of commitment and she has just released herself from the parental commitment.

Sławomira also prefers her new life and does not think about a serious relationship. After the experience of being alone and enjoying this, the departure of the children does not influence new decisions about the couple's arrangements:

> Sławomira: Yes, yes. To not spoil it, I think it must be that way. I'm saying, I wouldn't put up with him here in the long run either for sure. That I already know even today, yes?
> Interviewer: And why?
> Sławomira: Well, I think it's because of things like that because I'm used to being here on my own and **doing things my own way, and not having someone hanging around and maybe even wanting to introduce some rules of their own.** (C_PL_117, 55 y.o., one son, separated, not divorced, in a dating relationship)

Sławomira exemplifies the empty nest that let her develop her "female self" and a safe "herspace," which she is afraid could easily be lost.

Tamara and Sławomira have not experienced a change in their intimate status after the children's departure. What has changed is how they experience their intimate life and their attitude towards themselves—they admit prioritizing and appreciating the status of being alone in an empty nest with a dating relationship. Their children, living separately, gave them the opportunity to invite partners for sleepovers and to come back home at night without having to explain themselves. There is no longer any risk of the children meeting their mothers' boyfriends. The status of this type of recoupling is characterized by the missing trajectory step "Child introduction."

Dating Initiation → Empty Nest → Sleepover → Child Introduction → (Serious Involvement)

Both Agata and Grażyna are in new relationships with men that started before the children's departure. After this event, the relationships got more involved because of the amount of time they could devote to each other. When they share plans for the couple's rearrangements, they admit to also living apart in their empty nest phases because of the individual autonomy and intimacy it provides:

Agata: Wonderful. We travel, because my partner is, I would say, a globe-trotter. With him, I've started to spend a bit more time on myself and on pleasure and money on myself and not on other things. All the cultural opportunities—we go to the theatre, to the opera, to the ballet. He even goes with me to places he wouldn't necessarily go, but he goes. And unfortunately, I don't go with him where he would like to go, and he goes on his own. **And I only go where I like to go.** Also, maybe I'm not as nice as he is, but that's the result of this sacrifice in the marriage that I don't like too much anymore. **But he doesn't mind that I don't sacrifice too much. He doesn't require me to make sacrifices.** (C_PL_114, 52 y.o., divorced, in a new LAT relationship)

Grażyna: **There is room for intimacy here. It's just that our relationship is very intimate, and close.** We … I don't have a lot of experience of being in a relationship, but it's very different to my first relationship because we have time, we can lounge in bed until whatever time it is because it's very different. So that intimacy, that closeness, what I didn't have for many years, well I have a lot of that! The cuddling, the sex, all the things that are just so … all that relates to being in a relationship, well, we don't miss all that. At least I don't think so. Well, I don't miss it. We talk about it, it's not like I'm guessing. (C_PL_93, 53 y.o., 1 year in a new relationship LAT)

As financial and residential autonomy is something new and gained, the new relationship benefits from this. For Agata, the new relationship in the empty nest is planned under the name "No more sacrifices." For Grażyna, the arrangement of "living apart together" allows her to live at the stage of falling in love and dating. Compared to their previous marriages, which lacked intimacy and were full of sacrifices, new relationships after the departure of the children provide more time, space, and money for the women. What also changes in an empty nest is that the new relationship can be displayed more. The new partner is introduced to the children, friends, and the rest of the family. The potential for this type of recoupling is the next step: "Serious involvement."

Serious Involvement LAT → Empty Nest → Cohabitation → (Engagement/Remarriage)

Some women do not wait for the nest to be empty to get seriously involved in a new relationship. The living arrangements of such women in the majority were **Living Apart Together relationships—LAT.** The departure of the children was an important event to decide if a lasting LAT was only **a temporary arrangement** chosen for the time when the children were still at home and would change into cohabitation (or even remarriage) or if it were **a permanent form**.

The situation of living apart can be closely related to the children living at home. This was the case for Iwona, who waited until her youngest daughter moved out before moving in with Henryk. Henryk, in a way, replaced Iwona's daughters as a cure for the "emptiness." That is how the temporary LAT arrangement evolved into cohabitation. Iwona directly expresses the cure for the "emptiness" of the nest hidden in her new relationship:

> Iwona: Well there certainly isn't the loneliness of having someone there after all, yes? There is someone to talk to. You know, calling your daughters on the phone isn't the same, is it? And my daughters are young still, working and everything, so they don't have that much time either. What else? The confidence that I can still be with someone etc. The feeling of such joy, there's not that emptiness. (C_PL_105, widow, just married, retired)

The cases of (a) Christine and (b) Teresa present all the dynamics of transitions to recoupling with the empty nest context, where the LAT is a temporary arrangement that ends when the children move out (Christine) or when they are older and the relationship is "mature enough."

(a) Christine after divorce has the following sequence of transitions:

Full nest → Divorce → Dating Initiation→ Children introduction → Serious involvement LAT → **Empty nest** → Engagement → Remarriage → Cohabitation

Christine, 46 years old, divorced her husband after 18 years of marriage. Christine started her new relationship with Alexandre, 60 years old, 2 years after her divorce. He was going through a divorce at that time. At first, Christine wanted a partner for activities together, but not a spouse at home.

> Christine: I wanted to do a lot of things, he wanted to do a lot of things, so it was a good start. But I was very worried, I didn't want anyone in my life, so I was a bit, I was a bit reserved. (C_FR_3)

They began a long-distance relationship, taking advantage of the times when Christine's children were at their father's house to get together. After 10 months, they introduced each other to friends and their respective parents. After a year, they introduced each other to their respective children. Tensions soon arose with Christine's daughter over the status of her mother's partner:

> Christine: Because I didn't want to impose a man who wasn't their father on my children and I didn't want to impose children who weren't his children on Alexandre. And you know, recomposed couples are not so easy. My daughter was young, and she made it clear that he was an intruder. She told him straight out, but at one point she said to him: "but anyway, you're my rival". (C_FR_3)

Alexandre wanted to live with Christine, but she kept on refusing, not wanting to create tension with her children (and not wanting it for herself). The relationship continued by segmenting the time spent with the partner and the time spent with her children (or family gatherings with the grandparents). After 4 years, when Christine's son passed his baccalaureate and moved to Paris, Alexandre suggested living together again. The children were again a pretext for refusing:

Christine: Four years ago, but I still hadn't made up my mind because I wanted my children … We were getting the best out of each other, Alexandre, and I, and I wanted my children to be better off in terms of their studies and so on so that they would be more at home when we were living together. And in fact, that's what little by little … So, **I refused to live together twice.** It was risky, it was certainly … It could have ended our story. (C_FR_3)

Finally, when both children had moved out, Christine and Alexandre planned to buy and renovate a house in eastern France and live there together. At the moment of the interview, they were still living apart but had got married, and the decision to marry was made possible by the children's departure.

Christine: I think what changed that was the natural progression, that is, we didn't force things. When Alexandre was not well-received at the beginning, we did not force the system. I think that what has also changed is that my children have become young adults. They see it now with their adult eyes. I think they understood why I had separated from their father too, so that also made it easier to accept a new man in my life. I think my children are nice, they want me to be happy, so that's great, it's really … It's a wonderful thing because some children are selfish and it's true that it's also my selfishness to want to remake my life, **it's a form of selfishness.**
Interviewer: Selfishness?
Christine: Saying to yourself at a given moment in life "Well, when my children leave home, they won't give me their opinion. If they get married, if they go to live with someone, it's the same. If they're going to … If my son goes to work in Singapore tomorrow, I won't necessarily have any say in the matter and that's normal". So, I did the same thing in fact, it's a bit of a selfish decision to say "well I want to remake my life and I want to be happy, I want to feel good". I've never been unhappy, I've always left before being unhappy, I'm very positive, I'm cheerful and I want to feel good in my life. And that's part of this philosophy of life. And in fact, what has changed is that I think they have accepted that, and they want to please me and they see that I feel good, so I think they have accepted that. And my parents too. (C_FR_3)

Before the children left, Christine was first and foremost a mother and had a personal love life in parallel. But this love life was conditioned by the demands of the role of mother. After the children's departure, Christine could more directly affirm that she was acting for herself, that is, that her intimate life was no longer dependent on the opinion of the children, nor on the role of a mother. She could put herself first. The departure of the children was a moment of cleavage in the construction of the self.

Sometimes the children judge the mother's new love relationship negatively. The transition from a woman who was first a mother and spouse to a woman who has a new love life and lives by herself can be difficult for some children to accept. The women participating in the study who had such experiences admitted that they knew about their children's disagreement with their new relationship. Some had experiences of children choosing their father's side. Although the children's consent is desired, the mothers feel that they are free from family obligations and want to "live for themselves." They may legitimately feel "selfish," as Christine expressed earlier.

For those who have had a long-standing LAT relationship, which started before the children left, the romantic relationship may evolve more easily into cohabitation. The children are more accepting of their mother being surrounded and protected from the loneliness resulting from their departure.

(b) Teresa after getting divorced has a sequence of different transitions:

Full nest → Divorce → Dating Initiation (several partners) → Children introduction → Dating Maciej → Serious involvement LAT → Cohabitation → **Empty nest** → Serious commitment in the empty nest

Teresa divorced her husband very early in her life (a unique case from the sample). She conducted different relationships while her daughter was still living with her. She started the relationship with Maciej 8 years before the interview. After 5 years of LAT, Teresa and Maciej bought a new apartment and the three of them moved in there together. The LAT arrangement was then a temporary form of recoupling and evolved into cohabitation. First, during the full nest, cohabitation was a form of recomposed family. They lived together, all three of them, sometimes being visited by Maciej's sons. When the daughter moved out of the house, the cohabitation changed significantly. Teresa describes the changes introduced by the departure of Julia to their life as a couple in the empty nest.

> Teresa: Well, I think that if something has changed, then probably **the intimacy has moved out of the bedroom a bit**. Because before, the presence of my daughter, who's 24, was felt not only in her small room but in the

entire flat. Any intimate situations would take place in the bedroom, either late at night or early in the morning, having in mind that my daughter was there. Now, however, there's no need to worry, right? **There is no need to worry that someone the other side of the wall will feel embarrassed.** It's more Maciej who's loosened up because he's always been reluctant, "I'm not going to wear just pants around Julia, because she's a grown-up woman, and here's a guy in pants walking around the house in the morning", so he'd quickly put on a tracksuit or something, and now he's … Well, because I'm the one wearing a dressing gown, I'm always in a dressing gown. Maciej has loosened up and walks around in his pants in the morning, indeed. And we're not so careful about the order. There is something there. It's not that much of a mess, because it's not our nature, but it's a bit freer. **There's no need to set a good example.** (C_PL_106, 46 y.o. divorced after 4 years of marriage, in a relationship for 8y., living together for 3y.)

The departure of Teresa's daughter was the final step to changing the recoupling status into a couple living in "the empty nest." The everyday life practices described by Teresa show the increase in intimacy and increased freedom to display the couple.

Serious Involvement LAT→ Empty Nest → No Cohabitation/ Committed LAT

For some serious relationships which are created during the full nest phase, the LAT arrangements do not change after the children's departure. The status of no family obligations and the disappearance of constraints related to living with children do not necessarily lead to cohabitation. The balance of personal life may also be considered satisfactory in the long term, and there is a fear of losing it.

Fabienne, 55 years old, divorced her husband 3 years ago, after 30 years of living together. Her youngest son is 18 and comes back home every second weekend. Her new partner Fabrice is 65, has four children from two different marriages and now lives with his elderly mother. Fabienne and Fabrice have been in a relationship for 2 years and see each other every day. They do not live together, and they accept this choice, Fabrice does not want to leave his elderly mother alone and Fabienne refuses to look after her with him. Fabienne explained that she did not want to return to the situation she experienced for 30 years during her first marriage, even though her partner might have wanted to cohabit again. They meet every evening and then he goes back home, being a guest in her home with no domestic duties or obligations. The departure of the child does not change the situation. Fabienne protects herself from domestic obligations that would arise from living together. She likes the relationship but does not want it to be tainted by chores. Some of the women in a LAT relationship feel that it is a good balance between a stable relationship and freedom. The departure of the children does not alter the love contract.

> Fabienne: We don't live together … but, not uh, cohabiting we'll say, daily. I didn't want to do that at all, because … I didn't want to relive a situation that would be too similar … to my life as a couple, which lasted thirty years, you could say … to live with him, eh. So, I really didn't want to go through that again (…). And maybe he would have liked the other solution too, but in any case, given what I wanted, he … he acquiesced, so to speak, and he went along with it (laughs)! But he doesn't mind, eh … I think that otherwise …, he would have vetoed it, so here we are, we live, and we see each other every day, it suits us perfectly, it leaves us both the freedom, none of the constraints of daily life to manage together. Well, it's true that there may be financial advantages (laughs) in sharing expenses, **but for the moment it suits me perfectly.** (C_FR_4, 55 y.o., divorced, in a LAT relationship for 2 years)

Similarly, even though her daughters have left home, Marta's living situation has not changed. On the one hand, she is simply freer; the relationship with her new partner, Jan, does not have to be negotiated with her two daughters. On the other hand, Marta and Jan work in two distant locations. They both have a very active working life now, and they do not envisage moving to another place. Living apart has a positive effect on their relationship.

After her daughters moved out, the reduced involvement in domestic duties and practices of care resulted in more time that could be devoted to her new relationship. Her new partner was not involved in the domestic duties division because family practices were mainly executed by mother and daughters. The children's departure to study at universities in different cities made it possible to change their time management. The reduction in involvement in domestic chores and childcare practices gave time resources to the mother much less burdened by her maternal role (see Chaps. 1 and 12) and allowed her to devote more time to the relationship. The quality of the relationship has improved significantly although Marta and Jan continue to live "together but apart."

Marta: Certainly, since my daughters moved out, we spend more time with each other in general in this kind of romantic relationship, I would call it—oh yes. We give each other more time and we have more time—me because I tend to do that—to organise a space that is warm—some kind of soft light, candles, all sorts of things—it's like that. Before, it wasn't possible because the house was full—and the girls and often their partners, their friends—often there wasn't such intimacy then. Paradoxically, there were doors back then and it was less intimate than now without doors, but that's how it is sometimes. In general, I think the fact that my daughters have grown up means that we spend more time together [the two of us] and more time travelling. It doesn't have to be going abroad, although it can be, it's also short trips—we can go to the seaside, have a coffee in Dębki, go to the cliffs in Orłowo, or go shopping. It is a feeling of freedom and deciding 100% of our time, all the time—whether it is professional, private, or shared—in general always. (C_PL_107, 45 y.o., widow, in a LAT relationship).

The departure of the children strongly influenced the changes in the occupation of space in the home for both partners. The whole of Marta's apartment became a space open for the couple' s practices, influencing the increase of intimacy and giving space for the couple to be displayed at home.

Marta: In our full nest, weekends, for example, we liked to spend them in the kitchen—there's this classic worktop for various things. It's right there in the corner of the kitchen. I would prepare something for Sunday or Saturday, I'd have it ready in advance. We would sit at this table, we would talk, we would drink wine—we would eat something. And in fact, most of the time, when my daughters were living at home, we would just go to the kitchen. It was the best place for us at that time. But after **they moved out, it changed,** because we sort of moved our activities and our time together in the flat to the living room, to the big sofa, which used to be just a bedroom, really. Because we didn't really have my daughter in the living room with her boyfriend, and my other daughter in the other room chatting on the internet, because that's how it used to be, we had to separate that space somehow. Everyone had a minimum of privacy, even though we had a few rooms—now there are more rooms. And these rooms have completely changed their function. (C_PL_107, 45 y.o., widow, in a LAT relationship)

Marta and Jan like their independence. Neither of them wants to give up or change their job to move closer.

No Intimate Relationship → Empty Nest → Divorce → Dating Initiation (with Possible Further Phases)

For many women, it is only when their children leave home that they start a new relationship. The reduction of the maternal role allows them to move on to a new phase in their love life. Yolande and Claudia (now in LAT relationships / serious involvement) are examples of this approach. They didn't start any new relationship before the children moved out. After the children's departure, they entered new relationships, starting with "dating," although, in the case of Yolande, it took seven years of an empty nest to establish a new relationship.

Yolande is a 61-year-old woman. She got married at the age of 20 to an older man, Fabrice. They soon had a daughter and then a son. Yolande stayed married for the sake of her children but had no feelings for her husband. When her children left home, 15 years ago, Yolande decided to find a job.

> Yolande: I waited until my children finished their studies and were no longer at home, I decided to find work, oh, it wasn't easy because I was already almost 50 y.o., well I was over 40, 46 y.o., so it was hard to find work, but I found a job at Entreprise1, just for the winter season, 2–3 months. And when he found out that I was working there, he went to the shop to make a scandal. Well, he humiliated me in front of everyone and he didn't want me to work at all because if I worked, I was financially dependent and I could leave. I did a few seasons at Entreprise1 like that as a seasonal worker for 2–3 months, sometimes 6 months. And in the end, in 2003, the director saw that my situation was not good, so she gave me a permanent position, and it was from that moment on, well, roughly then, I decided to start divorce proceedings. (C_FR_2, 61 y.o., divorced, in a LAT relationship for 8 years)

After 32 years of marriage, she started divorce proceedings at a time when her husband was preparing to retire. She was afraid of living with her retired husband at home all the time not having time for herself, alone.

> Yolande: I decided to start divorce proceedings because I couldn't stay any longer, it was becoming unbearable, and I saw that he was going to retire and that when he was working during the day, I had a bit of freedom, I could see my friends, whatever, but once he retired, my life was, it was over.

So, I decided to leave, I told him after 32 years of marriage. (C_FR_2, divorced, in a LAT relationship for 8 years)

The departure of the children allows women like Yolande to regain a certain autonomy for themselves and make their own departure possible. Without children, they can more easily finance housing just for themselves. When the children have acquired residential autonomy, that is, when they are studying in a different town and everyday life does not impose daily duties such as cooking, cleaning, and doing laundry, mothers start to consider their children as autonomous adults and they gain time and space (see Chaps. 3 and 12).

Claudia is a 54-year-old woman. She is highly educated and has held positions of responsibility in companies. She met Sébastien in 1979. They got married in a church (which was important to her) and had three children. She gave up her job as a manager and took the competitive examination to become a teacher. She wanted to have more time to take care of her children and protect them. Despite many problems in their marriage, including periods of separation, their marriage lasted for 30 years. Once the children were gone, Claudia left the marital home and rented a small flat. The divorce was pronounced after 3 years of separation. Claudia, who has a very Catholic upbringing, insists that the children's departure was important to her divorce:

> Claudia: As long as I had the children at home, I would not have left. It wasn't possible in the grand scheme of things. I wouldn't have wanted to put them through that, even if they were experiencing something a little tense, of course. (C_FR_1, 54 y.o., in a LAT relationship for 4 years)

Claudia and Yolande found new partners and began a new emotional life, the start of which was marked by the departure of the children. These women had a sequential conception of their existence: they did not change their intimate life until the children had left, and then they could finally think about starting a new phase of their lives rather than deciding to stay in a together apart relationship (see Chap. 10).

Empty Nest as a Marker for Adult Children

The children's presence and their opinion turned out to be very important for many mothers when the nest was full when it comes to choosing a new partner, especially if it would mean living together. Children may either be in favor of the mother's new partner or treat him as an intruder. Mothers have been negotiating family boundaries with their children in mind. Decisions in a full nest about their romantic lives are influenced by the children's presence. Both the start of an intimate life and the disclosure of it or the creation of a serious relationship always happens in the context of the presence of the children at home. When the nest empties, the influence of children on mothers' decisions related to their intimate lives weakens. In many cases though, only once they have left, did they look favorably at the fact that their mother was not left alone. Some children encouraged their parents' love life by registering them on a dating website, for example, after their departure. Marzena's daughters validated their mother's choice of a new partner, but cohabitation and marriage came only after both daughters had moved out.

> Marzena: When it comes down to it, it was a bit of a funny situation, because when my husband died, I started going to this kind of seniors' club and I simply met Antoni there. But at the beginning, it was just … an acquaintance, a coffee somewhere, something. And then it started to develop in such a way that somehow some feelings started to come into play. And my daughters saw him here because I used to bring him home when my second daughter was still here. And they just liked him a lot, they said, yeah, 'mum, very nice guy' and a bachelor, because he had never had kids or anything. **And it just worked out that way.** (C_PL_105, widow, 62 y.o., 2 daughters, remarried after children moved out, retired)

Children around, in the full nest, may be seen as an obstacle to a possible "new intimate life". Once they are gone, their right to organize their mums' lives is weakened. Some women, like Grażyna, express it directly:

> Grażyna: The truth is that they [children] are adults, and they probably wouldn't have the courage or even the need to organise my life, because I never organised their lives, and I never told them what studies they should do. (…) I never organised their lives, so they don't organise my life either. You can see that there are […] conflicts, you could say. I mean something that one side or the other doesn't accept. But I don't have a problem with that, it's just that sometimes they will express their opinion. (C_PL_93, 53 y.o., 1 year in a new LAT relationship)

The departure of children symbolizes the end of a certain stage where there is no equivalent place for a new member, such as the mother's partner. After this event, everyone enters the phase where they can organize the intimate lives independently.

CONCLUSIONS

Analysis of transitions to recoupling in an empty nest showed that when the children leave home, it significantly affects the mothers' intimate lives. The moment of the empty nest complements the model of "Nine potential transitions in the postdivorce repartnering" (Anderson & Greene, 2005). First, we showed the complexity of creating life scenarios in a new couple after divorce, depending on when recoupling begins in the family's life. The moment when the children move out of the house proved to be an important event both for deciding to enter serious and committed relationships or for entering into the next phases of the relationship. Second, the lack of the possibility of having a child/children together distinguishes the group of women studied from those who still have this option. This allowed us to look at their choices regarding, for example, cohabitation in terms of their individual preferences as women. The role of a mother becomes more "latent" for them (see Chap. 3) and allows them to make choices which are less influenced by what the children "think" or what is "expected" by others. The change brought about by the children moving out usually entails changes in the form or quality of the relationship. Women begin a new intimate life after the children move out, or fully enjoy both new and serious relationships.

The empty nest is a turning point in the private lives of mothers insofar as it transforms their private commitments. It is an opportunity for them to think about themselves. For some of them, this is the moment when they can start new sentimental relationships which they had forbidden themselves from doing before. For others, it is a time to develop hidden LAT arrangements, love affairs, or informal relationships or to give them a new character thanks to greater independence from obligations to children. Temporary arrangements may change into permanent, cohabiting relationships or even marriages. Women learn to live their lives independently from their children. Many of them remain in LAT arrangements, particularly better educated, older women, with older children, and residents of urbanized areas, who are more likely to choose LAT permanently (De Jong Gierveld & Merz, 2013). These women seek to maintain a balance between different commitments (friendships, love, parenthood, work—cf. Giraud, 2020). The empty nest allows them to have greater comfort and less hiding from their partner, but these relationships remain a private, limited segment of their personal life and some women do not undertake the risk of losing it.

In many cases, no matter what the recoupling arrangement, the departure of adult children, by giving space, time, financial resources, and a sense of freedom resulted in a more serious commitment no matter the status of cohabitation (together or apart). The everyday life practices of both individuals and couples resemble the cases described in Chap. 9. Contrary to the "together apart couples" in Chap. 10, women in recoupling relationships might take advantage of an empty nest to switch from a parental role to a conjugal one, one they did not let themselves enter fully because of the children's presence at home.

It is important to note that Polish interviewees in our study married earlier, the main differences concern demographic variables (see Introduction). The Polish respondents married earlier and had children earlier. Consequently, they faced the situation of divorce or separation when they were younger compared to the age of the French women surveyed. Interestingly, however, the LAT configuration seems to be an equally popular solution for divorced women both in Poland and France. The observation of such a couple's living arrangement, therefore, becomes important in conducting longitudinal and comparative research on the family life course.

We realize that the above discussion shows one perspective; it is the narrative of a person who is experiencing the dynamics of change in the nest being its main occupant. The women from the study are the ones who remain in the nest alone with their children, sometimes exchanging flats for smaller ones. To see the picture of recoupling in its full light, we would also need the accounts of men entering relationships with such partners. Their perspective of their partner's "child-free" home would have shown more of what influences them to make such decisions. It would also be helpful to have the perspective of the children, who, having experienced moving out of the family home, would report on their relationship with their mother's intimate life. We did not get any deeper results from the interviews regarding the impact of the first failed marriage on the new relationship either. We can only surmise that they may influence how private life decisions are made with greater care and self-awareness.

REFERENCES

Aeby, G., & Gauthier, J.-A. (2021). The contribution of the life-course perspective to the study of family relationships: Advances, challenges, and limitations. In A. M. Castrén, V. Cesnuityte, I. Crespi, J. A. Gauthier, R. Gouveia, C. Martin, M. A. Moreno, & K. Suwada (Eds.), *The Palgrave handbook of family sociology in Europe* (pp. 557–574). Palgrave Macmillan.

Amato, P. R. (2010). Research on divorce: Continuing trends and new developments. *Journal of Marriage and Family, 72*(3), 650–666.

Amato, P. R., Booth, A., Johnson, D. R., & Stacy, J. R. (2007). *Alone together: How marriage in America is changing.* Harvard University Press.

Anderson, E. R., & Greene, S. M. (2005). Transitions in parental repartnering after divorce. *Journal of Divorce & Remarriage, 43*(3–4), 47–62. https://doi.org/10.1300/J087v43n03_03

Beaujouan, E. (2009). *Trajectoires conjugales et fécondes des hommes et des femmes après une rupture en France* [Thèse pour l'obtention du diplôme de Doctorat en Démographie, Université Panthéon-Sorbonne-Paris I]. Université Panthéon-Sorbonne-Paris I. Retrieved from https://www.theses.fr/2009PA010611

Bellamy, V. (2016). 123 500 divorces en 2014 Des divorces en légère baisse depuis 2010. *Insee.* Retrieved January 20, 2023, from https://www.insee.fr/fr/statistiques/2121566

Boguszewski, R. (2019). Rozwody w osobistych doświadczeniach Polaków. *CBOS.* Retrieved February 15, 2023, from https://www.cbos.pl/

Burkart, G., & Kohli, M. (1992). *Liebe, Ehe, Elternschaft. Die Zukunft der Familie.* R. Piper GmbH & Co.

Carranza, L. V., Kilmann, P. R., & Vendemia, J. M. C. (2009). Links between parent characteristics and attachment variables for college students of parental divorce. *Adolescence, 44,* 253–271.

Cooney, T. M. (2022). Introduction to special issue on "divorce and the life course". *Social Sciences, 11*(202), 1–4. https://doi.org/10.3390/socsci11050202

Davidson, K. (2001). Late life widowhood, selfishness and new partnership choices: A gendered perspective. *Ageing & Society, 21*(3), 297–317. https://doi.org/10.1017/S0144686X01008169

De Graaf, P. M., & Kalmijn, M. (2003). Alternative routes in the remarriage market: Competing-risk analyses of union formation after divorce. *Social Forces, 81,* 1459–1498.

De Jong Gierveld, J. (2004). Remarriage, unmarried cohabitation, living apart together: Partner relationships following bereavement or divorce. *Journal of Marriage and Family, 66*(1), 236–243. https://doi.org/10.1111/j.0022-2445.2004.00015.x

De Jong Gierveld, J., & Merz, E.-M. (2013). Parents' partnership decision making after divorce or widowhood: The role of (step)children. *Journal of Marriage and Family, 75*(5), 1098–1113. https://doi.org/10.1111/jomf.12061

de Singly, F. (2000). *Libres ensemble. L'individualisme dans la vie commune.* Nathan.

de Singly, F. (2021). The family of individuals: An overview of the sociology of the family in Europe, 130 years after Durkheim's first university course. In A. M. Castrén, V. Cesnuityte, I. Crespi, J. A. Gauthier, R. Gouveia, C. Martin, M. Moreno Mínguez, & K. Suwada (Eds.), *The Palgrave handbook of family sociology in Europe* (pp. 15–43). Palgrave Macmillan.

Demographic Yearbook. (2020). *UNSD.* Retrieved February 20, 2023, from https://unstats.un.org/unsd/demographic-social/products/dyb/dybsets/2020.pdf

Dewilde, C. (2003). A life-course perspective on social exclusion and poverty. *The British Journal of Sociology, 54*(1), 109–128. https://doi.org/10.1080/0007131032000045923

Duncan, S., & Phillips, M. (2010). People who live apart together (LATs) – How different are they? *The Sociological Review, 58*(1), 112–134. https://doi.org/10.1111/j.1467-954X.2009.01874.x

Elder, G. H., Jr. (1995). The life course paradigm: Social change and individual development. In P. Moen, G. H. Elder, & K. Luscher (Eds.), *Examining lives in context: Perspectives on the ecology of human development* (pp. 101–139). American Psychological Association.

Ermisch, J., & Siedler, T. (2008). Living apart together. In M. Brynin & J. Ermisch (Eds.), *Changing relationships* (pp. 29–43). Routledge.

Flaquer, L. (2021). Shared parenting after separation and divorce in Europe in the context of the second demographic transition. In A. M. Castrén, V. Cesnuityte, I. Crespi, J. A. Gauthier, R. Gouveia, C. Martin, M. Moreno Mínguez, & K. Suwada (Eds.), *The Palgrave handbook of family sociology in Europe* (pp. 377–398). Palgrave Macmillan.

Fraley, R. C., & Heffernan, M. E. (2013). Attachment and parental divorce: A test of the diffusion and sensitive period hypotheses. *Personality and Social Psychology Bulletin, 39*(9), 1199–1213. https://doi.org/10.1177/0146167213491503

Giraud, C. (2020). Relations non-cohabitantes après 50 ans et conjugalité. In M. Oris, T. Gnoumou, C. Bilampoa, & O. Ruxandra (Eds.), *Relations sociales dans la vieillesse: Solidarités et tensions* (pp. 15–24). AIDELF.

Gouveia, R., & Castrén, A. M. (2021). Redefining the boundaries of family and personal relationships. In A. M. Castrén, V. Cesnuityte, I. Crespi, J. A. Gauthier, R. Gouveia, C. Martin, M. Moreno Mínguez, & K. Suwada (Eds.), *The Palgrave handbook of family sociology in Europe* (pp. 259–278). Palgrave Macmillan.

Haskey, J. (2005). Living arrangements in contemporary Britain: Having a partner who usually lives elsewhere and living apart together (LAT). *Population Trends, 122*, 35–46.

Hughes, J. (2000). Repartnering after divorce. Marginal mates and unwedded women. *Family Matters, 55*, 16–21.

Langmeyer, A. N., Recksiedler, C., Entleitner-Phleps, C., & Walper, S. (2022). Post-separation physical custody arrangements in Germany: Examining sociodemographic correlates, parental coparenting, and child adjustment. *Social Sciences, 11*(3), 114. https://doi.org/10.3390/socsci11030114

Levin, I. (2004). Living apart together: A new family form. *Current Sociology, 52*, 223–240.

Lyssens-Danneboom, V., & Mortelmans, D. (2014). Living apart together and money: New partnerships, traditional gender roles. *Journal of Marriage and Family, 76*(5), 949–966.

Paprzycka, E., & Mianowska, E. (2019). Płeć i związki intymne – Strukturalne uwarunkowania. Trwałości pary intymnej. *Dyskursy Młodych Andragogów, 20*, 441–455. https://doi.org/10.34768/dma.vi20.38

Régnier-Loilier, A., Beaujouan, E., & Villeneuve-Gokalp, C. (2009). Neither single, nor in a couple: A study of living apart together in France. *Demographic Research, 21*, 75–108.

Reimondos, A., Evans, A., & Gray, E. (2011). Living-apart-together (LAT) relationships in Australia: An overview. *Family Matters, 87*, 43–55.

Roseneil, S. (2006). On not living with a partner: Unpicking coupledom and cohabitation. *Sociological Research Online, 11*, 1–14.

Stoilova, M., Roseneil, S., Carter, J., Duncan, S., & Philipps, M. (2017). Constructions, reconstructions and deconstructions of 'family' amongst people who live apart together (LATs). *The British Journal of Sociology, 68*(1), 78–96.

Turkle, S. (2011). *Alone together. Why we expect more from technology and less from each other*. Basic Books.

van Eeden-Moorefield, B., Pasley, K., Dolan, E. M., & Engel, M. (2007). From divorce to remarriage: Financial management and security among remarried women. *Journal of Divorce & Remarriage, 47*(3–4), 21–42.

Villeneuve-Gokalp, C. (1994). Après la séparation: conséquences de la rupture et avenir conjugal. In H. Leridon & C. Villeneuve-Gokalp (Eds.), *Constance et inconstances de la famille: Biographies familiales des couples et des enfants* (pp. 137–164). Les Cahiers de l'Ined.

PART III

The Self in 'The Empty Nest'

Without Children at Home: Transition to Herplaces and Hisplaces

Marianna Kostecka, Magdalena Żadkowska,
Bogna Dowgiałło, and Sophie David–Goretta

WOMAN AND MAN AT HOME

Many interdisciplinary studies demonstrate that home is an important space for developing the sense of self (Marcus, 1974; Gorman-Murray, 2008) and bonds (Low & Altman, 1992), as well as a dynamic space that changes due to many key life events (Łukasiuk & Jewdokimow, 2014; Woroniecka, 2014). Home also has different environmental and

M. Kostecka (✉)
Faculty of Sociology, Adam Mickiewicz University, Poznań, Poland
e-mail: markos10@amu.edu.pl

M. Żadkowska
Social Sciences Department (Institute of Sociology), University of Gdańsk, Gdańsk, Poland

Centre de recherche sur les liens sociaux (CERLIS, UMR 8070), Université Paris Cité, Paris, France
e-mail: magdalena.zadkowska@ug.edu.pl

© The Author(s), under exclusive license to Springer Nature Switzerland AG 2024
M. Żadkowska et al. (eds.), *Reconfiguring Relations in the Empty Nest*, Palgrave Macmillan Studies in Family and Intimate Life, https://doi.org/10.1007/978-3-031-50403-7_12

psychological dimensions in people's lives; what is also very important is that it does not depend upon traditional family structure for its meaning (Horowitz & Tognoli, 1982).

In modern western culture, the right to privacy is perceived as a human right. However, its long history is rooted in numerous social, economic, and technological changes, which have challenged the idea of home as a workplace or a place for family life. The boundaries between the public and private, between what is "strange" and what is" familiar", were organization of the home space (cf. Prost, 2000; Skowrońska, 2012: 150–153). The right to privacy in the home varies according to the roles that individuals play inside the social, cultural, and—more specifically—family system. Many researchers have analyzed the entanglement of privacy with gender ideologies and family roles (Allen, 1996; Madigan et al., 1990). Much attention has already been paid to the issue of power in the family home and intimate relations (Cromwell & Olson, 1977; Duch-Krzysztoszek, 2007; Ratecka, 2011; Krzaklewska & Ratecka, 2014).

The traditional narrative revolves around the idea of home as a woman's place, a "feminine site" (cf. Gorman-Murray, 2008: 369) and woman as a home-maker, emphasizing the importance of identity (woman as a housewife and a mother-at-home) and archetypal meanings (woman who is responsible for the "hearth and home") (Domosh & Seager, 2001; Chapman, 2004; Baydar, 2005; Gajewska et al., 2023). Numerous aspects of the relationship between women and home space have already been studied and deconstructed, showing the ambiguity of normative ways of understanding domesticity. The ambiguity lies in the restriction of women's roles to the private sphere, while at the same time excluding them from meaningful privacy at home, which organizes identity and a sense of autonomy. Thus, while women are commonly perceived as in control of managing the domestic space, they are also very frequently left without a private place of their own (Woolf, 1929; Allen, 1996; Madigan & Munro,

B. Dowgiałło
Social Sciences Department (Institute of Sociology), University of Gdańsk, Gdańsk, Poland
e-mail: bogna.dowgiallo@ug.edu.pl

S. David–Goretta
Centre de recherche sur les liens sociaux (CERLIS, UMR 8070), Université Paris Cité, Paris, France
e-mail: sophie.david.goretta@gmail.com

2002). The ambivalence is maintained in two ways. On the one hand in the form of expectations from the woman that she will maintain the family community and put the needs of other household members before her own, which are rooted in socio-economic and cultural patterns. On the other hand, in the internalization of these patterns, including the belief that if a woman exercises the right to privacy, the values of care and community will be compromised (DeVault, 1991; Allen, 1996). One of the influences on these beliefs is traditionally perceived femininity and masculinity, which organize the ways in which domesticity is understood.

In traditional societies, the division of roles was very clear, organized according to the binary divisions, such as "private", "wet," and "dark" (combined with woman and womanhood confined to the private home) and "public," "dry," and "light" (combined with man and manhood confined to the outdoors, public and its representative dimension) (Baydar, 2005; Bourdieu, 2007). Although contemporary homes lack such obvious categorization, certain archetypal divisions for a long time have been reflected in the occupation of herplaces and hisplaces, as well as within the division of household duties (for example, a woman's place in the kitchen, a man's place in the garage or car, a woman without her own room, a man in his own study). Thus, gender roles, supported by the architecture of the home, correspond with the right or exclusion from the right to privacy. Associating women with the home/private does not entail the exercise of the right to privacy, to have, for example, one's own room. Meanwhile men who are associated with the outdoors/public used to have broader access to spaces of solitude and independence such as workshops, basements, garages or gardens ("mancaves"), which affirm stereotypes of heterosexual masculinity (Miller, 2010; Moisio & Beruchashvili, 2016) and show the home as the scene for the "breadwinner" model (Tosh, 1998).

However, the traditional perception of homespace is nowadays challenged by rapid changes related to family life, housing cultures, and the cultural understanding of gender roles. Normative ways of understanding domesticity, in which the woman plays the role of home-maker and the man is captured as the breadwinner, are difficult to be sustained due to many social and cultural transformations. Different types of masculinity (e.g. caregiving), fatherhood (e.g. stay-at-home dads), concepts of domestic masculinities and masculine domesticities (Gorman-Murray, 2008), different activities of women in public life (e.g. multiple jobs), and motherhood (e.g. demystification of motherhood based on desirable sacrifice) contribute to changes in domestic imaginaries, the meanings of dwelling and domestic roles (Titkow, 2012; Żurek, 2016; Maciąg-Budkowska & Rzepa, 2017; Packalén Parkman, 2017; Włodarczyk, 2017). These changes have also led to New Woman and New Man models (Tosh, 1998; Gorman-Murray, 2008). "As an ideal partner for the 'New (Working) Woman', the New Man is intimately involved in the domestic sphere, doing his fair share of housework-parenting, cooking and cleaning. The New Man is, thus, a new model of hetero-masculinity molded through perceived greater participation in domestic activities and labor. As a result of his domestic masculinity, the home is also expected to be de-feminised, and housework de-gendered" (Gorman-Murray, 2008: 371). Thus, the place of women does not have to belong in an obvious and exclusive way to the domestic space. Moreover, the discourse of domesticity can no longer exclude men from it. Other relationships between masculinity and the home subverts normative imaginaries of home and "enabled men to negotiate alternative masculinities, where they could be expressive, emotive and engage in domestic labour and child care" (Gorman-Murray, 2008: 369).

Domestic Imaginaries: His and Her Perspective

The dominant understanding of the home is underpinned by the assumption that it is a place of privacy, comfort, and relaxation (cf. Allen, 1996: 54; Skowrońska, 2012). Even though the home, no matter the gender, is associated with "safety" and "privacy", the "feminine and masculine associations caused by the term 'home' are not the same, and this differentiation is largely anchored in different patterns of everyday life at home" (Budrowska, 2009b: 285). It is more of a male perspective to associate home not with work, but with a harbor, a place of rest and relaxation after work (Hansen Shaevitz, 1984; Titkow et al., 2004; Budrowska, 2009a, b), a respite from the world of stress (Gorman-Murray, 2008), with the so-called warm bath which he takes at home after a hard day (cf. Parsons, 1959). There is then a certain tension between relaxing family time and tiring working time. Some authors go so far as to claim that working men see their paternal obligations diminished by the values attached to work, even if it is still valued for "balancing the family": work represents security inside and outside the family system, a necessity that reinforces their identity as a man, father, and husband (Dulac, 1993, 1997). This tension is societal and is not intended to reduce fathers' ambitions to the strict world of work; it merely underlines the importance that society places on the proper conduct of the man's work, on the father, rather than on the aspects of fatherhood and homespace, even if this tension is less and less attested to.

The question of relaxation at home becomes problematic when it is linked to femininity. The increase of women's engagement in labor markets has not reduced their activity in the domestic space. Even though in France women spend less and less time on domestic work and more time on parenting, they do so significantly more often than men (cf. Champagne et al., 2015). In Poland, women's engagement in labor markets has led to a situation where many women have two jobs, one of which is unpaid (Titkow et al., 2004; Bożewicz, 2018). That is one of the reasons why the idea of home as a place to relax and unwind from the stresses of the outside world remains "truer" for men than for women (Madigan & Munro, 2002: 65; Budrowska, 2009a, b). In fact, many women can only relax at home when they have fully completed all the tasks related to domestic obligations. Since domestic work has the tendency to never truly be finished (Brach-Czaina, 1999), for many women the home is primarily a place of work (Budrowska, 2009a, b: 281).

It is worth mentioning that the idea of home as a place of work has recently been strengthened by working remotely, as a consequence of COVID-19 (Gouveia et al., 2021). In some cases, work from home will degenderize the home by being a place of work both for men and women, as well as reinforce the need of many women to create a working space at home (e.g. her study and home office). However, domestic obligations should be regarded as work even if it is unpaid and performed in the private sphere (Titkow et al., 2004; Coelho et al., 2021). The amount of time devoted to household duties differentiates families and couples by being an indicator of the position a woman occupies in them (Silvera, 2021).

Children's Moving Out and the Transition to One's Own (Sense of) Space

Entering into parenting roles does indeed change the home space. Sometimes these are small changes, like filling the living room with the baby's crib, toys, splotches, and sounds. Sometimes the changes are much bigger, like exchanging the apartment or house for a more spacious one or furnishing a separate room for the baby. It should be mentioned that changes do not appear only in material dimensions. Having a family is associated with new ways of negotiating space and rules of cohabitation, for example, in the form of temporal division of use of the living room ("time zoning"), which during the day is often a place of "invasive" presence of the child, while in the evenings a place of rest for the parents (Munro & Madigan, 1993; Madigan & Munro, 2002; Cieraad, 2013); in fact not only in the evenings. In many families, especially in those experiencing housing deprivation, when the child falls asleep in their own room, the parents return to the living room and fall asleep on the couch where friends were previously hosted (cf. Emilewicz, 2020).

The transition from full to empty nest often includes changes, such as emptying the child's room, additional square meters to be used in the house, and the absence of family members using the common spaces. All of them appear as an opportunity for parents to reclaim their space, as a chance to find herplace(s) and hisplace(s). Nevertheless, children's moving out does not necessarily result in a new study room or bedroom for one of the parents. This is especially true when it comes to families living in large houses, where there is no need to arrange additional and necessary space that previously belonged to a child (cf. Chaps. 5 and 7). However, what seems to unite many family stories—regardless of the size of the apartment and financial capabilities—are changes in domestic imaginaries (home as a place of work versus relaxation) and ways of reclaiming personal places at home (sometimes through the feeling that home without the children has mainly become a place of rest). Some may result in practices of renovating and redecorating the apartment that lead to gaining, for example, a separate room of their own. Some may only result in new uses of a common space, new rituals that foster the sense of "my own place," even if such a feeling only lasts for the duration of a long bath or a naked walk around the apartment that are possible when the children are not at home anymore (cf. Chap. 9).

So far, the empty nest stage has been broadly analyzed from the woman's perspective (Rubenstein, 2007; Wojciechowska, 2008; Gajewska et al., 2023). The reasons for emphasizing the female perspective in the empty nest research have often been explained by associating the female identity with a mother's and home-maker's role and with values such as sharing, helping others, sacrifice, or care (Chapman, 2004; Titkow, 2007; Kopciewicz, 2008; Maciąg-Budkowska & Rzepa, 2017; Rancew-Sikora & Skowrońska, 2022). However, as the domestic space is gendered, it is important to ask how the transition to the empty nest affects or is reflected in the changes analyzed from the perspective of both parents. This chapter demonstrates how the children's departure influences the creation of individual herplaces and hisplaces in Poland and France, mirroring the recomposition of new domestic roles. The changing event, that is, the children's departure, can influence both the space and the identity. Home creativity can challenge traditional and gendered uses of space and artifacts (Pink, 2004). As one "makes a home," one accumulates a sense of self (Gorman-Murray, 2008). Home without children enables "new" patterns of everyday life, styles of masculinity and femininity, and questions both normative imaginaries of home (cf. Gorman-Murray, 2008) and ways of feeling oneself at home, in one's own place.

Methods

This chapter is based on qualitative in-depth dyadic and individual interviews conducted in Poland and France. The empirical material contains 77 dyadic (corpus A) and 121 individual interviews (corpuses B and C); the sample consisted of 75 Polish women (26 took part in 2 interviews, dyadic and individual; 49 in one individual), 46 Polish men (26 took part in 2 interviews, dyadic and individual; 20 in one individual), 33 French women and 32 French men (all of them took part in one dyadic interview). We decided to include diverse groups of project participants both in Poland and in France, all united by the experience of the "empty nest" phase of life. The group also varied in terms of where they lived, both in terms of location—urban and non-urban and the size of houses and flats. We analyzed interviews conducted with women and men with the experience of long relationships (over 20 years of marriage), as well as interviews with women who had experienced divorce or death of their husband before the children had moved out from the family household.

Data analysis was carried out using Maxqda software. Coding was conducted by an international group of researchers (Polish and French) who first read, analyzed, and coded the transcriptions in their original language and then did the collaborative analysis of the findings in English.

Findings

Herplaces

Full-time mothering and home-maker roles associated with women's roles are often abandoned when children leave home. As a result of the child moving out, the material space of the house loses some of its objects, fills with new ones, and changes color; individual places gain new destinations and functions, some of them also eventually change their owner(s). Stories of children moving out are very often herstories of women in their own rooms and studies.

> Barbara: Also, **this desk**, which I am sitting at, I got it from my daughter—she left it, **I set myself up at it, organised myself**, I even have **my mess** on this desk, **I found myself**. Also, for me, **an empty nest means an increase in my privacy, my sanctuary**—that's how you can put it. (B_PL_69)

Children's rooms, however, have proven to have a much more diverse use. A family home without children is also filled with rooms for sports ("[…] I work out in my room, in my daughters' room I made a place for myself where I do yoga"), maintaining old interests and developing new ones ("right here where I'm sitting [my daughter's room] is my studio, because I paint for myself"). In addition to such broad pragmatic functions of one's own room, having it also has a highly social and psychological significance. **A room which previously belonged to a child may turn into a kind of backstage of a woman's daily life.** Women, after locking themselves in their own room, "dress out" the roles of mothers, housewives, and wives.

> Krystyna: But this is the room where I am currently.... I feel like I'm going to **be alone**. […] Moreover, sometimes I'll stay a little longer and read all the messages on my phone, well, here is where I feel like **no one is going to say "Krystynka, and where's this, and where's that?"**. It's kind of like an **escape** to this room. […] My son's room, well, a place where very nice things happen, because there is **relaxation, rest, isolation**. I am **simply alone** here. **It is like I'm not married here and I am not a mother, just like that, you know?** (B_PL_13G)

"Moving into" a child's room turns out to be an opportunity to create a kind of channel for relieving the daily tensions associated with working three jobs: wife, mother, and worker. It is a chance to escape both the caregiving roles that shrink a woman's privacy on a daily basis and the "busyness of everyday life" based on women performing most of the household chores. Finally, it is also an opportunity to reclaim those housing functions related to the idea of dwelling comfort that are not fulfilled by communal spaces (where there is always someone sitting, eating, listening to music, and so on). A woman's occupation of a child's room thus appears as an opportunity to improve her psychological well-being and the possibility to create a concept of herself in isolation from the culturally assigned, and often exploitative, role of mother, which was played intensively when the children were at home.

In addition to **having an opportunity to "escape"** from the obligations inherent in the traditional role of a mother, having one's own room encourages withdrawal from the communal areas where many tensions and power relations within the couple arise. A room of her own may then turn out to be a real "escape" from her partner and the role of wife currently being played. "Escape from a partner" is often more difficult to achieve and to assume while children are still living at home. The difficulties may arise from physical barriers, such as lack of space (e.g. separate rooms or bedrooms), but also from normative expectations that the couple should sleep together, spend time together, and generally perform their "couplehood" when the child is watching (cf. Chap. 10).

> Marzena: This is the kind of place where I **stay alone**, such as my.... well, I wouldn't call it a sanctuary, but well, my husband prefers to watch TV here, such programs that don't necessarily interest me. **Before I had to tolerate it somehow, and now I don't have to, I just lock myself in here. So here I am**. (B_PL_6G)

Thus, a room of one's own gives the basic right to refuse to participate in unfavorable situations and relationships in the space of the home, including the right to give up the labor women undertake to maintain the family community. Responses such as relief, escape, or rest suggest annoyance at the invisible emotional labor performed on a daily basis. The chance for women to regain their privacy after the children move out may also appear as a strong chance to improve their psychological well-being.

It is worth mentioning that women's attempts to reclaim their privacy and herplaces have not always been easy or smooth after the children move out. The oppressiveness of hegemonic maternal models is reflected in the narratives of some women recounting in positive terms the empty nest stage and the changes made in the child's room. These narratives were not without dilemmas. More or less successful attempts to transgress the norms of intensive motherhood, to transgress or negate the idea of self-sacrifice, evoked informal sanctions in the form of unpleasant emotions, negative self-criticism, and potential criticism from others, usually other mothers.

Ewelina: I will still say something like this—it will be unpopular.... **it's hard for me to admit it**, but I'll tell you this, I was actually **waiting for my second daughter to move out** as well, not forever, but in the sense that I had **such a need to run an independent life**. [...] **I don't know if I would say this to any friend**. (B_PL_59)

Dorota: I had this moment during those two months, the kids had moved out, of thinking **what a mean mother I am** (...). And after the two months I started feeling that hurrah, the house is mine, etc. At this point **I felt even worse, because I felt I should be in despair**. But (...) I felt that (...) I can make this room what I want, I can do something for myself (...) if there is a passion, there are activities, then there is no need to sit and wait. (B_PL_9G)

The belief that as a mother "I should have empty nest syndrome" (in Ewelina's words) is many times correlated with seeing oneself in the role of home-maker and room-keeper, which creates a tension with other roles, especially those facilitated by having space for oneself. Narratives in which the woman is seen as the person responsible for the "hearth and home" may prove to be a belief preventing changes in the child's space (e.g. the child's room), thus strengthening the need to keep a "place on earth" for them (cf. Chap. 5). In addition, the informal sanctions described earlier in the form of unpleasant feelings (e.g. guilt or bad conscience), self-criticism, and potential criticism from others are controlling tools for the performative potential in transforming the home space in accordance with the needs of a particular woman.

The intense maternal role played on a daily basis when the children were at home is often associated with an emerging need for rest and relaxation after the children have moved out. In our study, we also asked respondents directly about their preferred space at home. They most often mentioned places where they relax and spend their free time alone or as a couple. There are different ways to relax, one of them is taking a nap or lying on the sofa. It is difficult to find clear gender differences in the statements of respondents in relation to the type of places chosen for relaxation and recreation. However, the idea of relaxation itself seems to have a different meaning for women and men. Some female respondents, recalling stories of "lying on the sofa" or resting during the day, report at the same time **the uniqueness of these situations and their shortage in the full nest.**

Sandra: I remember my children one day came back from high school, we were in Jerusalem, it was the year Sophie was there, we had a big living room and we had the couch where I'm sitting today (...), and in fact I looked at my watch, I looked at my watch and said, "the kids are going to arrive soon, I'm going to lie down and wait for them" and in fact when they arrived, they opened the door and they saw the living room, they saw me, they stopped right away and said, "mom, what's going on? Why are you in bed?" And I said nothing, well, it's okay, I am waiting for you. And they said to me "but why are you lying down, what's going on?". And in fact I realized that my children had never seen me relaxing (laughs) and then I thought, oh yeah. And I said to myself, yeah, maybe now I'll have to...
　　Vincent: That you take naps.
　　Sandra: No, no, that I show them that I'm not just active. (A_FR_15)

The fact of sitting on the couch signifies the desire to take a moment for oneself. The sofa becomes a symbol of the entry to more personal moments, more focussed on oneself (deserved, with or without the consent of others).

Clarisse: There are the races at the end and Sunday afternoon **I want to sit on my couch and I don't want to be bothered** with 50,000 questions or to say no, **I want to be alone on Sunday afternoon.** If I feel like crocheting, I crochet, if I don't feel like crocheting I lie on my couch watching Netflix. That's how I like it now, but it's always been like that even when I was in my late teens I had my moments when I liked to be alone (...). (A_FR_10)

Maybe because of their age women talk about a need to stretch their legs, to read a book, or play a game. They now find time for these activities in between domestic duties.

Teresa: Because I like to go there to read a book even during the day, yes? I haven't marked the armchair, but there is one, even though it doesn't fit in with the interior design, I laugh that it's my alternative wardrobe, that there's a blouse here and some pants. **But when I put them away, I can sit down, stretch my legs out on the bed and read a book there, or play an electronic game by myself, or at least sit, think or lie down for a while.** (B_PL_7P)

Home as a place to relax and spend time on one's own terms is mentioned by Teresa as a reclaimed space for her and her husband after their daughters moved out of the house. When they lived there, it was not possible to relax freely, watch TV, think, play a game, lie down for a while, read books, or take a long bath. Changing the use of domestic space, including certain furniture or domestic appliances (such as a chair or a television), therefore means using them without limitations and according to one's needs. In a full nest, it was not possible to do the things she wanted to do in this way and to regain "time for herself." It turned out to be difficult especially during the day when the daughters were "everywhere, all over the house, and you tried to give them that space." "Doing home without children" is thus linked to a **change in the easier way of negotiating space and its use**, to having more time at one's disposal to immerse oneself in some relaxing practices for which, as Teresa said, "you finally have a space where you can do it." An example which confirms such an attitude towards domestic space is the bathroom:

> Interviewer: Okay, and this place now, here I see a lot of changes, this "wellness, home spa", is that just for you or do you and your husband both treat the place like that? Well, because there's certainly a bit of this space reclaimed, that it's not so crowded, right?
>
> Teresa: Well there is! Just the fact that you have more time, that I can dedicate my time to this, yes? And now you have a space to do that! So when I lie down in this bath, **I am immersed in a moment. Nobody knocks, "Mummy, hurry up, because…."**. Well, at the weekend it's still so hard for all of us together, but everyone can find a moment for themself, **it's no longer the case that we all have to be here at the same time**. Well, when it's a spa, you know, there has to be that time, but there's also time to lie down and there's somewhere to sit, somewhere to renew yourself. If you come back from a long walk, you can go in and sit down. (B_PL_7P)

"Time for myself" can be also transformed into time for professional work. In particular, women who are relieved of the responsibilities of motherhood can devote more time to their professional work or to developing their professional skills. As well as more time, there is now extra space that can be used as a workspace. For some women, this may be the first time they have had their own workspace.

> Dorota: Yes, and it's mine. **I never had room for it, it was always somewhere in the living room and then I had to roll it up when I came to do something.** And today I don't have to roll it up. (B_PL_9G)

In the Polish sample, the individual interviews took place during the lockdown caused by the COVID-19 pandemic. Many female respondents used this time to conceptualize and introduce the idea of an office at home.

> Maria: (…) and me, thanks to that… If I close it, I don't care then what happens there. I'm not going to go in there, I'm not going to climb up there. Well, we made such a move. Well, it involved, you know, a little bit of repainting here, redecorating. So that's how the change came about. So now Monica's room is an office. We use it in different ways for different things. Yes, it is now a study. We use it sometimes, mostly me. But sometimes like, for example, there is remote work, my husband was also in there. Or Monika's Internet did not work, she also came here. But, let's just say, this is an office mostly, well, occupied by me, whatever you call it. (B_PL_2P)

The return of some adult children (see Chap. 7) and the challenge of working remotely proved to be triggers for finalizing the idea of "**working herplaces**."

Hisplaces

The place occupied by men in the family universe is not as visible as the place occupied by women. For some male respondents, home remains a stage for women's home-making performance, so there is more evidence of "**having no space**" rather than "having hisplace." Even though the separate place does not exist for some men, the feeling of one's own space is achieved through particular use of furniture (e.g. a sofa) or activities (e.g. watching TV).

> Gérald: Béatrice [**his wife**] **needs to appropriate her house**… it's been like this since 1992 that we have been trying to have a fitted kitchen because … there you go … she wants her kitchen. **I don't care, I have a bed, a sofa, a TV and a computer and that's more than enough for me. I don't need anything more, I'd rather be a landlord of vehicles (…) than actually of a home.** (A_FR_14)

Another example of the man "having no space" scenario is Leszek. He mentions a small sofa in "her" space where he can lie down and just be close to Zofia, his wife, as long as she is not disturbed.

> Leszek: Well I have a small sofa downstairs and some sort of TV. I like to sit and lie down and be around Zosia. I think she likes it too, unless I snore. (B_PL_3P)

Before the children left, Leszek had no idea what his place in the empty nest would be. It was different in the case of his wife Zofia, an academic, for whom it had always been important to plan an office at home without the children, an office full of books. Leszek may also be in the process of planning his own place, a place which had never even thought of when the nest was full. **The empty nest stage flourishes with some men finding new ways of using personal spaces which they had not predicted.**

> Leszek: So there's kind of **no room for me**. I think. And, will it be in this big house? I don't know either. I just think, as you pointed out, **it will probably be somewhere outside the house, yes?** Sometimes it will be around the house, sometimes it will be in different rooms, sometimes it will be rather somewhere in between, I don't know, well, **we're simply going to plan it**, it will also be here somehow. But this particular space, I'm saying, I don't really have this space. (B_PL_3P)

Some men, like Piotr, Wojtek and Darek exemplify the type of **hetero-masculine domesticity**, a normative relationship between the man and his home, where "a man's home is his castle," a respite from the world of work (Gorman-Murray, 2008). Maybe there is no longer a warm bath waiting for him, but he takes the central place in the home, in the dining room, close to the table or by the TV set, both in a full and empty nest.

> Interviewer: And do you have a place in your flat where you like to spend as much time as possible alone?
>
> Piotr: Alone? **Of course, I have my own director's bed** with access to the TV and my computer on my lap and a phone next to it. It's well known that nowadays one source of information is not enough, you need three and preferably all on at once. (...) It's kind of a hut there, **the lazy man who doesn't do anything there,** that's the place, yes? (B_PL_11P)

Those men who represent the hetero-masculine identity and who are "left without a place of their own" do not even express the need to have one inside the home particularly. They feel that having separate rooms at home is not enough to meet their individual needs. However, the feeling of his-place is possible to be achieved through spaces of solitude, often combined with DIY places, so-called mancaves. These spaces are usually **located outside the central domestic space**, such as in basements or garages which affirm stereotypes of heterosexual masculinity.

Interviewer: Don't you feel a lack of a room? Wouldn't you like to have your own room?

Wojtek: No, I feel **the lack of a basement, this is what is missing here, 'cos you could always go there with a male friend for some beer and have some peace and quiet, no one would disturb you. And I had** [in the previous flat] **my garage there, so I could do little things, something arty-farty**.

Interviewer: A room wouldn't be good for that?

Wojtek: **Not really a room—the basement was good**, 'cos when you make a sound, everything can be heard. When the neighbor farts, you can hear it.

Researcher: Do you have your own place here? (…).

Wojtek: No, maybe in front of the TV, on the coach—other than that I do not have one… (A_PL_8G)

Darek: I will tell you in confidence that I fight for such a place all the time, but **there is no such place where I can hole up and get some peace and quiet**. There is no such place because we have a shared space, the living room is shared, without a door. The room we are in now is the only room where you can close the door and have a quiet conversation. But in turn, **it is not a room where you can think, relax**. Here there is a desk, a chair and all sorts of things associated with them that are **far from relaxing**. That's the kind of place—I'm working on it and I'll probably have a place like that. […] **it's going to be below ground, in the garage in the basement. There's a place where we have a projector and game equipment now. And I'm planning to make a place where you can watch a film or listen to music, or play a concert. That's what Im planning to do. There's also a fireplace down there, so I'm assuming that will be the space.** (B_PL_10G)

For many men, their space needs to be specially designed and carved out from the rest of the house, with clearly marked boundaries between home and "my place." Moreover, only in such an organized space is it possible for them to "relax fully" and gain "peace of mind." Additionally, Darek explains that relaxation and leisure in his home are based on his partners' different moods, which influence the way they spend their time at home.

The number of things she (the wife) does at home means he rests by himself.

> Darek: It would be nice to spend more time together, but it also comes down to how that time is spent. We don't do things like watching films or listening to music together, my wife has completely different expectations of music and films. She also has a slightly different character to me—I'm one of those people who, **when I have a free moment,I will sit down on the sofa and I can watch a whole film or listen to a whole concert. My wife will do a million other things in the meantime—so this kind of time, this kind of chillout, is hard to plan together.** (B_PL_10G)

Our sample does not consist only of men with "having no space" or "ideal mancave" scenarios. Another possible type of hisplace is a **"place for passion."** These kinds of spaces usually involve active leisure or manual work. Men collect the materials they need to carry out certain tasks in this space, making it their own. These moments are perceived by some male respondents as necessary and show the passion that drives them.

> Interviewer: And your room in the attic, Gérald, where you have all your equipment, do you go there often? Is it more a space for leisure? For work? Both?
> Gérald: It's for both leisure and work, well I've never considered it as a job it's... I've never counted the time I spend on music, I've always been passionate (...) (A_FR_1)

These spaces take on the **aspect of an individual sanctuary when it comes to making something with one's own hands, to find oneself through one's passion**. They require distance from other family members, both physically and symbolically.

> Tadeusz: Also music, the guitar, I even create music and write something. I also have time, and for that you need a lot of peace and quiet. (A_PL_2P)

The spaces that men take over are not spaces of conviviality where men and women, or men with their children, meet. They are rather individual spaces, to rest, to develop a passion. It can be a whole room or a specific place, but it is identified for a particular use. This place then becomes unique because it provides a feeling of personal place (even though male friends are often invited to such places). For Oliver, one's own place means to be alone, without his children or wife. Hisplace is the place where: "I want to be without Véronique" (A_FR_18).

There are also less traditional homes, where spaces are divided according to inhabitants' needs for rest and male respondents represent a new model of man where as a result of his domestic masculinity, **the home is de-feminized, and housework de-gendered** (Gorman-Murray, 2008: 371). Ryszard speaks of two sofas, placed side by side, where each sits alone and reads their book or at other times they watch a film together.

> Ryszard: Yes, as much as possible. I read things, my wife reads other things. We sit together **on two sofas, she on hers, me on mine.** Sometimes we watch the same things, the same films. (B_PL_4G)

A similar division is present in Jan's house. After work, with no one else at home, Jan rests in the bedroom and Halina on the sofa in front of the TV set. The empty nest situation lets them use all the space according to their resting preferences.

> Jan: Now I like my bedroom very much, I have my corner by the window **and when I come back from work quite tired I like to lie down on the bed in my bedroom with a newspaper or a book. My wife, on the other hand, has a huge sofa in the living room and this is her favorite place to rest.** Sometimes it is the case that we are actually separate, on the principle that I lie down upstairs in the bedroom and she lounges right there. I only put the back there, but there's this huge sofa and that's where my wife likes it. I don't watch TV at all, my wife watches a bit and it's good to watch TV from there, from that sofa. (B_PL_8P)

The de-feminized home and de-gendered housework may lead to a change in domestic roles. The partner who previously did not take on certain responsibilities can willingly and enthusiastically perform them in an empty nest. It is the case of male respondents who enter the kitchen stage, family actors who were absent from there before, during the full nest.

> Jan: [...] And often, even when my wife isn't here, I just bake buns, make some juice, some cream soups. I found a bit of a chef's talent in me, but only because this pot gives ready-made recipes. You only have to put things in the pot. Well, it is a kitchen accessory, but it makes you spend even more time in the kitchen. (B_PL_8P)

Although at the stage of a full nest it is mainly women who perform domestic tasks, men get involved to a greater extent in an empty nest (cf. Chap. 10). Women are also far more likely than men to be the ones to talk about the new division of household responsibilities in the empty nest. For example, Iwona admits:

> Iwona: As for chores, my husband has started doing more. He does the shopping—I do less and less, I don't do much shopping, I used to do more. And **now my husband will go and do the shopping, clean the kitchen, which used not to happen. The division has gotten so much better for me—I used to be more burdened with it all, I used to be overwhelmed with this work, the responsibilities for the kids, because if he always came back later, the kids were on my mind.** When they were at school, it was more or less when they finished, when they were smaller we spent a lot of time in the afternoon together. It wasn't my husband who did it, because he'd come back in the evening and he wasn't there more often. (A_PL_7G)

The cases of Jan and Ryszard are further examples of a de-feminized home and a de-gendered model of housework. Respondents admit that the reorganization of the nest after adult children's departure let them start to be involved in new practices of everyday life. However, during the transition to the "home without children," the parental households are sometimes reduced to the situation before parenthood. Mothers and fathers are released from their direct parenting roles and parental time binds. This gradual transition creates a context in which housework space and time allocation can be rearranged. It can take an idyllic form, in which partners not only share household duties but also do so with pleasure and out of love for the other person.

> Tadeusz: We sleep together, we wake up together, sometimes we wake each other up or encourage each other to get up. Then one of us goes to make breakfast, usually whoever gets up quicker—if someone wants take a bath, then the one who has more time makes breakfast. We do it interchangeably because I cook as well and it is not a problem. So we make breakfast and one person waits for the other. We come for breakfast, usually before 7 in the week, before work. We eat breakfast for a quarter of an hour. Then, when we have some time, we make ourselves a coffee. (A_PL_2P)

It may happen that the space that used to be associated with haste, work, and obligation has become a place where performing household tasks are no longer seen as a chore. Instead, it is now seen as an opportunity to spend quality time together, relaxing on the sofa while waiting to eat the meal the man and woman have cooked together (see Chap. 9). However, it can also become truly empty, with both spouses hiding in their own rooms and activities (see Chap. 10).

Discussion

The analysis of the in-depth interviews made it possible to observe that, mainly for women, the departure of an adult child is the key event in the life of the family that triggers creating a place of one's own at home. Moreover, in some cases the home without children is associated less with haste and obligations and more with relaxation. However, relaxation at home without children and the desire to have one's own place carries different meanings and functions for women and men. In the studied sample, the differences are evidently more pronounced between genders than between countries, Poland and France.

Giving up care, scheduled domestic chores, and intensive mothering is an awaited moment that causes relief and joy for many women. Furthermore, control over the space of the flat/house and in some cases gaining a room promotes taking care of one's own needs and "materialises" a feeling of intrinsic power or agency. For some women, getting out of intense day-to-day motherhood played-out daily will drive the performative potential in managing the space according to their needs and foster the annexation of a personal place (e.g. a room that no longer belongs to a child). Having one's own place indirectly enables one to reject the "pressure to empathise" to which women are socialized from an early age. At its core is the female model of identity, which is characterized by an orientation toward relationships with others, alignment with social roles and broad identification with them.

However, the room of her own has various functions. Besides being a space for dealing with "my stuff" (e.g. checking a phone, working remotely etc.), it is also a kind of "escape room" (from intense family life, playing social roles, household chores). The pressure of caring for a child and fulfilling the societal expectations of a mother can be a significant obstacle for some women seeking change in their home life. The "traditional" idea of a mother experiencing empty nest syndrome can also serve as a means of control, further restricting the potential for change. We have observed some informal sanctions in the form of, for example, bad conscience after occupying a daughter's or son's room. Thus it confirms that managing this space after the child has left is a problematic practice, especially for mothers who have many social and emotional obligations. However, within many home-making practices women find opportunities to build a specific space for themselves, a space of freedom, comfort, and rest. This is also the case of women who are not fully included in the processes of annexing the space for themselves. Finding privacy in the absence of a separate space is done through practices such as finding time for oneself while lying on the couch, stretching one's legs, or watching TV. Without children at home, women have a chance to regain their privacy, either in terms of a separate space (a room, study etc.) or isolated, relaxing practices (reading a book, playing a game). The regaining of privacy is also enhanced by the possibility of redefining the use of spaces and practices. This new set of rules allows for the unrestricted use of domestic space without the potential disturbance of others, and is tailored to the woman's individual needs and preferences. It can also lead to a greater sense of power and control over personal space in the home, even if it is not a story about her own room but a story about her afternoon nap.

The experiences of fathers indicate different ways in which men use the domestic space. We have observed traditional examples, with men in the full nesting phase treating the home as a family place, after work, home of which they are the "head." After all, "new masculinity" challenges the old, but does not always replace it. The children moving out raises questions about the continued fate of the space they occupy and new ways of using it, both together with their wives and separately. Some respondents seemed to use the time of change to activate themselves in the kitchen, for example, by participating in new degendered practices and rituals. For fathers who already participated in domestic practices during the full nest time, the domestic space seems to be tamer. They have a greater ease in negotiating both their own new corner and their new role as home-maker. Nowadays, thanks to changes related to New Man and New Woman models (Gorman-Murray, 2008), domesticity seems to be more inclusive for men. On the one hand, it is possible to maintain the "status quo" for a long time because it allows not to make changes in one's relationship or personal life, and this status is mirrored in an unchanged homespace. On the other hand, the changes occurring in the home reflect the new roles taken on by the inhabitants of the home and show their state of readiness to function in a changed, more empty space.

Comparing men and women, we have observed different approaches to the expanded space left by adult children and to changing the "homespace without children." When men change the practice or the child's space, they have no regrets. Women, on the other hand, introduce changes slowly, as if to check "what the children would think." Moreover, both women and men, especially those who do not have a separate room, find a sense of their own place in the home within control over many micro-spaces (e.g. personal desk space) and micro-practices (e.g. taking a long bath). However, women seem to do so with greater frequency. In a full nest, many of them faced limited privacy and blurred boundaries between "time/place for myself" and "time/place for family members." Thus, when transitioning to an empty nest, women experience such individual micro-practices and micro-spaces as more unique, as symbols of their own place. On the other hand, the vast majority of men in our sample express the need to have a specially designed, equipped, and separate space (preferably outside the home, e.g. garage, basement) to call their own. Such a "distribution" of her and hisplaces resembles the traditional division based on gender binaries: femininity associated with indoors and the private home, and masculinity associated with outdoors and the public. This statement suggests that some men may exhibit traits of dominant masculinity, but may not feel comfortable or fully integrated in their own homes, their "castles." For such men, living in a flat without access to the outdoors may be particularly challenging, as they have no external spaces to feel a sense of their own place. Moreover, in the case of men, the impact of the empty nest on the creation of individual places is less significant, whereas women experience directly how domestic space is changing or will change after the child has moved out. It is experienced more frequently through planning specific changes to the homespace, dilemmas in deciding what to do with a child's room, and looking forward to finally having their own room, bedroom, or study. The male need to have hisplace outside the house or apartment seems to be permanent and not directly triggered by the children's departure.

Nevertheless, there is also one general outcome—the home which does not revolve around children and their needs is a home where practices of relaxation and resting seem to be done more often and to be socially more acceptable, both by women and men who sometimes lie on the couch together.

REFERENCES

Allen, A. L. (1996). Privacy at home. The twofold problem. In N. J. Hirschmann & C. Di Stefano (Eds.), *Revisioning the political: Feminist reconstructions of traditional concepts in Western political theory* (1st ed., pp. 193–212). Westview Press.

Baydar, G. (2005). Figures of wo/man in contemporary architectural discourse. In H. Heynen & G. Baydar (Eds.), *Negotiating domesticity. Spatial productions of gender in modern architecture* (1st ed., pp. 30–46). Routledge.

Bourdieu, P. (2007). *Szkic teorii praktyki, poprzedzony trzema studiami na temat 37 etnologii Kabylów* (W. Kroker, Trans.). Kęty, Wydawnictwo Antyk Marek Derewiecki. (Original Work Published 1972).

Bożewicz, M. (2018). Kobiety i mężczyźni w domu. *CBOS.* Retrieved February 10, 2023, from https://www.cbos.pl/

Brach-Czaina, J. (1999). *Szczeliny istnienia.* Wydawnictwo eFKa.

Budrowska, B. (2009a). Krzątactwo codzienności a perspektywa "trzeciej socjologii". In B. Budrowska (Ed.), *Kobiety, feminizm, demokracja: wybrane zagadnienia z seminarium IFiS PAN z lat 2001–2009* (pp. 70–92). Wydawnictwo IFiS PAN.

Budrowska, B. (2009b). Kobiet codzienność krzątacza i męskie "gdzie jem i śpię", czyli z czym kojarzy się dom. In S. Rudnicki, J. Stypińska, & K. Wojnicka (Eds.), *Społeczeństwo i codzienność. W stronę nowej socjologii?* (pp. 278–304). Wydawnictwa Akademickie i Profesjonalne.

Champagne, C., Pailhé, A., & Solaz, A. (2015). Le temps domestique et parental des hommes et des femme: quels facteurs d'évolutions en 25 ans? *Économie et statistique, 478*(1), 209–242.

Chapman, T. (2004). *Gender and domestic life: Changing practices in families and households.* Palgrave Macmillan.

Cieraad, I. (2013). The family living room: A child's playpen? *Home Cultures, 10*(3), 287–314. https://doi.org/10.2752/175174213X13712175825557

Coelho, B., Maciel, D., & Torres, A. (2021). Gender, social class, and family relations in different life stages in Europe. In B. Coelho, D. Maciel, & A. Torres (Eds.), *The Palgrave handbook of family sociology in Europe.* Palgrave Macmillan. https://doi.org/10.1007/978-3-030-73306-3_3

Cromwell, R. E., & Olson, D. H. (1977). *Power in families.* Sage.

DeVault, M. L. (1991). *Feeding the family: The social organization of caring as gendered work.* The University of Chicago Press.

Domosh, M., & Seager, J. (2001). *Putting women in place: Feminist geographers make sense of the world.* Guilford Press.

Duch-Krzysztoszek, D. (2007). *Kto rządzi w rodzinie. Socjologiczna analiza relacji w małżeństwie.* Wydawnictwo IFiS PAN.

Dulac, G. (1993). Études féministes. Études masculines. In A. Turmel (Ed.), *Chantiers sociologiques et anthropologiques, actes du 51e congrès de l'ACSALF* (pp. 106–112). Méridien.

Dulac, G. (1997). Le complexe paternal. In G. Rondeau & J. Broué (Eds.), *Père à part entière* (pp. 13–23). Éditions Saint-Martin.

Emilewicz, J. (2020). Stan mieszkalnictwa w Polsce. *GOV.* Retrieved February 20, 2023, from https://www.gov.pl/web/rozwoj-technologia/raport-o-stanie-mieszkalnictwa

Gajewska, M., Herzberg-Kurasz, M., Żadkowska, M., Kostecka, M., & Dowgiałło, B. (2023). Room of her own: Remaking empty nest and creating herspaces in practices of Polish mothers whose children left home. *European Journal of Women's Studies, 30*(1), 7–21. https://doi.org/10.1177/13505068221110336

Gorman-Murray, A. (2008). Masculinity and the home: A critical review and conceptual framework. *Australian Geographer, 39*(3), 367–379. https://doi.org/10.1080/00049180802270556

Gouveia, R., Ramos, V., & Wall, K. (2021). Household diversity and the impacts of COVID-19 on families in Portugal. *Frontiers in Sociology, 6*(736714), 1–13. https://doi.org/10.3389/fsoc.2021.736714

Hansen Shaevitz, M. (1984). *The superwoman syndrome.* Random House.

Horowitz, J., & Tognoli, J. (1982). Role of home in adult development: Women and men living alone describe their residential histories. *Journal of Applied Family & Child Studies, 31*, 335–341.

Kopciewicz, L. (2008). Grzeczne dziewczynki, niegrzeczni chłopcy – wytwarzanie różnic rodzajowych w dydaktyczno-wychowawczej pracy szkoły. In M. Dudzikowa & M. Czerepaniak-Walczak (Eds.), *Wychowanie. Pojęcia, procesy, konteksty: interdyscyplinarne ujęcie, tom 4: Ku demokracji poprzez edukację* (pp. 349–392). Gdańskie Wydawnictwo Psychologiczne.

Krzaklewska, E., & Ratecka, A. (2014). Władza w intymnych związkach heteroseksualnych refleksja nad badaniem władzy w kontekście równości płci. *Acta Universitatis Lodziensis. Folia Sociologica, 51*, 149–167.

Low, S. M., & Altman, I. (1992). Place attachment : A Conceptual Inquiry. In I. Altman & S. M. Low (Eds.), *Place attachment* (pp. 1–12). Springer US. https://doi.org/10.1007/978-1-4684-8753-4_1

Łukasiuk, M., & Jewdokimow, M. (Eds.). (2014). *Socjologia zamieszkiwania.* Wydawnictwo Naukowe Sub Lupa.

Maciąg-Budkowska, M., & Rzepa, T. (2017). Jaka jest "idealna matka?". Rozumienie roli matki przez współczesne kobiety. *Annales Universitatis Marie Curie Skłodowska, 30*(3), 93–106.

Madigan, R., & Munro, M. (2002). "The more we are together": Domestic space, gender and privacy. In T. Chapman & J. Hockey (Eds.), *Ideal homes? Social change and domestic life* (pp. 61–72). Taylor & Francis e-Library.

Madigan, R., Munro, M., & Smith, S. J. (1990). Gender and the meaning of the home. *International Journal of Urban and Regional Research, 14*(4), 625–647. https://doi.org/10.1111/j.1468-2427.1990.tb00160.x

Marcus, C. C. (1974). The house as symbol of the self. In J. Land, C. Burnette, W. Moleski, & D. Vachon (Eds.), *Designing for human behavior* (pp. 130–146). Dowden, Hutchinson & Ross.

Miller, T. (2010). The birth of the Patio Daddy-O: Outdoor grilling in postwar America. *Journal of American Culture, 33*(1), 5–11.

Moisio, R., & Beruchashvili, M. (2016). Mancaves and masculinity. *Journal of Consumer Culture, 16*(3), 656–676. https://doi.org/10.1177/1469540514553712

Munro, M., & Madigan, R. (1993). Privacy in the private sphere. *Housing Studies, 8*, 29–45. https://doi.org/10.1080/02673039308720748

Packalén Parkman, M. A. (2017). Macierzyństwo bez lukru i retuszu. Wizerunek Matki Polki w literaturze polskiej po roku 2000 i blogach. *Postscriptum Polonistyczne, 2*(20), 63–83.

Parsons, T. (1959). The social structure of the family. In R. N. Anshen (Ed.), *The family: Its functions and destiny*. Harper & Row.

Pink, S. (2004). *Home truths: Gender, domestic objects and everyday life* (1st ed.). Routledge.

Prost, A. (2000). Granice i obszar prywatności In A. Prost, & G. Vincente (Eds.), *Historia życia prywatnego, t. 5: Od I wojny światowej do naszych czasów* (K. Skawina, Trans.). Ossolineum.

Rancew-Sikora, D., & Skowrońska, M. (2022). Adult children move out: Family and reflections on parental self-sacrifice at the moment of transition. *Sociological Research Online, 28*(1), 136078042110650. https://doi.org/10.1177/13607804211065050

Ratecka, A. (2011). Niedokończona egalitaryzacja: O władzy w polskich małżeństwach. In K. Slany, B. Kowalska, & M. Ślusarczyk (Eds.), *Kalejdoskop genderowy: W drodze do poznania płci społeczno-kulturowej w Polsce* (pp. 255–270). Wydawnictwo Uniwersytetu Jagiellońskiego.

Rubenstein, C. (2007). *Beyond the mommy years: How to live happily ever after... After the kids leave home*. Springboard Press.

Silvera, R. (2021). Reconnaître le travail domestique, sans le rémunérer pour autant. *Travail, Genre et Sociétés, 46*, 189–193.

Skowrońska, M. (2012). "U siebie jestem sobą" – autentyczność i samorealizacja jako ważne narracje na temat domowej przestrzeni. *Kultura i Społeczeństwo, 56*(4), 149–116.

Titkow, A. (2007). *Tożsamość polskich kobiet. Ciągłość, zmiana, konteksty*. Wydawnictwo IFiS PAN.

Titkow, A. (2012). Figura Matki Polki. Próba demitologizacji. In R. Hryciuk & E. Korolczuk (Eds.), *Pożegnanie z Matką Polką? Dyskursy, praktyki i reprezentacje macierzyństwa we współczesnej Polsce* (pp. 27–48). Wydawnictwo Uniwersytetu Warszawskiego.

Titkow, A., Duch-Krzystoszek, D., & Budrowska, B. (2004). *Nieodpłatna praca kobiet: Mity, realia, perspektywy.* Wydawnictwo IFiS PAN.

Tosh, J. (1998). New men? The bourgeois cult of home. In G. Marsden (Ed.), *Victorian values. Personalities and perspectives in nineteenth century society* (2nd ed., p. 77–88). Routledge.

Włodarczyk, E. (2017). Misja mama. Wyzwania i trudności. In E. Włodarczyk (Ed.), *W trosce o macierzyństwo* (pp. 53–68). Wydawnictwo Naukowe UAM.

Wojciechowska, L. (2008). *Syndrom pustego gniazda. Dobrostan matek usamodzielniających się dzieci.* Wydawnictwo Instytutu Psychologii PAN.

Woolf, V. (1929). *A room of one's own* (1st ed.). Hogarth Press.

Woroniecka, G. (2014). "Ja" czy "my" w przestrzeni? Doświadczenia i klasyfikacje w sytuacjach współzamieszkiwania. In M. Łukasiuk & M. Jewdokimow (Eds.), *Socjologia zamieszkiwania* (pp. 37–62). Wydawnictwo Naukowe Sub Lupa.

Żurek, A. (2016). Przymus kreowania ról rodzinnych. In I. Przybył & A. Żurek (Eds.), *Role rodzinne. Między przystosowaniem a kreacją.* Wydawnictwo Naukowe Wydziału Nauk Społecznych UAM.

CHAPTER 13

Navigating Emotional Terrain: Women's Experiences of Loss and Gain

Bogna Dowgiałło, Christophe Giraud,
and Magdalena Herzberg-Kurasz

INTRODUCTION

The departure of a child from the parental home may mark a turning point in the identity of parents, particularly mothers, who traditionally assume a more central role than fathers in the daily care of children. According to Strauss (1992), such turning points represent critical incidents that compel individuals to recognise that they are no longer the same as they used to be (Strauss, 1992: 149). Redefining identities and roles raises the questions: what do I feel and why do I feel it?

B. Dowgiałło (✉) • M. Herzberg-Kurasz
Social Sciences Department (Institute of Sociology), University of Gdańsk,
Gdańsk, Poland
e-mail: bogna.dowgiallo@ug.edu.pl; magdalena.herzberg-kurasz@ug.edu.pl

C. Giraud
Centre de recherche sur les liens sociaux (CERLIS, UMR 8070), Université Paris
Cité, Paris, France
e-mail: christophe.giraud@parisdescartes.fr

M. Żadkowska et al. (eds.), *Reconfiguring Relations in the Empty
Nest*, Palgrave Macmillan Studies in Family and Intimate Life,
https://doi.org/10.1007/978-3-031-50403-7_13

The emotional experiences of women during this stage of life are complex and characterised by ambiguity and fluidity (Hiedemann et al., 1998; Beaupré et al., 2006; Sheriff & Weatherall, 2009; Dare, 2011). Women may experience positive, negative, and ambivalent emotions (Mitchell & Lovegreen, 2009), which can change and develop as they step into a new role (Gajewska et al., 2023). Within this chapter, we undertake a more comprehensive examination of five emotional patterns that emerged from women's accounts. They were associated with the departure of their children from home, and the resulting outcomes, perceived as either losses or gains. Specifically, we explore the patterns of grief, frustration, pride/ guilt, relief, and pleasure.

THEORETICAL PERSPECTIVE ON EMOTIONS

According to the symbolic interactionist perspective, emotions are meaningful objects to be interpreted, controlled, used, or managed by social actors, who are engaged in understanding themselves and managing others' impressions of them (Thoits, 1989). We share the basic premises of the sociology of emotions, which claims that emotions are not purely uncontrolled, as proposed by Hochschild (1979) in her concept of the sentient actor, and are never separable from the social context. In fact, emotions are seen as signalling people's engagement with others and their cultural membership, reflecting the social norms, values, and beliefs of a particular society. Social actors use the available vocabulary of sentiments as an interpretive resource to negotiate their identities and statuses (Gordon, 1981). The way people label and interpret bodily sensations has social sources and social consequences. Shott (1979) argues that physiological emotional arousal is ambiguous enough to be labelled in a variety of ways.

Symbolic interactionist analyses possess a unique capacity to illuminate two essential dimensions. Firstly, these analyses can probe how the micro-level feelings of individuals diffuse "upward" to reconstruct or reinforce current social structures. Secondly, they can examine the "downward" impact of culture, structure, and social institutions in shaping the individual's emotions (Shott, 1979). "Feeling" and "display rules" (Hochschild, 1979) can be followed, disregarded, negotiated, and internalised to varying extents. Emotional rules dictate what emotions individuals should feel and how they should be expressed and prescribe the intensity and duration of these emotions. Mapping the universe of beliefs about emotions (e.g. women feel loss when their children leave or women feel excited about their children's departure) can illuminate the larger tensions and dynamics at play within a society.

WOMEN'S EMOTIONS IN THE POSTPATERNAL PHASE

Emotions are influenced and even shaped by "the volatile stuff of culture: norms, language, stereotypes, metaphors, symbols" (Illouz, 1997: 6) and the concept of an empty nest might be regarded as an important element of "the stuff." The "empty nest" is commonly associated with loss, as it implies the loss of parental roles and the loss of "cosiness" of the family space (de Singly, 2021). Mazzucco (2006) calls the departure of adult children from the household an important "loss" event in midlife. According to Borland (1982), the loss of intimate and frequently enacted roles may diminish the reaffirmation of the self-concept and place role identities in jeopardy, leading to empty nest syndrome: depression, an identity crisis, confusion, and a lowered sense of well-being. Although the "empty nest" and "empty-nest syndrome" refer to distinct concepts, the former signifies a stage in family life while the latter describes negative reactions towards the transition. Notably, these terms are often used interchangeably, as the empty-nest phase is commonly regarded as problematic (Kearney, 2002; Dare, 2011).

Although social scientists have recently shifted their focus from solely examining the negative effects of the empty nest (Mitchell & Wister, 2015; Mitchell, 2016;) and have found that empty nesters may experience a higher sense of well-being compared to "full nesters" (Grover & Dang, 2013), their findings hardly transcend the associations present in an empty nest "decline narrative" (Gullette, 2002: 557). The metaphor of the empty nest continues to be widely recognised and colloquially employed as an interpretation of the post-parental loss (Mazzucco, 2006) and "contributed to the pessimistic view of this developmental phase" (Bouchard, 2014: 70). It places particular emphasis on social expectations regarding the vague sense of emptiness experienced by parents, especially mothers in the empty-nest period (Mitchell & Lovegreen, 2009; Badiani & De Sousa, 2016).

On the other hand, "loss events" can be interpreted in positive terms. Barnett and Baruch (1985) argue that the impact of losing a role depends on the nature of that role. Roles are not alike with respect to their effects on role overload, role conflict, or anxiety. The role of a mother is often associated with strain, as it requires more obligations than privileges. This suggests that the transition to the post-parental stage may be beneficial, as it can bring relief. However, the concept of "relief" does not allow for the full realisation of the benefits of post-maternity. Role strain relief theory implies that something negative has disappeared rather than something good being added. This is in line with McQuaide's (1998) observation that most research studies on women in midlife tend to focus solely on the problems that women face and neglect the opportunities that this stage of life can bring. In this regard, the perspective of gain seems novel and may resonate with demographic trends such as increasing growth in the older population, referred to as the "Silver Tsunami" (Calasanti, 2020). Calasanti (2020) argues that it is crucial to recognise and fight against both the continued depictions of the elderly as decrepit and unattractive, as well as the social practices that facilitate these representations. Furthermore, a growing recognition has emerged that views women with non-resident offspring as being released to pursue new activities and opportunities, rather than as being prematurely aged by culture (Gullette, 2002: 555). As "there is an exuberance in these women that is hard to miss, along with a sense of personal authority and agency." (Stewart & Ostrove, 1998: 119), referring to them as empty nesters might not be accurate (see Bouchard, 2014). Gullette (2002) suggests talking about "post-maternal" women who, instead of fearing "empty nest" syndrome, look forward to it. In other words, this stage of life might be seen as an opportunity (Karp et al., 2004) as women start to perceive themselves as more autonomous, socially active, and as partners for their non-resident children, among other self-identifications (see Gajewska et al., 2023).

Although there is extensive literature on women's emotions during the post-parental stage, Mitchell and Lovegreen (2009) argue that there is still a need to delve deeper into understanding how women make sense of this experience. This is especially important given the evolving social expectations and emotional ideologies referring to women with non-resident children, which can significantly influence how this experience is framed and reframed.

Method

Within the framework of this chapter, we analysed 40 in-depth individual interviews (Poland Corpus B) and 43 dyadic interviews (DDI) with couples (Poland and France, Corpus A), both in urban and rural settings.

In the chapter, we give a voice to women by exploring their narratives about emotions. It is worth mentioning that we did not reach those states of arousal that had not yet been subject to "emotional identification" (Rosenberg, 1990: 6). Instead, we concentrated on women's accounts of affect and the ways they make meaning of situations and episodes connected with letting the children go. Our primary focus was on the accounts connected with the change understood as a loss and/or a gain caused by the process. Analysing the sections of the interviews in which women talked about their emotional reactions towards their children's departure allowed us to distinguish five emotional patterns: grief, frustration, pride/guilt, relief, and pleasure.

FINDINGS

Speaking of Loss: Grief

Loss connected with the children's departure was primarily associated with their absence. Silent and empty homes evoke a kind of mourning atmosphere. Indeed, the participants reported similar phases, emotions, and coping strategies as those outlined in the literature on bereavement. According to Boss (2007), after the death of a significant other, people may experience the continued "presence" of the deceased. Shortly after the children leave, the participants may feel the physical presence of their beloved ones.

> Sandra: For 6 months I could hear the elevator at night and for me it was actually her coming home. And it was a bit difficult. And then for Gaël, well, it was a little bit the same, I could hear noise in the room (…) I would look to see if Gaël was there, but he wasn't. (A_FR_15)

As "loss ambiguity" (Boss, 2007) may hamper coping with it, according to Worden's (1991) model of grief, the first task in the process of grieving is accepting the reality of the loss. In our study, women shared similar strategies for coping, which involved first acknowledging their loss. For example, Barbara could not resist entering her daughter Ania's room, even though it made her acutely aware of how much she missed her.

> Barbara: And at Ania's place, when I arrive, there's also her big bed, I've made myself comfortable on it, but I miss it when I come in in the evening

after work and go into Ania's room and the bed is empty. She always slept there and always said "hello mama" and good night. Now we say goodnight on the phone, sleep well, etc., but something's missing—these are the intimate places, like the bed—it's really a private sphere and you really miss it when you enter the room. (B_PL_69)

The second task, which involves working through the pain of grief and dealing with the feelings (Worden, 1991), was also clearly visible, as women reflected on their emotions and described this time as terrible and their feelings as strong and unbearable. Working through the pain means allowing yourself to feel it no matter how difficult it may be. Although Ela felt very bad, she started to deal with her feelings and look for their causes.

Ela: I wasn't completely ready for it. But maybe it's just the way it is with me that always, ever since Mariusz was born, those moments when he was more independent—I was very uncomfortable with it. When I stopped feeding him, there was a moment when I burst into tears because I was saying, I'm a bad mother because I don't have breastmilk, he's less mine because maybe there's something else. He started walking—oh gosh, he's less and less dependent on me, he can go and get something on his own. So I was always quite emotional about the fact that his development was really making him less dependent on me, and I was really sad and angry about that. And the fact that he left so suddenly probably compounded the fact that I experienced it so much. (A_PL_1P)

Ela understands that her attachment style plays a role in her intense emotional reaction. Parents who are overprotective may struggle to separate from their child, discourage their independence, and exhibit controlling behaviours (Thomasgard & Metz, 1997). Women's working through the pain could provide valuable insights into the nature of the loss.

The loss might be dramatic as the absence of the significant others is interpreted as identity loss. Especially women with high commitment to the identity of a mother may experience an emotional void, as Valérie does, who feels as if a part of herself is missing since her child left.

Valérie: (…) it is something that you feel, it is beyond words, it is physiological what, it is a part of you nevertheless which disappears. (A_FR_6)

Children's departure may also be interpreted as the closing of a certain period in a woman's life and the loss of her self-concept at the same time.

For example, Francoise, like many other women, became aware of her own ageing and not being young anymore:

> Fabienne: The silence in the house. Uh.... The feeling of having grown old all of a sudden for me. That's it. (A_FR_2)

As women mentioned, grieving is non-linear and involves ups and downs of emotions. Typically, the most intense feelings of sorrow and suffering happen during the initial few months after the loss, but gradually subside with time. Nevertheless, memories of the lost attachment may trigger periodic emotional suffering.

Lofland's (1985) work on the social shaping of grief highlights the existence of strict norms that prescribe the timing and duration of grief. Participants in the study also referred to the specific periods when mourning began and ended while discussing social expectations regarding the intensity and duration of grief. Marzena says "she cried for 2 weeks" (A_PL_6G). Women tended to express their grief openly, which was in accordance with cultural scripts of mourning rituals. However, women's free expression of grief was limited when the children were present. For instance, Sandra engaged in emotion and worked hard to conceal her tears and despair in front of her daughter. She cried alone, concealed, so as not to let her daughter witness her tears (A_FR_15).

Speaking of Loss: Frustration

Scherer (1994: 28) argues that frustration is a pervasive and universal emotion since all living organisms, at any stage of their developmental process, can encounter obstacles that block their ability to fulfill their needs or accomplish their objectives. Frustration becomes especially apparent in situations where individuals are unable to openly express their anger due to cultural, psychological, or situational factors. The fact that women did not often mention anger in their descriptions of emotional reactions could imply that anger is not a culturally patterned response. A sense of helplessness in the face of the children's departure appeared to resonate more strongly with the women's experiences.

According to the participants, the feeling of loss was related to the enforced change in their performance of the role of a mother. Women described a range of chores associated with caring for their families while their children were still living at home, such as cooking, doing laundry, and driving the kids around. However, when their children left home, these aspects of the parental role disappeared and some mothers felt a sense of meaningless.

> Bogumiła: (…) To me it was nice when it was a full house, so noisy, and all these problems, like I can't find my sock or who's going to pick me up somewhere, or why can't I stay over at my friend's house. These were things that made one's life meaningful. Now (…) no one is going to notice if I'm sitting here or not (…) I feel I'm not needed. (A_PL_10G)

Bogumiła's observations align with the role loss hypothesis, which suggests that the termination of a role that has provided parents, particularly mothers, with a sense of fulfillment, may result in a decline in their well-being (see White & Edwards, 1990). However, the departure of children should not be viewed as a complete loss of the parental role but rather as a loss of the ability to adequately fulfill role-related duties, as role performance is always linked to a counterrole. The participants noted that stepping away from the role of having a dependent child could impact their ability to care for their children effectively. The most challenging experience mentioned by the participants was losing control over their children, which may have already started during the launching period. Maria recalled that she "had to worry" because she was unable to exert any control over their children. Meanwhile, she was expected to meet the unrealistic expectation that her children's safety was her sole responsibility, leading to frustration.

> Maria: (…) the last years were very stressful for me, at least, because my children were driving cars, coming home very late, and when there were weekends, I just didn't sleep at night. It was very difficult for me, their growing up—it was a difficult time for me and I had to worry about it. Although there weren't any major problems, just waiting at night to see if they would come back if nothing had happened if there had been be an accident—that made me very tired. (B_PL_70)

Some women experienced frustration just after their children's departure, as they felt blocked from adequately caring for them. This was especially noticeable when the departure occurred earlier than expected and the mother felt that this care was still needed.

Interviewer: And how did you experience it? Because it's not very common to leave at 16, it's more common at 18 when you're of age.

Fabienne: Well, I had a bad experience, I had a bad experience. Moreover, I had not seen... Well, he was an intern. I hadn't seen him in his dormitory, well I saw him when I was in Rennes a year later. And the fact that I couldn't see where he lived. It made me very anxious. (A_FR_2)

The experience of loss occurred in both literal terms, when mothers confronted the physical absence of a child, and in more abstract terms, when the loss manifested as frustration due to a diminished sense of control over role performance. How mothers coped with this feeling depended on individual factors, including the time that had elapsed since their children moved out and the need for control, as well as other roles and responsibilities the women were engaged in at that particular moment.

Speaking of Gain and Loss: Pride/Guilt

According to Cooley's work on the looking-glass self (Cooley, 1964), humans are continuously experiencing self-feelings (affects evoked by self-evaluation). They form an image of themselves by looking at the responses of others towards them, and this image always includes a sense of how others are judging their actions. If individuals perceive that others have a positive evaluation of them, they feel proud, but if they sense a negative evaluation, they experience shame. If someone violates the moral (especially religious) tradition, he or she experiences guilt as a result, and it may lead them to seek punishment as a way to make up for their wrongdoing. This punishment, in turn, serves as a means of atonement, or a way to seek forgiveness and restore their moral standing in the eyes of the community. In other words, violating moral standards and feeling guilty about it may create a desire for punishment as a form of penance and an attempt to regain moral rectitude (see Kemper, 2006: 98–99).

Pride was connected with the fact that both children and mothers decided to make an effort and succeeded in overcoming (or at least facing) the difficulties and hardships of their separation. Sandra recalls the time when her daughter was about to leave. Ambivalent emotions of sadness and pride and happiness accompanied it:

Sandra: "Why are you crying, Mom?" and I couldn't talk to her, and I smiled at her and packed her suitcase. And she said "I understand it's because I'm leaving" and she said "I don't understand why you have red eyes all the time" and it's a bit of a difficult moment but ... I told her "don't worry, I'm so proud, you have to go, you have to go, I'm so proud, don't worry, but it's just that you're my first baby, you're leaving and that's it, but I'm so happy and everything." (A_FR_15)

While there is undoubtedly a sense of sadness and loss as this event marks the end of a significant phase in their lives, mothers also recognise and support their children's need for independence. They take pride in the parenting work they have done to prepare their children for life on their own, even if they miss their presence at home, as expressed by Anna:

Anna: When she moved out, on the one hand we felt such sadness—you know it's going to be empty without the children, but on the other hand we found such pride that practically all of our daughters—almost all of them—have found love, have children, are happy—such pride. And also that they have started to live on their own. (B_PL_62)

The feeling of pride is not automatically gained, but is instead dependent on meeting societal expectations. This requires a mother to let go of a child who is capable of managing their own life effectively. It is a challenging task, but necessary for a parent to feel proud of their child's accomplishments. According to Mitchell (2010), positive emotions are often associated with a child's perceived success in their development, which can be exhibited through the maintenance of strong relationships with their parents and the demonstration of good citizenship.

The process of a child leaving the family home was frequently viewed as a benchmark for maternal success. If everything went well, it was considered a demonstration of good mothering and a reason for maternal pride. However, any problems that arose during the process could trigger feelings of guilt for the mother. Thus, the sense of pride associated with this milestone was precarious and could easily be lost. Alicja acknowledges that her despair after her son's early departure (at the age of 18) might have resulted from her seeing herself as a bad mother and blaming herself for the situation.

Interviewer: And what was the reason for that? What were you afraid of, or was it too fast?
    Alicja: I don't know how to analyse it like that now. I don't think I've ever made such an analysis. But I would rather say that I was probably guilty

of being such a bad mother, that my child had moved out of the house. (B_PL_24)

In that sense, a child's departure might mean losing one's face as a mother.

Speaking of Gain: Relief

The departure of children from the home may have resulted in a "phew" feeling among mothers who had previously experienced role overload. Relief arose from a comparison between the situation before and after the departure, and an appreciation of the improved circumstances. The reduction in responsibilities that comes with the children leaving the nest aligns with the predictions of role strain theory (White & Edwards, 1990). According to Angèle, relief is experienced mainly by those women who felt frustration before:

> Angèle: When they are teenagers, you just can't take it anymore. So maybe it's also because I didn't organise the tasks at home well. But you can't take all the logistics, the laundry, the food. And on top of that, since they're teenagers, they leave in all directions, you never know if they're here, what time they'll be back, if they'll be back in one, two or three hours. It becomes a mess, and you can't take it anymore. (A_FR_19)

The participants reported experiencing relief in various areas, including family budgets, spatial organisation of the house, time management, personal relations, and the work environment. Some couples, for the first time in their lives, were able to enjoy a separate bedroom and no longer had to wait in line to use the bathroom (see Chap. 13).

Improved time management could have an impact beyond the family sphere. Julia, whose youngest son now resides in a boarding school, is able to devote herself to her work without being exposed to the stress that was previously a result of the necessity to reconcile her roles as a mother and a professional.

> Julia: I just didn't have any more responsibilities, so I didn't have to rush home, because I knew Borys was there, I just knew that I could work quietly, because he was at this school, I'm here at work in the afternoon. I didn't have to rush for his sake. He wasn't that little, but you always know that the child is alone at home and you're at work. No matter how big or small they are. (A_PL_32G)

It is also important to consider the emotional relief that can result from the fact of physical separation. When a woman is separated from her child, it can lead to a sense of detachment from her child's problems. This detachment can then lead to reduced stress, as the parent may feel less responsible for their child. Less stress also comes from less responsibility for a child and a kind of emotional distancing, as Marzena puts it: "Out of sight, out of heart, you know."

The sense of relief experienced by women after the physical separation from their child can be so intense that they perceive their child's departure as a gain. This was the case with Angèle and her first daughter, as their relationship had been particularly strained:

> Angèle: Oh yeah, yeah they were thrilled! Honestly, Elena was ruining our lives. She was so stressful we couldn't take it anymore. Romane told me: "Mom, either she leaves or I leave, but I can't take it anymore." So honestly, we were all happy that she was leaving. It's sad, but it's the truth.
>
> Yves: Oh no. You speak for yourself, I was very sad that she was leaving.
>
> Angèle: Yeah, except for her father, I think me, Romane and Lothaire were happy that she was leaving. (A_FR_19)

For some couples, the departure may be viewed as a chance to enhance their relationship. The differences in their parenting approach, which used to be a source of constant conflict, may eventually disappear.

> Krystyna: We certainly have more peace between us now. Because sometimes it happens that one parent allows it, and the other one says come on—and now there's no such thing. So it's good, now it's really, as far as our relationship is concerned, it's good. (A_PL_13G)

Thus the departure might be interpreted as beneficial for the couple.

Speaking of Gain: Pleasure

Regaining control over one's life may not only provide a sense of relief but also elicit pleasure. According to Krajewski: "Pleasure is the result of such satisfaction of needs in which the individual is aware of their nature, has a distance from them, decides how to satisfy them and chooses the objects that fulfil them, has complete control over the process of fulfilling a particular need" (Krajewski, 2005: 33). It suggests that pleasure arises from the satisfaction of needs in a way that allows the individual to have complete control over the process of fulfilling those needs.

The sensation of pleasure is distinct from that of relief, but they are linked and rely on each other. It can be viewed as a novel approach to engaging in activities that were once disliked. For example, Zofia now derives pleasure from cooking, as she has the freedom to do it in a way that suits her:

> Zofia: There was a lot of everything in the kitchen; I did the cooking; I felt...
> I generally don't like cooking, so now, when it's just me and my husband, I cook every two days; and when I cook, it's a pleasure for me. Back then, I mostly felt this burden and this duty to get the shopping done. (B_PL_9P)

Women reported experiencing new everyday pleasures, such as sitting comfortably in an armchair without being interrupted or enjoying a peaceful morning coffee alone (see Chap. 12). Some participants even expressed that their lives with non-resident children were more enjoyable overall. They spoke about the pleasure of meeting with their non-resident children and having conversations as equals.

> Marzena: (...) It's not only the longer it goes on, this separate flat of ours, but also the fact that she's becoming, well, an adult. (A_PL_6G)

They emphasised feeling less pressure and obligation, with domestic tasks becoming more flexible and optional, and having more quality time for themselves. Additionally, they were able to pursue tasks based on their personal preferences. While they stressed the importance of peace and the need for rest, they also talked about new perspectives opening up. Overall, their experiences highlighted the benefits of having more autonomy in their lives.

It is important to note that the women's experiences did not imply that they felt entirely released from their roles as mothers. Rather, their mothering responsibilities seemed to have become more tailored to their individual needs, abilities, and preferences, resulting in a more enjoyable experience. When speaking about her children's visits, Maria emphasised that she managed to find pleasure both in their arrival and in their departure:

Maria: (…) I am happy when they come, but I am also happy when they leave. I think it's already been years, my husband and I have our habits and we also feel older and we have our systematic life arranged. And it's nice when someone comes and messes things up for a few days or a week, but then you're glad when you get back to it. That peace of mind is very important to us. (B_PL_70)

The case of Maria taking pleasure in both the arrival and departure of her children exemplifies the newfound joys associated with the empty nest phase.

CONCLUSION

The transition to an empty nest can be an emotional time for women as they are saying goodbye to the role of a mother of dependent children and are faced with a new phase of their lives. The circumstance of children leaving home marks a transition to a more distant parenting role and calls forth a reinterpretation of one's fundamental life roles. Because the emptying of the family nest—if only temporarily—also typically coincides with parents' "middle age," letting go of children is an important age marker. In this chapter, we primarily explore the emotions women feel when letting go of their children, specifically focusing on those related to the changes perceived as either losses or gains resulting from this process.

By analysing the segments of the interviews where women shared their emotional reactions to their children leaving home, we were able to discern five distinct emotional patterns that emerged in both the Polish and French data sets. Although the frequency of these patterns differed, the qualitative nature of our research precludes us from drawing quantitative conclusions. We may hypothesise that French women are more prone to experiencing maternal pride, whereas Polish women may experience more maternal guilt due to Poland being a more religious country, but this requires further empirical testing to validate. Our findings do not imply that every woman experiences the same set of emotions. Instead, it indicates that there is a consistency in accounting for their emotional states. This similarity suggests the existence of strong cultural norms and expectations regarding emotions that are associated with this particular phase of life. The women's understanding of emotions was shaped by a process of navigating through the perception of a given situation as either a loss (empty nest perspective) or a gain (post-maternal perspective) related to the departure of the children. These perspectives were not mutually exclusive. The feeling of loss and gain can become intertwined, leading to a sense of ambiguity or ambivalence. Such ambivalence might be described in sociological terms as the presence of conflicting societal norms and values within a specific social relationship (Connidis & McMullin, 2002) and is often observed when children leave home (Karp et al., 2004; Gajewska et al., 2023). Navigating this complexity can be challenging. Women may feel both grief, frustration, pride, relief, and pleasure. On the one hand, the feeling of loss may be apparent when one or more family members are missing, resulting in a loss of identity and role loss for a woman. On the other hand, these apparent losses can also be viewed as opportunities, such as the departure of children serving as a turning point in life. Women, in particular, may experience newfound freedom and discover pleasurable experiences without the weight of maternal guilt.

References

Badiani, F., & De Sousa, A. (2016). The Empty Nest syndrome: Critical clinical considerations. *Indian Journal of Mental Health, 3*(2), 135–142. https://doi.org/10.30877/ijmh.3.2.2016.135-142

Barnett, R. C., & Baruch, G. K. (1985). Women's involvement in multiple roles and psychological distress. *Journal of Personality and Social Psychology, 49*(1), 135–145. https://doi.org/10.1037/0022-3514.49.1.135

Beaupré, P., Turcotte, P., & Milan, A. (2006). When is junior moving out? Transitions from the parental home to independence. *Canadian Social Trends, 82*, 9–15.

Borland, D. C. (1982). A cohort analysis approach to the empty-nest syndrome among three ethnic groups of women: A theoretical position. *Journal of Marriage and the Family, 44*(1), 117–129. https://doi.org/10.2307/351267

Boss, P. (2007). Ambiguous loss theory: Challenges for scholars and practitioners. *Family Relations, 56*(2), 105–110. https://doi.org/10.1111/j.1741-3729.2007.00444.x

Bouchard, G. (2014). How do parents react when their children leave home? An integrative review. *Journal of Adult Development, 21*, 69–79. https://doi.org/10.1007/s10804-013-9180-8

Calasanti, T. (2020). Brown slime, the silver tsunami, and apocalyptic demography: The importance of ageism and age relations. *Social Currents, 7*(3), 195–211. https://doi.org/10.1177/2329496520912736

Connidis, I. A., & McMullin, J. A. (2002). Sociological ambivalence and family ties: A critical perspective. *Journal of Marriage and Family, 64*(3), 558–567. https://doi.org/10.1111/j.1741-3737.2002.00558.x

Cooley, C. H. (1964). *Human nature and the social order.* Schocken Books.

Dare, J. S. (2011). Transitions in midlife women's lives: Contemporary experiences. *Health Care for Women International, 32*(2), 111–133. https://doi.org/10.1080/07399332.2010.500753

de Singly, F. (2021). The family of individuals: An overview of the sociology of the family in Europe, 130 years after Durkheim's first university course. In A.-M. Castrén, V. Česnuitytė, I. Crespi, J.-A. Gauthier, R. Gouveia, C. Martin, A. M. Mínguez, & K. Suwada (Eds.), *The Palgrave handbook of family sociology in Europe* (pp. 15–43). Palgrave Macmillan.

Gajewska, M., Herzberg-Kurasz, M., Żadkowska, M., Kostecka, M., & Dowgiałło, B. (2023). Room of her own: Remaking empty nest and creating herspaces in practices of Polish mothers whose children left home. *European Journal of Women's Studies, 30*(1), 7–21.

Gordon, L. S. (1981). The sociology of sentiments and emotions. In M. Rosenberg & R. H. Turner (Eds.), *Social psychology: Sociological perspectives* (pp. 562–569). Basic Books.

Grover, N., & Dang, P. (2013). Empty nest syndrome vs empty nest trigger: Psychotherapy formulation based on systemic approach – A descriptive case study. *Psychological Studies, 58*(3), 285–288. https://doi.org/10.1007/s12646-013-0207-9

Gullette, M. M. (2002). Valuing "postmaternity" as a revolutionary feminist concept. *Feminist Studies, 28*(3), 553–572.

Hiedemann, B., Suhomlinova, O., & O'Rand, A. M. (1998). Economic independence, economic status, and empty nest in midlife marital disruption. *Journal of Marriage and the Family, 60*(1), 219–231. https://doi.org/10.2307/353453

Hochschild, A. R. (1979). Emotion work, feeling rules, and social structure. *American Journal of Sociology, 85*(3), 551–575.

Illouz, E. (1997). *Consuming the romantic utopia: Love and the cultural contradictions of capitalism.* University of California Press.

Karp, D. A., Holmstrom, L. L., & Gray, P. S. (2004). Of roots and wings: Letting go of the college-bound child. *Symbolic Interaction, 27*(3), 357–382. https://doi.org/10.1525/si.2004.27.3.357

Kearney, S. M. (2002). *Exploring the empty nest transition.* Wayne State University. Retrieved March 3, 2023, from https://drnissani.net/mnissani/SE/kearney.htm

Kemper, T. D. (2006). Power and status and the power-status theory of emotions. In J. E. Stets & J. H. Turner (Eds.), *Handbook of the sociology of emotions* (pp. 87–113). Springer.

Krajewski, M. (2005). *Kultury kultury popularnej.* Wydawnictwo Naukowe Uniwersytetu im. Adama Mickiewicza.

Lofland, L. H. (1985). The social shaping of emotion: The case of grief. *Symbolic Interaction, 8*(2), 171–190.

Mazzucco, S. (2006). The impact of children leaving home on the parents' wellbeing: A comparative analysis of France and Italy. *Genus, 62*(3/4), 35–52.

McQuaide, S. (1998). Women at Midlife. *Social Work, 43*(1), 21–31. https://doi. org/10.1093/sw/43.1.21

Mitchell, B. A. (2010). Happiness in midlife parental roles: A contextual mixed methods analysis. *Family Relations: An Interdisciplinary Journal of Applied Family Studies, 59*(3), 326–339. https://doi.org/10.1111/ j.1741-3729.2010.00605.x

Mitchell, B. A. (2016). Happily ever after? Marital satisfaction during the middle adulthood years. In J. Bookwala (Ed.), *Couple relationships in the middle and later years: Their nature, complexity, and role in health and illness* (pp. 17–36). American Psychological Association. https://doi.org/10.1037/14897-002

Mitchell, B. A., & Lovegreen, L. D. (2009). The empty Nest Syndrome in midlife families: A multimethod exploration of parental gender differences and cultural dynamics. *Journal of Family Issues, 30*(12), 1651–1670. https://doi.org/10. 1177/0192513X09339020

Mitchell, B. A., & Wister, A. V. (2015). Midlife challenge or welcome departure? Cultural and family-related expectations of empty Nest transitions. *The International Journal of Aging and Human Development, 81*(4), 260–280. https://doi.org/10.1177/0091415015622790

Rosenberg, M. (1990). Reflexivity and emotions. *Social Psychology Quarterly, 53*, 3–12.

Scherer, K. R. (1994). Toward a concept of 'Modal emotions. In P. Ekman & R. J. Davidson (Eds.), *The nature of emotion: Fundamental questions* (pp. 25–31). Oxford University Press.

Sheriff, M., & Weatherall, A. (2009). A feminist discourse analysis of popular-press accounts of postmaternity. *Feminism & Psychology, 19*(1), 89–108. https:// doi.org/10.1177/0959353508098621

Shott, S. (1979). Emotion and social life: A symbolic interactionist analysis. *American Journal of Sociology, 84*(6), 1317–1334.

Stewart, A. J., & Ostrove, J. M. (1998). Women's personality in middle age. Gender, history, and midcourse corrections. *American Psychologist, 53*(11), 1185–1194.

Strauss, A. (1992). Turning points in identity. In C. Clark & H. Robboy (Eds.), *Social interaction: Readings in sociology* (4th ed., pp. 149–155). St. Martin's Press.

Thoits, P. A. (1989). The sociology of emotions. *Annual Review of Sociology, 15*, 317–342.

Thomasgard, M., & Metz, W. P. (1997). Parental overprotection and its relation to perceived child vulnerability. *American Journal of Orthopsychiatry, 67*(2), 330–335. https://doi.org/10.1037/h0080237

White, L. K., & Edwards, J. N. (1990). Emptying the nest and parental well-being: An analysis of National Panel Data. *American Sociological Review, 55*, 235–242.

Worden, J. W. (1991). *Grief counselling and grief therapy: A handbook for the mental health practitioner*. Routledge.

CHAPTER 14

Struggling with Limitations, Creating New Possibilities: Perspective of Men Experiencing the Empty Nest

Radosław Kossakowski, Natasza Kosakowska-Berezecka, and Sophie David–Goretta

Introduction

Current modalities of manhood (and fatherhood) are torn between the old, classic model of the income provider (Quéniart, 2004) and a more modern trend that allows for the disclosure of emotions and care practices (mostly connected to child care and home duties) (cf. Schoppe-Sullivan &

R. Kossakowski (✉) • N. Kosakowska-Berezecka
Social Sciences Department (Institute of Sociology), University of Gdańsk, Gdańsk, Poland
e-mail: radoslaw.kossakowski@ug.edu.pl; natasza.kosakowska-berezecka@ug.edu.pl

S. David–Goretta
Centre de recherche sur les liens sociaux (CERLIS, UMR 8070), Université Paris Cité, Paris, France
e-mail: sophie.david.goretta@gmail.com

© The Author(s), under exclusive license to Springer Nature Switzerland AG 2024
M. Żadkowska et al. (eds.), *Reconfiguring Relations in the Empty Nest*, Palgrave Macmillan Studies in Family and Intimate Life, https://doi.org/10.1007/978-3-031-50403-7_14

Fagan, 2020). However, studies on changing or emerging fatherhood and manhood schemes are rarely devoted to men experiencing empty nests. In this chapter, we would like to fill an existing gap in this area. Ageing has usually been analysed in a completely de-contextualised way and, therefore, many studies have ignored important developmental and personal reference points (Diehl et al., 2014). Therefore, shedding light on the experience of ageing in men while being faced with an empty nest constitutes an important, novel, and insightful ageing context. We would thus like to present and analyse the trajectories of male identity that emerge from an empirical study on men experiencing the empty nest. It is clear that the experience of an empty nest coincides with other important aspects of men's lives: ageing, assessment of achievements, and acceptance of limitations (Scher, 1992). We analyse how the children leaving 'the nest' influences not only the relationship between the children and the father, or, for example, the wife and husband (as presented in other chapters of our book) but how it potentially forces the reconstruction of the identity of the man and the father that takes place in the lives of the respondents. Analysis of the interviews shows that the effect of the empty nest in men raises questions about passing away and the need to reformulate their current lives. Some respondents are confronted with the fact that the possibilities of crossing new boundaries and new achievements have significantly reduced; some respondents, however, see the new situation as a space for the pursuit of new passions and interests.

Our chapter will focus on the individual narratives of men experiencing empty nest syndrome. The individual statements of the respondents will sometimes be set in a broader context to present their meaning fully. It is important to note that although all respondents share the experience of an empty nest, many other variables—age, professional career, and so on—often distinguish them from one another. The chapter is divided into the following sections. First, we present the relevant background dedicated to masculinity derived from existing studies on masculinities. They mostly concern traits that are socially highly desired for men to avoid being 'not-real' men. Using them, we highlight those thematic motifs that allow us to understand the experience of the respondents. The second, and most important, aim of the chapter is to introduce the narratives of the men interviewed.

MASCULINE IDENTITY IN THE CONTEXT OF DIFFERENT DEVELOPMENTAL TASKS

According to Connell (1987), masculinity can be defined as a social construct describing what it means to be a man at a certain time and place and which traits and behaviours man needs to avoid to manifest his prescribed and proscribed masculinity traits (cf. also Bosson et al., 2022). Most often these are: showing weakness and not acting from a position of strength in relation to other men; not being strong enough (Goodey, 1997; Connell, 2002: 94); reluctance or inability to have sex with women (e.g. due to impotence or depression); lack of initiative-taking in sexual relations with women; lack of behavioural risk-taking (Vandello et al., 2008; Tyler & Fairbrother, 2013). These behaviours are often associated with ageing—a stage that the men in our sample enter when experiencing an empty nest. In addition to avoiding the aforementioned non-masculine types of behaviour, men must also suppress and reject displays of emotion and vulnerability associated with femininity (Genoe & Singleton, 2006). It is suggested that men are more restricted than women in maintaining their socially dictated gender role in fear of the contempt they might face should they deviate into an unacceptable feminine role or fail in a masculine one (Messner, 1998; Courtenay, 2000). Connell (1993) suggests that only 10% of men can and do measure up to the hegemonic version of masculinity—and this is especially true for older men. Old age is associated with a loss of strength, autonomy, and physical and mental resiliencies (Bennett, 2007) that ostensibly contradict the standards of hegemonic masculinity. Ageing men must struggle to maintain a culturally accepted masculine identity as the Western ideal of manliness ends with middle age (Spector-Mersel, 2006).

On the other hand, the precarious manhood theory posits that manhood is widely conceptualised as a social status that is hard to earn, easy to lose, and must be proven repeatedly via action (Vandello et al., 2008; Bosson et al., 2021). This theory suggests that the precariousness of their gender status leads men to experience higher levels of social anxiety and greater motivation to compensate than women, sometimes by engaging in risky or aggressive behaviour, when their gender status is challenged and not confirmed (Vandello & Bosson, 2013). Using quantitative methods to examine the cross-cultural prevalence of precarious manhood beliefs in 62 nations covering 13 world regions and representing over 33,400 respondents, it was proved that precarious manhood is a universal construct present across the 6 continents (Bosson et al., 2021).

Overall, we can see that research on masculinity has largely ignored the experience of older men, reflecting the absence of a gendered prescription for ageing men in our society (Spector-Mersel, 2006; Thompson, 2008). Ageing is associated with loss of independence and affects various health behaviours, including diet, dependence, recovery from injury, physical activity, and mental deterioration (Smith et al., 2007). Men face unique health disparities from women, such as shorter overall life spans, higher mortality from 12 of the 15 leading causes of death, and a greater lifetime risk of developing cancer (Mahalik et al., 2007)—especially in countries where manhood is precarious (Vandello et al., 2023).

When confronted with a health threat, men have the choice of denying the threat, modifying risk factors and health behaviours in an attempt to alleviate the threat, or seeking professional help. Galdas et al. (2005) reviewed the literature on men's health-seeking behaviour and proposed 'traditional masculine behaviour' as an explanation for delays among men who experience illness-seeking help. Addis and colleagues suggest that men's help-seeking behaviour—or lack thereof—is a direct product of masculine gender-role socialisation and social constructionism (Bertakis et al., 2000; Addis & Mahalik, 2003). Many of the tasks associated with seeking help from a health professional, such as relying on others, admitting a need for help, or recognising and labelling an emotional problem, conflict with the messages men receive about the importance of self-reliance, physical toughness, and emotional control. How men navigate the decision to seek help likely depends on a certain reconciliation between contradicting self-perceptions of strength and weakness.

In the case of our study, men need to acknowledge that they are ageing but also need to embrace the fact that the children are leaving the family home. These two events constitute an important context of studying masculine identity. Although the impact of this experience on the relationship between fathers and children is described in another chapter, it is difficult to separate it from the narrative of men's identities. It is also worth noting that there is little research on the male experience of empty nest syndrome (Bouchard, 2014). Some research indicates that there is, for example, no distinction between the emotional reaction of fathers and mothers to the empty nest. However, there are studies that show that the experience of emotions related to an empty nest is different for men and for women (see e.g. Boss et al., 1987). Women's and men's emotions differ as the way they perform their parenthood is strongly gendered—gender stereotypes prescribe and proscribe different behaviours to women and men—for example, allowing mothers more freedom to express their emotions, while at the same time limiting men's (Van Lissa et al., 2019). The development of the 'new' construction of fatherhood is still complicit with many standards of traditional masculinity. This is particularly apparent in fathers' firm disassociation from the 'feminine style' of parenting. It could thus be hypothesised that such strategies enable fathers to maintain a masculine identity in the context that was usually associated with traditional masculinity. As the data in Chap. 4 (dedicated to the relationships between fathers and children) in the first part of the book shows, Polish and French fathers do not generally express extreme emotional attitudes when the children leave their family homes (however, there are some cases of longing and loneliness). Rather, they try to continue to perform the roles and functions associated with traditional models of masculinity. It can therefore be assumed that a key aspect in the context of masculine identity will not so much be the children leaving for the respondents but the sense of time passing and the need to confront the consequences that result from this impermanence. Therefore, the analyses presented in this chapter are built around the following question: whether the passing of time and the awareness of ageing will affect the respondents' sense of threat to their masculinity. All the more so, Polish society still seems to require men—regardless of age—to conform to norms associated with traditional, hegemonic masculinity. French society also contributes to the creation of stereotypes, grouping representations around gender. These gender stereotypes describe the characteristics of one group in opposition to the other. The 'stereotype threat' (Duru-Bellat, 2016) explains a gendered organisation, each person referring to representations. However, we can now observe a decline in adherence to gender stereotypes, as France is less attached to the traditional division of labour (Papuchon, 2017).

FINDINGS

Emotional Awareness of Ageing

The situation in which adult children leave the 'nest' to start an independent life is a distinctive, albeit natural, stage in the lives of both individuals and the family environment. It is something that respondents perceive as a natural process, a stage of life. This interpretation runs through most of the respondents' statements—and the fathers we interviewed see this as a source of reflexivity concerning the process of ageing. Male respondents contextualise their children's leaving the family home in terms of an awareness of the passing of time and the ageing process (it is crucial to add that comments dedicated to the relationship between the experience of the empty nest and awareness of ageing were also expressed by mothers; see more on this subject in the chapter on female emotions).

> Wiesiek: I mean I think it is also a bit of a perspective, maybe it is related to the children' departure, that a person starts to think about what they still have to live for, yes? What one still wants to do in life and where? Sometimes he starts to look at this prospect that one day he won't be working, there's going to be retirement or something like that. (B_PL_1P)

The departure of the children makes respondents aware of a new era. Gérald, the father of two daughters, speaks about their departure as a representation of the time passing:

> Gérald: And then I have to tell you, it was a blow when they left but afterwards, we organised our life. (A_FR_14)

However, it should be underlined that the example of Gérald is a rare case when interviews with French fathers are analysed. It is connected to the fact that in the French sample, it was hard to detect a relationship between the empty nest experience and the process of ageing in the men's narratives. What was, however, evident, was that some fathers, relieved of their parental role, appreciated the children's departure.

In some cases, deeper reflections on individual identity can be detected. This point resonates particularly strongly with the following statement:

> Tadeusz: It is that first moment when you start to realise that you are already old. And then somewhere around birthdays—gosh, that's the worst. And the fact that the child moves out—I mean it is normal I guess, but I think it is connected with the fact that you start to realise that you are old, that you're getting older—that it starts to add up. They moved away, I am 50 here. And I think it's also … it is all cumulative and so with these separations that cause emotions somehow—it is just that when you put it all together, it even seems to me that some of the emotions that are associated with getting older can be pushed in, that here my child has moved out, it is horrible. (B_PL_2P)

The above quote does not only indicate that men experiencing the empty nest are aware of the changes affecting their families and themselves. This quote contradicts common opinions and research reports that a real man should not express emotions, leaning only towards rational attitudes and explanations of reality (Montes, 2013). This quote may indicate a departure from the construct of hegemonic masculinity imposing certain behaviours and attitudes on men such as emotional constraints and feeling weak. The quotation is also significant (it is worth emphasising that it is not the only one, as other respondents also indicated an emotional component in the context of experiencing the passing of time and ageing) for the reason that our respondents—men aged 50 or more—were generally brought up in traditional families. We, therefore, assume (some biographical elements appeared in the interviews, although the biographical narratives were primarily dedicated to the respondents' relationship and marriage histories rather than their biographies) that they were raised in a traditional environment that required men either not to experience emotions or not to express them. A fragment of a statement expressed by a respondent from Gdańsk confirms, moreover, how strong the emotions men can experience in an empty nest situation are:

> Franciszek: This is when (…) that there was no one to open your mouth to. There were all sorts of strange feelings … And that's where this kind of sadness came from, that there was no one at home. When the kids were there, maybe it was also a bit different. And that's where the depression came from—I don't know if it was depression, but such a mental gloom. (B_PL_9G)

Sometimes the ageing process is explained very rationally, almost textbook-like, according to a rational interpretation of the knowledge of biology and man. It is worth adding that the respondent who shared the emotive side of passing and ageing also 'fulfilled' the male pattern in terms of a distanced and emotionless description:

> Wiesiek: (…) it all comes down to the fact that we are getting older. Maybe I'm overstating it, but it's all dammit, some of these problems, dilemmas, it's all to do with the fact that people are beginning to realise that it's closer rather than further away. Well, because it's a bit like that biologically—we're animals, reproduction is finished and that's it. (B_P_1P)

Depending on the personal story, the empty nest phase may raise awareness of ageing for fathers. The cultural and gender context influences the strategies that men use to deal with the change.

The Limitations

Awareness of the passing of time and the ageing process is only one side of the situation in which our interviewees find themselves. However, surprisingly, most of the interviewees who recognise the importance of their age do not see their situation as limiting their life choices and opportunities. Instead, one of the statements relates to how age affects bodily limitations. We present this one case not in order to illustrate any existing pattern among the interviewees; our aim, in this case, is to analyse a rather radical experience of the passing of time and the shrinking of possibilities in this context. This case is also notable for the fact that the focus on one's limitations dominated over other aspects of the empty nest experience. This concerns sporting activities and how they are perceived as a space for pushing one's limits and breaking records—even if it is in amateur sports. The following passage is part of a dialogue between a researcher and a respondent:

> Interviewer: But you also look at this passing in the context of sporting opportunities, that as a very active person, for whom...
> Wiesiek: Yes, yes...
> Interviewer: That's the kind of limitations you see, that you are not going to do what you would have done a few years ago?
> Wiesiek: I can see that.
> Interviewer: That's the kind of thing that's so heartbreaking, depressing?
> Wiesiek: I think it's terrible. For me it's terrible. Simply—because it feels like—it compounds all the negative emotions, with everything. Here's a child, here's this, moving out, a round birthday, something here, something there, physical limitations are starting to give signs somewhere. And all of this adds up to negative emotions for me.
> Interviewer: Do you have any ideas for how to get out of this? Maybe you are planning something else?
> Wiesiek: I haven't even thought about it. Even if the possibilities are getting smaller and smaller—someone also told me not to worry so much, because a lack of regression is progression, but it's a bit hard to accept. (B_P_1P)

The above case is distinctive in that the respondent primarily sees the dark side of ageing in terms of physical activity. His statement goes against existing research, most of which reports the positive impact that sport has on older people. In general, sporting activity allows such people to distance themselves from the problem of the ageing body, challenge age-appropriate norms and disassociate themselves from the aged stereotype, and set new goals (Jenkin et al., 2017). Sport is not a tool to negate the fact of the ageing body, but it empowers older people. It is noteworthy that, unlike the respondent quoted above, those respondents who practise some form of physical activity (most often it is cycling or long walks) mention it in positive terms—as an activity empowering their current life. In the case of our respondent, if one treats sport as a means to prove oneself, and break one's limits, then ageing seems to lead to deprivation of an important source of power, potentially masculine power. Many respondents also emphasise that the children leaving the family nest has meant that they have more time for such activities:

> Erwan: Yeah, I do more sports, more outings and also some work in the house that we hadn't had time to do: small jobs. Well, a little painting, repairs, small details, small jobs, and more time. (A_FR_40)

In this case, it seems that the difference results from the ambitions that individuals associate with the importance of sport in the context of individual development and power as a man. In this sense, the above passage shows the freedom to do individual activities offered by the children leaving.

Creating New Possibilities

The above cases cannot be taken as representative, even for a qualitative sample. Indeed, in other interviews, men were much more likely to mention positively evaluated ways of coping with their situation, for example, by setting further plans for the future for themselves.

> Leszek: But I also see that I still have a lot of potential and a lot of possibilities, and I also see people around me who are 20 years younger than me and don't have the energy and the drive, to put it colloquially. I know I'll still have to pull it off or I won't be able to do it anymore, it depends. But I know that in order to provide some kind of welfare and to be able to pass

these things on to my children, my grandchildren, I should work for another 15 years, then I think I will close all the things, and then let them worry about it, and we will have done our job. (B_PL_3P)

This statement fits into the tradition of masculinity trajectory in which a man does not step out of the breadwinner role, even if his children are now grown up and independent, but the prospect of supporting grandchildren is on the horizon. This attitude fits with the father's roles described in Chap. 4, which refer to certain ways of helping children after they have left the family home. However, the discussed case of a private entrepreneur from Poznań who devotes a lot of time and energy to running a business is not straightforward, as the sense of family duty is mixed in his case with a sense of the need to do something for himself, to think about his own needs:

Leszek: I'm already thinking about the grandchildren, I'm thinking about making a dugout and there will be a Hobbit house and already there from that angle … although I would like to realise something for myself first. I'm saying that for me, the priority would be an outdoor sauna and a jacuzzi because I love the sauna, but I've never had the opportunity. (B_PL_3P)

This quote indicates that the respondent is trying to reconcile the dilemma of helping family members with the need to pursue his own needs and passions. Finally, in the course of the interview, there are hints in his statement about how he would like to spend his time in the future when the need to help his children and grandchildren will not be so pressing.

Leszek: I'd like our whole professional life to end somewhere around 60, I'd like (…) to have peace and quiet here. I would also like Zofia [wife] to slow down a bit with her professional work. And in such a perspective. We don't plan now, well, also because of the situation. We love travelling, we love going out, I love spending time together with Zofia. Well, we have planned that if we have enough money, we will buy a camper and we will make some future trips in the camper, some here in the neighbourhood, Poland, then Europe, and then maybe somewhere further. (B_PL_3P)

This case is interesting, as it reveals the dilemmas unfolding in the respondent's consciousness concerning masculine duties and roles. On the one hand, he still feels a certain pressure to care for and support his children and grandchildren, while on the other hand, he has a sense of his own need for self-fulfilment. The respondent tries to find the 'golden mean'—reconciling family responsibilities with his own needs. It is worth mentioning that elsewhere he indicates that when he decided (a decision jointly made with his wife) to build a house outside the city, the concept and design of the construction envisaged room for family members (children, future grandchildren, but also distant relatives), but he also planned—as can be seen in the above quotes—special places for others to spend time. Perhaps this case provides the impetus for a type of 'modern-traditional' father who (further research would be necessary to verify such an assumption), although pursuing old scripts for the man (the breadwinner), also begins to see space for self-development that earlier generations of men did not put into practice (see Chap. 12 for more details).

Most of the respondents, as they are professionally active men, had no problem with indicating the activities they would be involved in after the children left the family home. In most cases, the thing concerned the continuation of certain trajectories: the performance of professional roles and possibly increasing space for hobbies and leisure activities. Occasionally, there were also statements in which men appreciated the very fact of having free time and the quiet time they could enjoy in an empty nest:

> Interviewer: Do you also like a bit of time like that? Alone at home?
>
> Robert: I like it, yes, I like it. If it had to be, say, 5 days a week, that I would spend most of my time at home alone, that wouldn't suit me, no? But with the amount that I have at the moment, as much as possible, there is no problem at all. (B_PL_13G)

Statements concerning the new opportunities that arise after the children leave home very often refer precisely to more free time, which can be used in various ways. In addition to professional responsibilities, which are still an important element in the identity trajectories for the interviewed men (see the next paragraph for details), it is precisely the fact that this 'new' free time can be used as a space for self-development or to expand the possibilities of spending time with a partner. This is mentioned by one of the interviewees:

> Zbyszek: And with my wife, I do like 3.5 to 4 km, and in the evening I do another 5 km and that's time alone by myself. With that, I dedicate it to some podcasts, to education, to English too ... During such walks,

depending on what kind of day I have had, I either have more English or more global information or about food. (B_PL_5G)

Otherwise, free time allows for doing all those things that there was no time for before, and by doing so, the respondent avoids the emptiness and boredom that can sometimes occur when the working period ends and the children have left the family home long ago:

> Ryszard: Because I have so many activities, I'm dealing with so many things that were always put off, I don't have time to be bored—that's what I would say. (…) because before, when I was working, I would leave for work at 8 a.m. and come back at, say, 7 p.m. So practically the whole day was away from home and when I arrived home, the last thing I felt like doing was reading—I just had to relax, I would take the remote control in my hand and that was it. Occasionally a walk of some sort, a few screws here and there and that was it. And now I have more time, I read more, I spend my time more pleasantly and I cut coupons. (B_PL_4G)

For men active on the labour market, the empty nest stage means more time for personal activities and the entry into pre-pensionary phase when they allow themselves to ease off from the breadwinner challenges they faced during the full nest years.

Work that Fills an Empty Nest

The children's departure from the family home is easier to experience when other aspects of life's routine remain the same. The impact the children's leaving has on the relationship between partners (e.g. husband and wife) is described in other chapters of our book. The departure of children affects, among other things, the re-experiencing of the relationship. For most of the interviewed men, an important element that maintains the routine of life is the continuation of work life. Work makes it possible not to confront the empty nest as significantly as for those who spend their days at home. This is clearly emphasised by a respondent from Gdańsk:

> Krzysztof: It's like with people who retire—as long as you are working, those eight hours are filled, but after that, they say, you can get worn out, so why should I get up in the morning? And especially I will be alone, why do I need to get dressed, why do I need to do anything? I'll be walking around in my pyjamas all day—that's how I'd understand it, this fear of what's

going to happen, that it's going to have to be done in a new way, and I wouldn't have any idea how to do it, what to do with this void that's going to be created, how to manage it. That's how it seems to me. (B_PL_3G)

Another example demonstrates that work fills not only an empty nest but also the whole life of the respondent:

> Darek: No, but I miss out a little here because I'm very involved in my work and I spend too much time at work. And I don't have time for myself at all—and for holidays, as it should be, to rest for a fortnight ... And the working day is one that starts at 7 am—I am at work at 7 am and I finish after 6 pm, like now, or even a bit longer. The only plus is that during the day I can regulate my own working hours and get different things done if I'm needed on the phone—that's no problem. But in general, I sit at work all the time. (B_PL_10G)

Many studies show the enormous importance of work for men's identities, and this applies to men at different stages of their career as well as those who have retired (Berdahl et al., 2018; Gradman, 1990). This relates to the great importance that work has in maintaining the role of breadwinner and protector of the 'herd' and 'nest'. For respondents, work is a source of satisfaction and an important part of the life agenda:

> Józef: It's just that I work normally. (…) I like to work. I mean there has to be a sacred balance between the amount of work and the amount of rest. That's more or less how it works for me at the moment, 3/4 of a month at work and a week off, that's such a positive state of affairs for me. (B_PL_8P)

Our study mainly discussed the trajectories of working men. Whether they were employers or employees had a dominant influence on how the majority of them dealt with the empty nest phase.

Conclusions

For both parents, the children moving out of the family home is an important change. This chapter has dealt with how men experience this situation (women's experiences are described in another chapter in the volume). As we have shown, this situation correlates with the broader context of ageing and passing, which can be unique if we look at it through the lens of masculine identity. According to Precarious Manhood Theory (Vandello & Bosson, 2013), manhood requires validation and can be easily threatened—for example, by the experience of one's weakness—which is the case of manhood at the onset of ageing and our participants' experiences. There is also an awareness associated with these processes in the statements of our respondents. Men also experience emotions in this context, which in a way goes against dominant standpoints (but also some research findings) about the emotionless nature of masculinity. Respondents may not have expressed these emotions in a highly expressive way, but their narratives included expressions of anxiety, and fear on the one hand, but also of serenity and a sense of fulfilment on the other.

The passing of time and an awareness of ageing encourage the respondents to reflect, sometimes evoking the feeling that certain opportunities are limited and that space for development are significantly reduced. On the other hand, however, many respondents see the new situation as an opportunity to create new possibilities. Some start practising new activities (or increase their frequency) and change their current habits (e.g. nutrition). It should be noted that the majority of respondents are still employed, so their situation is somewhat different from those who remain permanently at home. Therefore, they continue to function in the familiar trajectories of their life routines so they can more easily cope with empty nest syndrome. Obviously, it is not possible to draw statistical generalisations from qualitative data, but it is reasonable to propose some generalisations of a theoretical nature.

A significant number of respondents came from a class-specific stratum (representatives of the middle class, albeit a diverse one), and the conclusions are somewhat restricted. It is evident, however, that most of the men's stories are optimistic ones. These are stories of men for whom everything was generally 'as it should be': the children were raised, most often with a good education, and in the cases studied there were no harmful events (extreme violence or, for example, alcoholism, or broken contact with the children for whatever reason), although in this aspect research vigilance and distance should be maintained—during the research we did not have access to complete family histories. However, in general, the analysed stories followed an accepted (and anticipated) pattern in which a child leaving appears as a natural stage in the life of the family. The male respondents were therefore able to confront a fairly 'standard' situation—and this was an important variable for exploring their identity narratives in a fairly uncluttered way.

These narratives convince us that although a child leaving does not leave men indifferent and evokes emotions (also difficult ones), they cope quite well with the whole situation. It is not seen as threatening their congruity as men—it is therefore evident that most of the cases analysed seem to empirically confirm existing research findings in literature on what a man 'should do' (Vandello et al., 2023). While the passing of time may make issues of male identity more relevant, this does not imply a radical change from what is culturally expected of men. In many cases, respondents remain faithful to traditionally constructed models of masculinity. There are, of course, polar cases (a desperate struggle with fading opportunities vs. a courageous dissection of the emotional state), but as a general rule, the respondents' identities do not transcend cultural norms, they rather stick to them and perceive ageing as a limitation to fulfilling male prescriptions. They seem to be more content with a less restrained life, allowing themselves to express emotions of sadness and emptiness linked to the fact that their children have left the 'nest'. However, they don't feel less manly. This is supported by the fact that most of them are still economically active and therefore do not have the time to experience the new family situation.

REFERENCES

Addis, M. E., & Mahalik, J. R. (2003). Men, masculinity, and the contexts of help seeking. *American Psychologist, 58*, 5–14.

Bennett, K. M. (2007). 'No sissy stuff': Towards a theory of masculinity and emotional expression in older widowed men. *Journal of Ageing Studies, 21*, 347–356.

Berdahl, J. L., Cooper, M., Glick, P., Livingston, R. W., & Williams, J. C. (2018). Work as a masculinity contest. *Journal of Social Issues, 74*(3), 422–448. https://doi.org/10.1111/josi.12289

Bertakis, K. D., Azari, R., Helms, J., Callahan, E. J., & Robbins, J. A. (2000). Gender differences in the utilization of health care services. *Journal of Family Practice, 49*, 147–152.

Boss, P., Pearce-McCall, D., & Greenberg, J. (1987). Normative loss in mid-life families: Rural, urban, and gender differences. *Family Relations, 36*(4), 437–443.

Bosson, J. K., Jurek, P., Vandello, J. A., Kosakowska-Berezecka, N., Olech, M., Besta, T., & Bender, M. (2021). Psychometric properties and correlates of precarious manhood beliefs in 62 nations. *Journal of Cross-Cultural Psychology, 52*, 231–258. https://doi.org/10.1177/0022022121997997

Bosson, J. K., Wilkerson, M., Kosakowska-Berezecka, N., Jurek, P., & Olech, M. (2022). Harder won and easier lost? Testing the double standard in gender rules in 62 countries. *Sex Roles, 87,* 1–9. https://doi.org/10.1007/s11199-022-01297-y

Bouchard, G. (2014). How do parents react when their children leave home? An integrative review. *Journal of Adult Development, 21,* 69–79.

Connell, R. W. (1987). *Gender and power: Society, the person and sexual politics.* Polity Press.

Connell, R. W. (1993). The big picture: Masculinities in recent world history. *Theory and Society, 22,* 597–623.

Connell, R. W. (2002). On hegemonic masculinity and violence: Response to Jefferson and Hall. *Theoretical Criminology, 6*(1), 89–99. https://doi.org/10.1177/136248060200600104

Courtenay, W. H. (2000). Constructions of masculinity and their influence on men's well-being: A theory of gender and health. *Social Science & Medicine, 50,* 1385–1401.

Diehl, M., Wahl, H. W., Barrett, A. E., Brothers, A. F., Miche, M., Montepare, J. M., Westerhof, G. J., & Wurm, S. (2014). Awareness of aging: Theoretical considerations on an emerging concept. *Developmental Review: DR, 34*(2), 93–113. https://doi.org/10.1016/j.dr.2014.01.001

Duru-Bellat, M. (2016). À l'école du genre. *Enfances & Psy, 69,* 90–100.

Galdas, P. M., Cheater, F., & Marshall, P. (2005). Men and health help-seeking behaviour: Literature review. *Journal of Advanced Nursing, 49,* 616–623.

Genoe, R. M., & Singleton, J. F. (2006). Older men's leisure experiences across their lifespan. *Topics in Geriatric Rehabilitation, 22,* 348–356.

Goodey, J. (1997). Boys don't cry: Masculinities, fear of crime and fearlessness. *The British Journal of Criminology, 37*(3), 401–418. Retrieved from http://www.jstor.org/stable/23637949

Gradman, T. J. (1990). *Does work make the man: Masculine identity and work identity during the transition to retirement.* The RAND Corporation.

Jenkin, C. R., Eime, R. M., Westerbeek, H., O'Sullivan, G., & van Uffelen, J. G. G. (2017). Sport and ageing: A systematic review of the determinants and trends of participation in sport for older adults. *BMC Public Health, 17*(976), 1–20.

Mahalik, J. R., Burns, S. M., & Syzdek, M. (2007). Masculinity and perceived normative health behaviors as predictors of men's health behaviors. *Social Science & Medicine, 64,* 2201–2209.

Messner, M. A. (1998). The limits of 'the male sex role': An analysis of the men's liberation and men's rights movements' discourse. *Gender & Society, 12,* 255–276.

Montes, V. (2013). The role of emotions in the construction of masculinity: Guatemalan migrant men, transnational migration, and family relations. *Gender & Society, 27*(4), 469–490.

Papuchon, A. (2017). *Rôles sociaux des femmes et des hommes L'idée persistante d'une vocation maternelle des femmes malgré le déclin de l'adhésion aux stéréotypes de genre*. Retrieved March 13, 2023, from https://www.insee.fr/fr/statistiques/2586467?sommaire=2586548

Quéniart, A. (2004). A profile of fatherhood among young men: Moving away from their birth family and closer to their child. *Sociological Research Online, 9*(4), 1–11. https://doi.org/10.5153/sro.976

Scher, M. (1992). The empty Nest father. *The Journal of Men's Studies, 1*(2), 195–200. https://doi.org/10.3149/jms.0102.195

Schoppe-Sullivan, S. J., & Fagan, J. (2020). The evolution of fathering research in the 21st century: Persistent challenges, new directions. *Journal of Marriage and Family, 82*, 175–197.

Smith, J. A., Braunack-Mayer, A., Wittert, G., & Warin, M. (2007). 'I've been independent for so damn long!' Independence, masculinity and aging in a help seeking context. *Journal of Ageing Studies, 21*, 325–335.

Spector-Mersel, G. (2006). Never-aging stories: Western hegemonic masculinity scripts. *Journal of Gender Studies, 15*, 67–82.

Thompson, E. H., Jr. (2008). Gender matters: Aging men's health. *Generations: Journal of the American Society on Aging, 31*(1), 5–8.

Tyler, M., & Fairbrother, P. (2013). Bushfires are 'men's business': The importance of gender and rural hegemonic masculinity in Australian understandings of bushfire. *Rural Studies, 30*(2), 110–119.

Van Lissa, C. J., Keizer, R., Van Lier, P. A. C., Meeus, W. H. J., & Branje, S. (2019). The role of fathers' versus mothers' parenting in emotion-regulation development from mid-late adolescence: Disentangling between-family differences from within-family effects. *Developmental Psychology, 55*(2), 377–389.

Vandello, J. A., & Bosson, J. K. (2013). Hard won and easily lost: A review and synthesis of theory and research on precarious manhood. *Psychology of Men & Masculinity, 14*(2), 101–113. https://doi.org/10.1037/a0029826

Vandello, J. A., Bosson, J. K., Cohen, D., Burnaford, R. M., & Weaver, J. R. (2008). Precarious manhood. *Journal of Personality and Social Psychology, 95*, 1325–1339.

Vandello, J. A., Wilkerson, M., Bosson, J. K., Wiernik, B. M., & Kosakowska-Berezecka, N. (2023). Precarious manhood and men's physical health around the world. *Psychology of Men & Masculinities, 24*(1), 1–15.

APPENDIX: CHARACTERISTICS OF PARTICIPANTS

Country	Corpus	Couple code	Name	Gender	Age	Number of children	When did the last child move out?	Profession	Voivodeship	Education
PL	A	A_PL_1G	Agnieszka	F	52	3	Less than half a year ago	Manager, NGO	Pomorskie	Tertiary
PL	A	A_PL_1G	Jan	M	55			Artisan/own business	Pomorskie	Tertiary
PL	A	A_PL_2G	Celina	F	49	1	Less than half a year ago	Sales and services	Pomorskie	Secondary
PL	A	A_PL_2G	Adam	M	49			Sales and services	Pomorskie	Secondary
PL	A	A_PL_3G	Magdalena/Magda	F	56	1	Less than half a year ago	Teacher	Pomorskie	Tertiary
PL	A	A_PL_3G	Krzysiek/Krzysztof	M	50			IT specialist	Pomorskie	Tertiary
PL	A	A_PL_4G	Basia/Barbara	F	54	2	4,5 years ago	Teacher	Pomorskie	Tertiary
PL	A	A_PL_4G	Ryszard	M	56			Lawyer	Pomorskie	Tertiary
PL	A	A_PL_5G	Teresa	F	52	2	7 years ago	Manufacturing industry	Pomorskie	Secondary
PL	A	A_PL_5G	Zbyszek	M	56			Missing data	Pomorskie	Secondary
PL	A	A_PL_6G	Marzena	F	60	1	4 years ago	Teacher	Pomorskie	Tertiary
PL	A	A_PL_6G	Maciej	M	59			Academic teacher	Pomorskie	Tertiary
PL	A	A_PL_7G	Iwona	F	51	2	1 year ago	Teacher	Pomorskie	Tertiary
PL	A	A_PL_7G	Konrad	M	50			Sales and services	Pomorskie	Tertiary
PL	A	A_PL_8G	Maria	F	47	3	1 year ago	Sales and services	Pomorskie	Primary
PL	A	A_PL_8G	Wojtek/Wojciech	M	48			Sales and services	Pomorskie	Vocational
PL	A	A_PL_9G	Dorota	F	54	2	1 year ago	Business and administration	Pomorskie	Tertiary
PL	A	A_PL_9G	Franciszek	M	59			Sales and services	Pomorskie	Tertiary
PL	A	A_PL_10G	Bogumiła	F	50	2	Intention to move out	Manager, business and administration	Pomorskie	Tertiary
PL	A	A_PL_10G	Darek	M	51			Artisan	Pomorskie	Secondary

		ID	Name	Gender	Age	No.	Move out	Occupation	Region	Education
PL	A	A_PL_11G	Małgorzata	F	49	2	3 years ago	Sales and services	Pomorskie	Secondary
PL	A	A_PL_11G	Wiktor	M	49			Sales and services	Pomorskie	Secondary
PL	A	A_PL_12G	Anna	F	48	1	3 years ago	Sales and services	Pomorskie	Secondary
PL	A	A_PL_12G	Marcin	M	49			Retired/former manager	Pomorskie	Secondary
PL	A	A_PL_13G	Krystyna	F	50	2	Intention to move out	Civil servant	Pomorskie	Tertiary
PL	A	A_PL_13G	Robert	M	55			Analyst	Pomorskie	Tertiary
PL	A	A_PL_14G	Missing data	F	56	4	Intention to move out	Teacher	Pomorskie	Tertiary
PL	A	A_PL_14G	Tadeusz	M	56			Sales and services	Pomorskie	Secondary
PL	A	A_PL_1P	Ezlbieta/Ela	F	49	1	3 years ago	Lawyer	Pomorskie	Tertiary
PL	A	A_PL_1P	Wiesław/Wiesiek	M	50			Engineer	Wielkopolskie	Tertiary
PL	A	A_PL_2P	Tadeusz	M	53	2	1 year ago	Manager	Wielkopolskie	Tertiary
PL	A	A_PL_2P	Maria	F	50			Doctor	Wielkopolskie	Tertiary
PL	A	A_PL_3P	Zofia	F	44	2	Intention to move out	Academic teacher	Wielkopolskie	Tertiary
PL	A	A_PL_3P	Leszek	M	45			Entrepreneur	Wielkopolskie	Tertiary
PL	A	A_PL_4P	Mieczysław	M	53	2	2 years ago	Academic teacher	Wielkopolskie	Tertiary
PL	A	A_PL_4P	Irena	F	53			Office assistant	Wielkopolskie	Tertiary
PL	A	A_PL_5P	Danuta	F	51	1	Intention to move out	Own business	Wielkopolskie	Secondary
PL	A	A_PL_5P	Henryk	M	45			Own business	Wielkopolskie	Secondary
PL	A	A_PL_6P	Halina	F	46	2	Intention to move out	Art and culture	Wielkopolskie	Secondary
PL	A	A_PL_6P	Marek	M	45			Artisan	Wielkopolskie	Secondary
PL	A	A_PL_7P	Grzegorz	M	49	2	1 year ago	Office assistant	Wielkopolskie	Secondary
PL	A	A_PL_7P	Teresa	F	48			Office assistant	Wielkopolskie	Secondary
PL	A	A_PL_8P	Halina	F	58	2	2 years ago	Doctor	Wielkopolskie	Secondary
PL	A	A_PL_8P	Jan	M	62			Doctor	Wielkopolskie	Secondary
PL	A	A_PL_9P	Zofia	F	50	1	3 months ago	Manager, NGO	Wielkopolskie	Tertiary
PL	A	A_PL_9P	Andrzej	M	50			Engineer	Wielkopolskie	Tertiary
PL	A	A_PL_10P	Ewa	F	52	2	Just moving out	Office assistant	Wielkopolskie	Secondary
PL	A	A_PL_10P	Józef	M	68			Entrepreneur, retired	Wielkopolskie	Secondary

(continued)

(continued)

Country	Corpus	Couple code	Name	Gender	Age	Number of children	When did the last child move out?	Profession	Voivodeship	Education
PL	A	A_PL_11P	Elżbieta/Ela	F	51	2	1 year ago	Doctor	Wielkopolskie	Secondary
PL	A	A_PL_11P	Piotr	M	49			Engineer, supervisory position	Wielkopolskie	Secondary
PL	A	A_PL_12P	Kazimierz	M	59	2	3 years ago	Analyst	Wielkopolskie	Tertiary
PL	A	A_PL_12P	Krystyna	F	57			Doctor	Wielkopolskie	Tertiary
PL	A	A_PL_21G	Żaneta	F	59	4	2 years ago	–	Pomorskie	Secondary
PL	A	A_PL_21G	Łukasz	M	66			–	Pomorskie	Secondary
PL	A	A_PL_22G	Justyna	F	62	5	5 months ago	Social worker	Pomorskie	Secondary
PL	A	A_PL_22G	Miłosz	M	67			Physical worker	Pomorskie	Primary
PL	A	A_PL_23G	Monika	F	56	2	2 years ago	Physical worker	Pomorskie	Missing data
PL	A	A_PL_23G	Józef	M	65			Driver	Pomorskie	Secondary
PL	A	A_PL_24G	Honorata	F	52	1	2 years ago	Office assistant	Pomorskie	Secondary
PL	A	A_PL_24G	Mirek/Mirosław	M	61			Driver	Pomorskie	Tertiary
PL	A	A_PL_26G	Magdalena/Magda	F	46	3	2 years ago	Sales and services	Pomorskie	Secondary
PL	A	A_PL_26G	Stanisław	M	51			Driver	Pomorskie	Vocational
PL	A	A_PL_27G	Jadwiga	F	44	2	2 years ago	Artisan	Pomorskie	Tertiary
PL	A	A_PL_27G	Cezary	M	47			Mechanic	Pomorskie	Primary
PL	A	A_PL_28G	Regina	F	44	2	2 years ago	Sales and services	Pomorskie	Vocational
PL	A	A_PL_28G	Jeremi	M	48			Public services	Pomorskie	Secondary
PL	A	A_PL_29G	Felicja	F	Missing data	Missing data	Missing data	Missing data	Pomorskie	Missing data
PL	A	A_PL_29G	Gustaw	M				Missing data	Pomorskie	Missing data
PL	A	A_PL_30G	Irmina	F	62	1	19 years ago	Art and culture	Pomorskie	Tertiary
PL	A	A_PL_30G	Ksawery	M				Artisan	Pomorskie	Vocational

PL	A	A_PL_31G	Zdzisława	F	53	1	3 years ago	Public services	Pomorskie	Secondary
PL	A	A_PL_31G	Gracjan	M	69			Public services	Pomorskie	Tertiary
PL	A	A_PL_32G	Julia	F	60	3	6 years ago	Teacher	Pomorskie	Tertiary
PL	A	A_PL_32G	Zenon	M	56			Entrepreneur	Pomorskie	Tertiary
PL	A	A_PL_33G	Wioleta	F	62	2	5 years ago	Nurse	Pomorskie	Secondary
PL	A	A_PL_33G	Wiesław	M	53			Entrepreneur	Pomorskie	Secondary
PL	A	A_PL_21P	Magdalena/Magda	F		3	6 years ago	Civil servant	Wielkopolskie	Tertiary
PL	A	A_PL_21P	Mrek/Mirosław	M	59			Sales and services	Wielkopolskie	Tertiary
PL	A	A_PL_22P	Kazimiera	F	54	2	4 years ago	Teacher	Wielkopolskie	Tertiary
PL	A	A_PL_22P	Tomasz	M	59			Manager	Wielkopolskie	Tertiary
PL	A	A_PL_23P	Franciszka	F	63	3	Missing data	Teacher	Wielkopolskie	Missing data
PL	A	A_PL_23P	Jerzy	M	65			Artisan, retired	Wielkopolskie	Vocational
PL	A	A_PL_24P	Marzena	F	46	3	6 years ago	Teacher	Wielkopolskie	Tertiary
PL	A	A_PL_24P	Ryszard	M	49			Entrepreneur	Wielkopolskie	Tertiary
PL	B	B_PL_1G	Agnieszka	F	52	3	Less than half a year ago	Manager, NGO	Pomorskie	Tertiary
PL	B	B_PL_1G	Jan	M	55			Artisan/own business	Pomorskie	Tertiary
PL	B	B_PL_2G	Celina	F	49	1	Less than half a year ago	Sales and services	Pomorskie	Secondary
PL	B	B_PL_2G	Adam	M	49			Sales and services	Pomorskie	Secondary
PL	B	B_PL_3G	Magdalena/Magda	F	56	1	Less than half a year ago	Teacher	Pomorskie	Tertiary
PL	B	B_PL_3G	Krzysiek/Krzysztof	M	50			IT specialist	Pomorskie	Tertiary
PL	B	B_PL_4G	Basia/Barbara	F	54	2	4,5 years ago	Teacher	Pomorskie	Tertiary
PL	B	B_PL_4G	Ryszard	M	56			Lawyer	Pomorskie	Tertiary
PL	B	B_PL_5G	Teresa	F	52	2	7 years ago	Manufacturing industry	Pomorskie	Secondary
PL	B	B_PL_5G	Zbyszek	M	56			Missing data	Pomorskie	Secondary
PL	B	B_PL_6G	Marzena	F	60	1	4 years ago	Teacher	Pomorskie	Tertiary

(continued)

(continued)

Country	Corpus	Couple code	Name	Gender	Age	Number of children	When did the last child move out?	Profession	Voivodeship	Education
PL	B	B_PL_7G	Iwona	F	51	2	1 year ago	Teacher	Pomorskie	Tertiary
PL	B	B_PL_7G	Konrad	M	50	2		Sales and services	Pomorskie	Tertiary
PL	B	B_PL_9G	Dorota	F	54	2	1 year ago	Business and administration	Pomorskie	Tertiary
PL	B	B_PL_9G	Franciszek	M	59	2		Sales and services	Pomorskie	Tertiary
PL	B	B_PL_10G	Bogumiła	F	50	2	Intention to move out	Manager, business and administration	Pomorskie	Tertiary
PL	B	B_PL_10G	Darek	M	51	2		Artisan	Pomorskie	Secondary
PL	B	B_PL_11G	Małgorzata	F	49	2	3 years ago	Sales and services	Pomorskie	Secondary
PL	A	A_PL_11G	Wiktor	M	49	2		Sales and services	Pomorskie	Secondary
PL	B	B_PL_12G	Anna	F	48	1	3 years ago	Sales and services	Pomorskie	Secondary
PL	B	B_PL_12G	Marcin	M	49	1		Retired/former manager	Pomorskie	Secondary
PL	B	B_PL_13G	Krystyna	F	50	2	Intention to move out	Civil servant	Pomorskie	Tertiary
PL	B	B_PL_13G	Robert	M	55	2		Analyst	Pomorskie	Tertiary
PL	B	B_PL_14G	Hanna	F	56	4	Intention to move out	Teacher	Pomorskie	Tertiary
PL	B	B_PL_14G	Tadeusz	M	56	4		Sales and services	Pomorskie	Secondary
PL	B	B_PL_1P	Ezlbieta/Ela	F	49	1	3 years ago	Lawyer	Wielkopolskie	Tertiary
PL	B	B_PL_1P	Wiesław/Wiesiek	M	50	1		Engineer	Wielkopolskie	Tertiary
PL	B	B_PL_2P	Tadeusz	M	53	2	1 year ago	Manager	Wielkopolskie	Tertiary
PL	B	B_PL_2P	Maria	F	50	2		Doctor	Wielkopolskie	Tertiary
PL	B	B_PL_3P	Zofia	F	44	2	Intention to move out	Academic teacher	Wielkopolskie	Tertiary
PL	B	B_PL_3P	Leszek	M	45	2		Entrepreneur	Wielkopolskie	Tertiary
PL	B	B_PL_4P	Mieczysław	M	53	2	2 years ago	Academic teacher	Wielkopolskie	Tertiary
PL	B	B_PL_4P	Irena	F	53	2		Office assistant	Wielkopolskie	Tertiary
PL	B	B_PL_7P	Grzegorz	M	49	2	1 year ago	Office assistant	Wielkopolskie	Secondary
PL	B	B_PL_7P	Teresa	F	48	2		Office assistant	Wielkopolskie	Secondary

PL	B	B_PL_8P	Halina	F	58	2	2 years ago	Doctor	Wielkopolskie	Secondary
PL	B	B_PL_8P	Jan	M	62	2		Doctor	Wielkopolskie	Secondary
PL	B	B_PL_9P	Zofia	F	50	1	3 months ago	Manager, NGO	Wielkopolskie	Tertiary
PL	B	B_PL_9P	Andrzej	M	50	1		Engineer	Wielkopolskie	Tertiary
PL	B	B_PL_10P	Ewa	F	52	2	Just moving out	Office assistant	Wielkopolskie	Secondary
PL	B	B_PL_10P	Józef	M	68	1		Entrepreneur, retired	Wielkopolskie	Secondary
PL	B	B_PL_11P	Elżbieta/Ela	F	51	2	1 year ago	Doctor	Wielkopolskie	Secondary
PL	B	B_PL_11P	Piotr	M	49	1		Engineer, supervisory position	Wielkopolskie	Secondary
PL	B	B_PL_12P	Kazimierz	M	59	2	3 years ago	Analyst	Wielkopolskie	Tertiary
PL	B	B_PL_12P	Krystyna	F	57	2		Doctor	Wielkopolskie	Tertiary
PL	B	B_PL_41	Ania/Anna	F	Missing data	3	Not collected	Missing data	Not collected	Missing data
PL	B	B_PL_69	Bożena	F	44	2	Not collected	Doctor	Not collected	Tertiary
PL	B	B_PL_43	Joanna	F	53	2	Not collected	Art and culture	Not collected	Tertiary
PL	B	B_PL_46	Katarzyna/Kasia	F	44	3	Not collected	Own business	Not collected	Secondary
PL	B	B_PL_47	Elżbieta/Ela	F	68	2	Not collected	Teacher	Not collected	Tertiary
PL	B	B_PL_49	Maria	F	54	2	Not collected	Architect	Not collected	Tertiary
PL	B	B_PL_51	Edyta	F	45	2	Not collected	Sales and services	Not collected	Tertiary
PL	B	B_PL_52	Honorata	F	63	2	Not collected	Teacher	Not collected	Tertiary
PL	B	B_PL_54	Magdalena/Magda	F	65	2	Not collected	Missing data	Not collected	Tertiary
PL	B	B_PL_57	Antonina	F	50	1	Not collected	Teacher	Not collected	Tertiary
PL	B	B_PL_59	Ewelina	F	52	2	Not collected	Teacher	Not collected	Tertiary
PL	B	B_PL_60	Irena	F	52	3	Not collected	Entrepreneur	Not collected	Tertiary
PL	B	B_PL_61	Mariola	F	55	1	Not collected	Teacher	Not collected	Tertiary
PL	B	B_PL_62	Anna	F	65	3	Not collected	Homemaker	Not collected	Secondary
PL	B	B_PL_63	Marek	M	59	1	Not collected	Own business	Not collected	Tertiary
PL	B	B_PL_64	Alicja	F	44	2	Not collected	Own business	Not collected	Tertiary

(continued)

(continued)

Country	Corpus	Couple code	Name	Gender	Age	Number of children	When did the last child move out?	Profession	Voivodeship	Education
PL	B	B_PL_69	Barbara	F	49	2	Not collected	Nurse	Not collected	Secondary
PL	B	B_PL_70	Weronika	F	50	2	Not collected	Teacher	Not collected	Secondary
PL	B	B_PL_75	Henryk		60	1	Not collected	Academic teacher	Not collected	Tertiary
PL	B	B_PL_25N	Elżbieta/Ela	F	56	2	7 years ago	Physical worker	Not collected	Secondary
PL	C	C_PL_84	Konstancja	F	49	2	Not collected	Missing data	Not collected	Tertiary
PL	C	C_PL_85	Dorota	F	54	3	Not collected	Manager	Not collected	Missing data
PL	C	C_PL_88	Bogna	F	50	2	Not collected	Nurse	Not collected	Tertiary
PL	C	C_PL_90	Kinga	F	51	4	Not collected	Unemployed	Not collected	Secondary
PL	C	C_PL_93	Grażyna	F		2	Not collected	Teacher	Not collected	Tertiary
PL	C	C_PL_95	Stanisława/Stasia	F	59	4	Not collected	Sales and services	Not collected	Secondary
PL	C	C_PL_96	Hanna	F	57	2	Not collected	Finance and administration	Not collected	Tertiary
PL	C	C_PL_98	Ewa	F	55	2	Not collected	Teacher	Not collected	Tertiary
PL	C	C_PL_105	Marzena	F	62	2	Not collected	Finance and administration	Not collected	Tertiary
PL	C	C_PL_106	Teresa	F	46	1+1	Not collected	Sales and services	Not collected	Tertiary
PL	C	C_PL_107	Marta	F	45	2+1	Not collected	Teacher	Not collected	Tertiary
PL	C	C_PL_108	Krzysztof	M	57	1+1	Not collected	Entrepreneur	Not collected	Tertiary
PL	C	C_PL_111	Tamara	F	57	2	Not collected	Art and culture	Not collected	Tertiary
PL	C	C_PL_113	Natasza	F	57	3	Not collected	Teacher	Not collected	Tertiary
PL	C	C_PL_114	Agata	F	52	2	Not collected	Finance and administration	Not collected	Tertiary
PL	C	C_PL_116	Jakub	M	46	1+1	Not collected	Public services	Not collected	Tertiary
PL	C	C_PL_117	Sławomira	F	55	1	Not collected	Liberal profession	Not collected	Tertiary
PL	D	D_PL_201	Maryla	F	49	1	Returned	Doctor	Not collected	Tertiary

PL	D	D_PL_202	Zofia	F	45	2	Returned	Finance and administration	Not collected	Tertiary
PL	D	D_PL_203	Arkadiusz	M	58	1	Returned	Academic teacher	Not collected	Tertiary
PL	D	D_PL_204	Irena	F	43	2	Returned	Culture and education	Not collected	Tertiary
PL	D	D_PL_205	Asia	F	52	3	Returned	Sales	Not collected	Tertiary
PL	D	D_PL_205	Tadeusz	M	53		Returned	Services	Not collected	Tertiary
PL	D	D_PL_206	Anna	F	47	2	Returned	Doctor	Not collected	Tertiary
PL	D	D_PL_207	Aneta	F	52	2	Returned	Missing data	Not collected	Tertiary
PL	D	D_PL_207	Mariusz	M	52		Returned	Missing data	Not collected	Tertiary
PL	D	D_PL_208	Maciej	M	50	2	Returned	Own business	Not collected	Tertiary
PL	D	D_PL_209	Sandra	F	43	3	Returned	Entrepreneur	Not collected	Tertiary
PL	D	D_PL_210	Grażyna	F	54	1	Returned	Teacher	Not collected	Tertiary
PL	D	D_PL_210	Grzegorz	F	56		Returned	Architect	Not collected	Tertiary
PL	D	D_PL_211	Teresa	F	47	1	Returned	Civil servant	Not collected	Tertiary
PL	D	D_PL_211	Wójciech	M	52		Returned	Teacher	Not collected	Tertiary
PL	D	D_PL_212	Joanna	F	50	2	Returned	Sport and recreation	Not collected	Secondary
PL	D	D_PL_213	Żaneta	F	45	2	Returned	Finance and administration	Not collected	Tertiary
PL	D	D_PL_214	Karolina	F	48	1	Returned	Sales and services	Not collected	Secondary
FR	A	A_FR_1	Delphine	F	52	2	Intention to move out	Missing data	Not collected	Not collected
FR	A	A_FR_1	Gérald	M	54			Art and culture	Not collected	Not collected
FR	A	A_FR_2	Florence	F	62	2	7 years ago	Teacher	Not collected	Not collected
FR	A	A_FR_2	Fabrice	M	64			Manager	Not collected	Not collected

(continued)

(continued)

Country	Corpus	Couple code	Name	Gender	Age	Number of children	When did the last child move out?	Profession	Voivodeship	Education
FR	A	A_FR_4	Clarisse	F	60	3	10 years ago	Sales and services	Not collected	Not collected
FR	A	A_FR_4	Sébastien	M	60			Technician	Not collected	Not collected
FR	A	A_FR_5	Juliette	F	57	2	Missing data	Sales and services	Not collected	Not collected
FR	A	A_FR_5	Claude	M	59			IT specialist	Not collected	Not collected
FR	A	A_FR_6	Valérie	F	53	2	3 years ago	Academic teacher	Not collected	Not collected
FR	A	A_FR_6	Eric	M	54			Academic teacher	Not collected	Not collected
FR	A	A_FR_7	Cynthia	F	54	4	Missing data	Doctor	Not collected	Not collected
FR	A	A_FR_7	Bruno	M	53			Engineer	Not collected	Not collected
FR	A	A_FR_8	Charlotte	F	52	3	Intention to move out	Teacher	Not collected	Not collected
FR	A	A_FR_8	Olivier	M	48		(other already left)	Finance and administration	Not collected	Not collected
FR	A	A_FR_10	Clarisse	F	54	3	Intention to move out	Childcare at home	Not collected	Not collected
FR	A	A_FR_10	Eric	M	54		(other already left)	Sales and services	Not collected	Not collected

FR	A	A_FR_11	Delphine	F	53	1	1 year ago	Manager	Not collected	Not collected
FR	A	A_FR_11	Didier	M	50			Sales and services, supervisory position	Not collected	Not collected
FR	A	A_FR_12	Clarisse	F	59	3	9 years ago	Social worker	Not collected	Not collected
FR	A	A_FR_12	Jean-Paul	M	64			Retired, sales and services	Not collected	Not collected
FR	A	A_FR_13	Eric	M	54	4	1 year ago	Teacher	Not collected	Not collected
FR	A	A_FR_13	Delphine	F	Missing data			Office and administration	Not collected	Not collected
FR	A	A_FR_14	Béatrice	F	53	2	3 years ago (but returned)	Finance and administration	Not collected	Not collected
FR	A	A_FR_14	Béatrice	M	53			Driver	Not collected	Not collected
FR	A	A_FR_15	Sandra	F	46	2	2 years ago	Homemaker	Not collected	Not collected
FR	A	A_FR_15	Vincent	M	54			Manager	Not collected	Not collected
FR	A	A_FR_16	Angèle	F	52	2	5 years ago	Manager	Not collected	Not collected
FR	A	A_FR_16	Thierry	M	52			Public services	Not collected	Not collected
FR	A	A_FR_17	Patricia	F	57	1	3 years ago	Nurse	Not collected	Not collected
FR	A	A_FR_17	Patricia	M	55			Social worker	Not collected	Not collected

(continued)

(continued)

Country	Corpus	Couple code	Name	Gender	Age	Number of children	When did the last child move out?	Profession	Voivodeship	Education
FR	A	A_FR_18	Véronique	F	62	3	1 year ago	Finance and administration	Not collected	Not collected
FR	A	A_FR_18	Pascal	M	60			Engineer	Not collected	Not collected
FR	A	A_FR_19	Véronique	F	52	3	3 years ago	Engineer	Not collected	Not collected
FR	A	A_FR_19	Sylvain	M	54			Manager	Not collected	Not collected
FR	A	A_FR_20	Fabienne	F	50	1	1 year ago (but returned, intend to move out again)	Manager	Not collected	Not collected
FR	A	A_FR_20	Francis	M	51			Finance and administration	Not collected	Not collected
FR	A	A_FR_21	Angélique	F	53	3	Missing data (but returned)	Finance and administration	Not collected	Not collected
FR	A	A_FR_21	Max	M	53			Manager	Not collected	Not collected
FR	A	A_FR_22	Estelle	F	53	2	3 years ago	Teacher	Not collected	Not collected
FR	A	A_FR_22	Frédéric	M	56			Technician	Not collected	Not collected
FR	A	A_FR_24	Christine	F	48	4	Intention to move out (the first already left)	Sales and services	Not collected	Not collected
FR	A	A_FR_24	Roger	M	51			Driver	Not collected	Not collected

FR	A	A_FR_26	Delphine	F	57	2	1 year ago (but returned)	Physiotherapist	Not collected	Not collected
FR	A	A_FR_26	Didier	M	55			Physiotherapist	Not collected	Not collected
FR	A	A_FR_27	Claudia	F	53	2	Intention to move out	Teacher	Not collected	Not collected
FR	A	A_FR_27	Guillaume	M	60			Retired	Not collected	Not collected
FR	A	A_FR_29	Sabrina	F	49	2	3–6 months ago	Business and administration	Not collected	Not collected
FR	A	A_FR_29	Jérémy	M	49				Not collected	Not collected
FR	A	A_FR_32	Laurence	F	54	3	2 years ago	Office assistant	Not collected	Not collected
FR	A	A_FR_32	Mounir	M	58				Not collected	Not collected
FR	A	A_FR_35	Ambre	F	52	2	Less than 6 years ago	Teacher	Not collected	Not collected
FR	A	A_FR_35	Max	M	54			Manager	Not collected	Not collected
FR	A	A_FR_36	Sabrina	F	53	2	Intention to move out (the other already left)	Civil servant	Not collected	Not collected
FR	A	A_FR_36	Alexandre	M	58			Technician	Not collected	Not collected
FR	A	A_FR_37	Valérie	F	50	3	Intention to move out (left but returned; the other two have not left yet)	Missing data	Not collected	Not collected
FR	A	A_FR_37	Vincent	M	52			Missing data	Not collected	Not collected

(continued)

(continued)

Country	Corpus	Couple code	Name	Gender	Age	Number of children	When did the last child move out?	Profession	Voivodeship	Education
FR	A	A_FR_39	Nour	F	53	3	1/2 year ago	Missing data	Not collected	Not collected
FR	A	A_FR_39	Sofiane	M		3	1/2 year ago	Missing data	Not collected	Not collected
FR	A	A_FR_40	Carole	F	53	2	2 years ago	Manager	Not collected	Not collected
FR	A	A_FR_40	Erwan	M	51			Art and culture	Not collected	Not collected
FR	A	A_FR_41	Inès	F	50	2	Left but returned	Nurse	Not collected	Not collected
FR	A	A_FR_41	Guillaume	M	50			Physical worker	Not collected	Not collected
FR	A	A_FR_43	Sabrina	F	49	3	Intention to move out	Teacher	Not collected	Not collected
FR	A	A_FR_43	Max	M	50		(first one already left)	Manager	Not collected	Not collected
FR	A	A_FR_44	Marie-Dominique	F	56	2	4 years ago	Business and administration	Not collected	Not collected
FR	A	A_FR_44	Jean-Luc	M	55			IT specialist	Not collected	Not collected

Printed by Printforce, United Kingdom

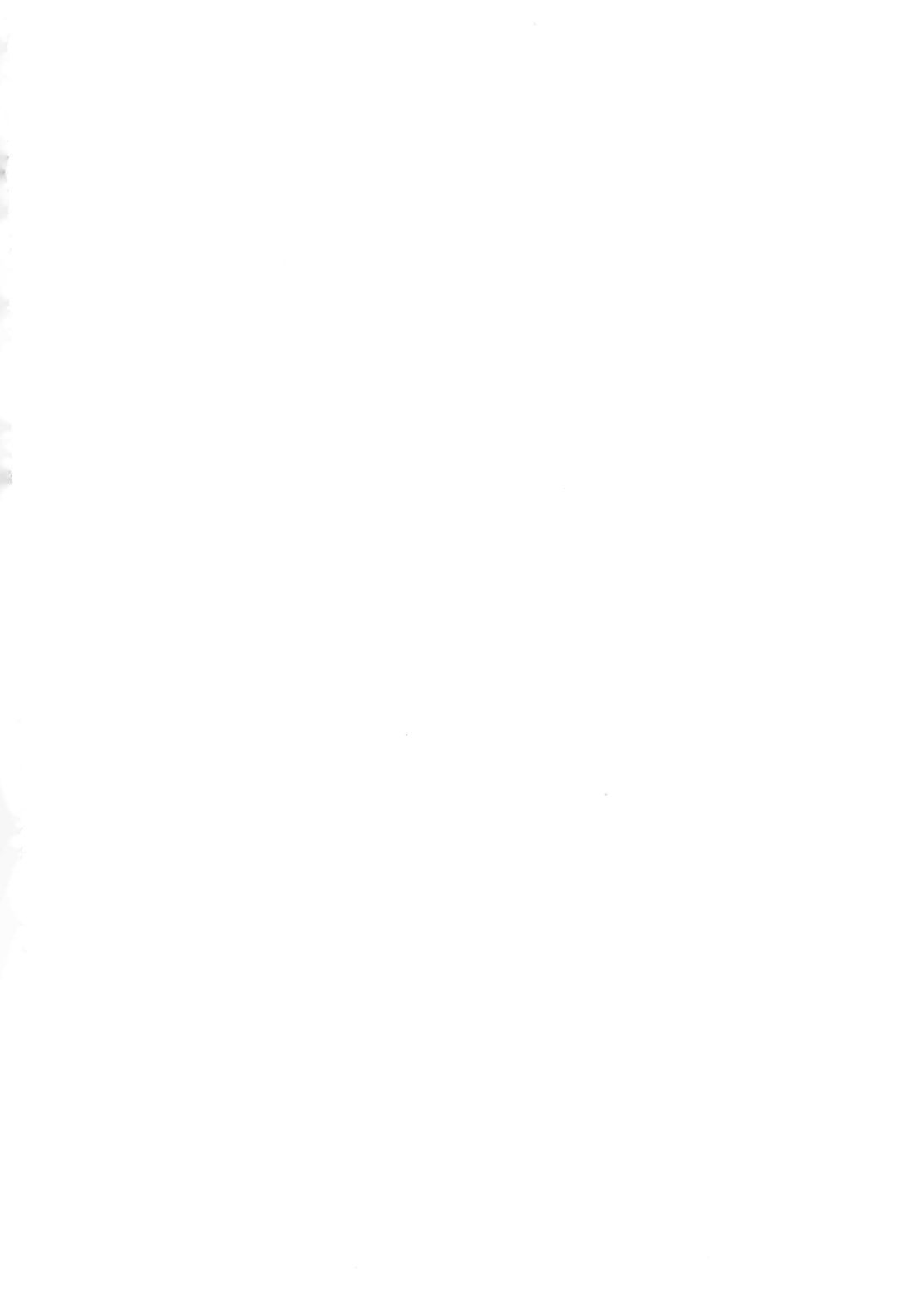